The Handbook of Clinically Tested Herbal Remedies

Volume 2

The Handbook of Clinically Tested Herbal Remedies

Volume 2

**Part III: Botanical Profiles—
Product and Clinical Trial Information
(Grape Seed–Valerian and Herbal Formulas)**

Marilyn Barrett, PhD
Editor

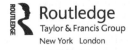

Routledge
Taylor & Francis Group
New York   London

First published by
The Haworth Press, Inc., 10 Alice Street, Binghamton, NY 13904-1580.

First issued in paperback 2013

This edition published 2013 by Routledge
711 Third Avenue, New York, NY 10017
2 Park Square, Milton Park, Abingdon, Oxon OX14 4RN

Routledge is an imprint of the Taylor & Francis Group, an informa business

TR: 8.9.04.

PUBLISHER'S NOTE
This book has been published solely for educational purposes and is not intended to substitute for the medical advice of a treating physician. Medicine is an ever-changing science. As new research and clinical experience broaden our knowledge, changes in treatment may be required. While many potential treatment options are made herein, some or all of the options may not be applicable to a particular individual. Therefore, the author, editor and publisher do not accept responsibility in the event of negative consequences incurred as a result of the information presented in this book. We do not claim that this information is necessarily accurate by the rigid scientific and regulatory standards applied for medical treatment. **No Warranty, Expressed or Implied, is furnished with respect to the material contained in this book. The reader is urged to consult with his/her personal physician with respect to the treatment of any medical condition.**

Cover design by Marylouise E. Doyle.

Photography by Linda Nikaya.

Library of Congress Cataloging-in-Publication Data

The handbook of clinically tested herbal remedies, volumes 1 and 2 / Marilyn Barrett, editor.
    p. ; cm.
Includes bibliographical references and index.
ISBN 0-7890-1068-2 Volumes 1 and 2 (hard : alk. paper)
ISBN 0-7890-2723-2 Volume 1 (hard : alk. paper)
ISBN 0-7890-2724-0 Volume 2 (hard : alk. paper)
ISBN 978-0-415-65246-9 (paperback)
    1. Herbs—Therapeutic use—Handbooks, manuals, etc. [DNLM: 1. Plant Preparations—Handbooks. QV 39 H2362 2004] I. Barrett, Marilyn.
RM666.H33H363 2004
615'.321—dc22

              2003025270

CONTENTS

VOLUME 1

VOLUME 2

PART III: BOTANICAL PROFILES—
PRODUCT AND CLINICAL TRIAL INFORMATION
(Grape Seed–Valerian and Herbal Formulas)

ABOUT THE EDITOR

Marilyn Barrett, PhD, is founder and principal of Pharmacognosy Consulting, whose mission is to provide a scientific foundation for botanical medicine. She was awarded a PhD in pharmacognosy from the School of Pharmacy, University of London, UK, in 1985 and a BA in botany from the University of California, Berkeley, CA, in 1977.

Since 1994, Dr. Barrett has provided scientific information and technical expertise to manufacturers, associations, and government concerning medicinal plant products through her consulting business. She is a member of the United States Pharmacopeia Committee of Experts for Dietary Supplements Information, an external advisory board member for the University of California at Los Angeles Center for Dietary Supplements (an NIH-funded center) and a consultant to the Office of Dietary Supplements in preparation of their botanical fact sheets. Dr. Barrett served on a working group for the Institute of Medicine of the National Academy of Sciences Committee developing a Framework for Evaluating the Safety of Dietary Supplements. She is a member of the American Botanical Council Advisory Board, the American Herbal Pharmacopoeia and Therapeutic Compendium Technical Advisory Board, and the American Herbal Products Association's Scientific Advisory Board.

Dr. Barrett has published over 30 publications in peer-reviewed journals and a booklet titled *Reference on Evaluating Botanicals* for the Council for Responsible Nutrition, in 1998. More information is available on her Web site at <www.pharmacognosy.com>.

EDITOR'S NOTE

The purpose of this book is informational. It is not intended as a guide to self-medication or as a substitute for the advice of a health practitioner.

The production of this book was partially supported by a grant from The Haworth Press. No monetary assistance was provided by any manufacturer whose product is, or is not, included in the book.

This book is not meant to promote any product(s) in particular. The purpose of the book is to examine the scientific data supporting the efficacy of herbal preparations. As therapeutic equivalence of these products has not been proven, examining the clinical evidence cannot be done without profiling individual products.

Manufacturers who wish to submit their product(s) for inclusion in future editions of this book should contact the editor via e-mail at <marilyn@pharmacognosy.com> or via the Internet at <http://www.pharmacognosy.com>.

PART III:
BOTANICAL PROFILES—
PRODUCT AND CLINICAL TRIAL
INFORMATION
(Grape Seed–Valerian and Herbal Formulas)

Grape Seed

Other common names: **European grape; wine grape**
Latin name: *Vitis vinifera* **L.** [Vitaceae]
Plant part: **Seed**

PREPARATIONS USED
IN REVIEWED CLINICAL STUDIES

The grape plant is a woody, perennial vine that produces fruit from which juice, raisins, and wine are produced. Pigments and tannins in grapes contribute to the color and taste of the fruit. The tannins are polymers of the polyphenols catechin and epicatechin. Other names for these polymers are procyanidins, leucoanthocyanins, procyanidolic oligomers, and oligomeric proanthocyanidins (OPCs). The strong antioxidant properties of the OPCs have sparked interest in their therapeutic use. OPCs are concentrated in the skins of red grapes, but are even more abundant in the seeds. A patented process has been developed that produces a highly concentrated extract of polyphenols from crushed grape seeds (Bombardelli and Morazzoni, 1995).

Endotelon® contains a grape seed extract (LeucoSelect®) that is a 100-fold concentrate standardized to 95 percent polyphenols (80 to 85 percent OPCs). Endotelon is manufactured by Sanofi-Synthelabo in France using the LeucoSelect extract produced by Indena S.p.A in Italy. The LeucoSelect extract is incorporated into products distributed in the United States by Thorne Research (O.P.C.-100) and Bluebonnet Nutrition Corporation (Grape Seed Extract).

LeucoSelect™-phytosome® is a proprietary formulation made by Indena S.p.A. in Italy that combines the LeucoSelect extract with soy phospholipids in a ratio of one to two. This combination is reported by Indena to improve the bioavailability of grape procyanidins.

Proclandiol is manufactured by Bruschettini s.r.l. in Italy and contains a fermented grape seed product for which we could find very little specification. This product is not available in the United States.

GRAPE SEED SUMMARY TABLE

Product Name	Manufacturer/ U.S. Distributor	Product Characteristics	Dose in Trials	Indication	No. of Trials	Benefit (Evidence Level-Trial No.)
Endotelon®	Sanofi-Synthelabo, France (Indena S.p.A., Italy)/None	Grape seed extract containing 80 to 85% OPCs (LeucoSelect®)	150 mg daily; range 100 to 300 mg daily	Chronic venous insufficiency	3	Yes (II-2) Trend (II-1)
				Capillary fragility	3	Trend (III-1) Undetermined (III-2)
				Postoperative edema	1	Trend (III-1)
				Vision	1	Yes (II-1)
LeucoSelect™- phytosome®	Indena S.p.A., Italy/Indena USA Inc.	LeucoSelect™ extract plus phospholipids	600 mg daily	Antioxidant activity	1	MOA (III-1)
Procianidol	Bruschettini s.r.l., Italy	Fermented product	300 mg daily	Vision	1	Trend (II-1)

*Products sold in the United States that contain the Indena LeucoSelect® extract as a single ingredient are listed here. The extract in these products has been tested clinically, but the final formulation has not.

Product Name   **Manufacturer**
O.P.C.-100   Thorne Research
Grape Seed Extract   Bluebonnet Nutrition Corporation

SUMMARY OF REVIEWED CLINICAL STUDIES

Most of the clinical studies on grape seed preparations have focused on benefits to the circulatory system. The studies described in this section explore the possible benefit of grape seed preparations in treating venous insufficiency, capillary fragility, edema, and visual contrast sensitivity due to glare, as well as antioxidant properties.

The procyanidins in grape seed extracts are thought to help maintain normal blood capillary function through their antioxidant, free-radical scavenging activity. In addition, the procyanidins inhibit the enzymes involved in the degradation of collagen, elastin, and hyaluronic acid, the main structural components of the matrix that surrounds the capillaries. Capillaries are the small blood vessels that allow for the exchange of fluid, nutrients, and blood cells between the blood and surrounding tissues. An increase in the permeability of the capillaries leads to an increase in fluid and blood cells in the tissues surrounding the capillaries. This decrease in capillary resistance, also called capillary fragility, can cause bleeding under the skin (purpura) sometimes observed as pinpoint black and blue spots (Dartenuc, Marache, and Choussat, 1980).

Chronic venous insufficiency is a term applied to a syndrome resulting from insufficient circulation to the legs and feet. Symptoms can include edema, bluish discoloration of the skin, and ultimately ulcers. Treatment can include elastic support stockings, drugs, or surgery (Schulz, Hänsel, and Tyler, 2001).

The circulatory system supports vision through the capillaries that deliver blood to the retina of the eye. The effect of grape seed extracts on recovery of vision after exposure to strong light or glare has been tested in a few studies. The procyanidins are thought to assist in the regeneration of rhodopsin, a visual pigment depleted by glare (Corbe, Boissin, and Siou, 1988).

Endotelon

Chronic Venous Insufficiency

Three good-quality trials focused on the effect of Endotelon on venous insufficiency in the legs. A large, placebo-controlled study, including 357 subjects with venous insufficiency in the legs, reported improvement in a clinical symptom composite score consisting of heaviness or fatigue, itching (paresthesia), nocturnal leg cramps, leg agitation, and subjective edema. A benefit compared to placebo was observed following administration of 300 mg per day for two months, and increased benefit when treatment was extended for three months (Henriet, 1988). A smaller study, with 50 participants, compared the effects of 150 mg Endotelon to 450 mg Diosmine (a semisynthetic bioflavonoid) for one month. Endotelon appeared to benefit patients sooner (at day 9 compared to day 14) and to be more effective than Diosmine (Delacroix, 1981). This study would have been strengthened by the addition of a placebo group. A placebo-controlled trial, also with 50 patients diagnosed with venous insufficiency, showed significant benefit compared to placebo following treatment with 150 mg per day for 45 days. The trial used thermography (the use of heat to assess circulation) and rheography (the use of electrical impedance to measure blood volume) measurements as end points. Both measurements indicated statistical improvements in arterial and venous tone with treatment compared to placebo (Paitel, 1981).

Capillary Fragility

Three poorly described, small, placebo-controlled trials explored the effect of Endotelon on vascular resistance. One trial included 25 subjects with either hypertension or diabetes, and used a dose of 150 mg per day for one to three months. It reported a trend toward increasing capillary resistance (from 14.6 to 18.0 cmHg as measured using a capillarodynamometer) with treatment and no change with placebo (Lagrue, Olivier-Martin, and Grillot, 1981). Another trial included 37 subjects with capillary fragility who were given a dose of 100 mg grape seed extract or placebo per day for 15 days. The Endotelon group showed greater improvement than the placebo group, as measured using an angiosterrometer. The fact that some subjects had normal capillary resistance to begin with, along with other inadequacies in the methodology, meant the possible benefit of treatment was not determined by this study (Dartenuc, Marache, and Choussat, 1980). The third trial included two sets of subjects: patients with venous insufficiency and healthy subjects who took aspirin to experimentally induce a reduction in capillary resistance. Both sets of participants were given either 150 mg Endotelon per day or placebo for one month. The authors reported improvement in both sets of participants following treatment with Endotelon compared with placebo (Dubos, Durst, and Hugonot, 1980). However, the number of subjects was judged too small, 30 in total, by our reviewer, Dr. Mary Hardy, for such a complex four-part design.

Postoperative Edema

A rather unique study explored the effect of Endotelon on post-operative edema caused by face-lift operations. Treatment was 300 mg per day for five days before surgery and for five days after surgery. The postoperative edema resolved more quickly in the treatment group (11.4 days) compared with the placebo group (15.8 days), according to the subjective evaluation of the physician. The volume of the edema did not differ in the two groups (Baruch, 1984).

Vision

A trial with 95 subjects without any major retinal or ophthalmological pathology studied the effect of Endotelon on visual contrast sensitivity. The trial was designed to imitate exposure to glare from video display units or traffic headlights while driving. Subjects received either 200 mg per day or nothing for five weeks. Visual recovery from glare, both general retinal glare and night vision glare, as a function of time, was significantly better in the treatment group compared to the baseline and the control group (Corbe, Boissin, and Siou, 1988).

LeucoSelect-phytosome

Antioxidant Activity

A small, placebo-controlled trial including a total of 20 healthy young students measured antioxidant activity in the plasma following one dose of 300 mg of LeucoSelect-phytosome or placebo and again after five days of treatment. After one dose of grape seed extract, the antioxidant activity in the serum of subjects increased for a period of 30 minutes to three hours. No effect was observed following administration of placebo. Similar results were obtained following five days of treatment (Nuttall et al., 1998).

Procianidol

Vision

The trial with 75 subjects using video display units for at least six hours daily were divided into three treatment groups. One group (50 subjects) received 100 mg Procianidol capsules three times daily. The second group (ten subjects) received 100 mg bilberry anthocyanosides three times daily. The third group (15 subjects) received placebo. Following two months of treatment, a statistically significant increase in contrast sensitivity was observed in all ten points of the contrast sensitivity curve in the Procianidol group, six points of the curve for the bilberry group, and two points of the curve for the placebo group. No change was observed in visual acuity or chromatic sense (Fusi et al., 1990). A criticism of the latter trial was the unequal distribution of subjects.

ADVERSE REACTIONS OR SIDE EFFECTS

The preceding trials did not find any serious adverse effects with any of the products. When mentioned, the side effects, which did not differ from placebo, were gastric discomfort, nausea, headaches, and dizziness.

REFERENCES

Baruch J (1984). The effects of Endotelon on postoperative edema: Results of a double-blind study vs. placebo in thirty-two patients. *Annales de Chirurgie Plastique et Esthetique* 29 (4): 393-395.

Bombardelli E, Morazzoni P (1995). *Vitis vinifera L. Fitoterapia* 66: 291-317.

Corbe C, Boissin JP, Siou A (1988). Chromatic sense and chorioretinal circulation: Study of the effect of O.P.C (Endotelon). *Journal Français d'Ophtalmologie* 11 (5): 453-460.

Dartenuc JY, Marache P, Choussat H (1980). Capillary resistance in geriatrics: Study of a microangioprotector = Endotelon. *Bordeaux Medical* 13: 903-907.

Delacroix P (1981). Double-blind trial of Endotelon in chronic venous insufficiency. *Revue de Medecine* 27/28: 1793-1802.

Dubos G, Durst G, Hugonot R (1980). Capillary resistance evolution, spontaneously or artificially lessened by action of a capillaro-toxic substance in aged people. *Extrait de Geriatrie* September: 302-305.

Fusi L, Czimeg F, Pesce F, Germogli R, Boero A, Vanzetti M, and Gandiglio G (1990). Effects of procyanidolic olygomers from *Vitis vinifera* in subjects working at video-display units. *Annali di Ottalmologia e Clinica Oculistica* 116: 575-584.

Henriet JP (1988). Endotélon® dans les manifestations fonctionnelles de l'insuffisance veineuse périphérique: Etude EIVE [Endotelon® in the functional disorders caused by peripheral vascular insufficienty]. *Actualité Médicales Internationales—Angiologie* 5 (74): n.p.

Lagrue G, Olivier-Martin F, Grillot A (1981). A study of the effect of procyanidolic oligomers on capillary resistance in the hypertension and certain nephropathies. *La Semaine des Hopitaux Paris* 57 (33-36): 1399-1401.

Nuttall SL, Kendall MJ, Bombardelli E, Morazzoni P (1998). An evaluation of the antioxidant activity of a standardized grape seed extract, Leucoselect. *Journal of Clinical Pharmacy and Therapeutics* 23 (5): 385-389.

Paitel D (1981). Rheographic and thermographic study of the effects on peripheral hemodynamics of an endotheoliotrophic, double blind versus placebo study. *Vie Medicale* 11: 776-783.

Schulz V, Hänsel R, Tyler VE (2001). *Rational Phytotherapy: A Physicians' Guide to Herbal Medicine*, Fourth Edition. Trans. TC Telger, Berlin: Springer-Verlag.

DETAILS ON GRAPE SEED PRODUCTS AND CLINICAL STUDIES

Product and clinical study information is grouped in the same order as in the Summary Table. A profile on an individual product is followed by details of the clinical studies associated with that product. In some instances, a clinical study, or studies, supports several products that contain the same principal ingredient(s). In these instances, those products are grouped together.

Clinical studies that follow each product, or group of products, are grouped by therapeutic indication, in accordance with the order in the Summary Table.

Index to Grape Seed Products

Product Profile: Endotelon®

Manufacturer	**Sanofi-Synthelabo, France (Indena S.p.A., Italy)**
U.S. distributor	**None**
Botanical ingredient	**Grape seed extract**
Extract name	**LeucoSelect™**
Quantity	50 mg
Processing	Plant to extract ratio 100:1.
Standardization	95% polyphenols (80-85% oligomeric proanthocyanidins)
Formulation	Tablet

Source(s) of information: Dartenuc, Marache, and Choussant, 1980; information provided by Indena USA, Inc.

Product Profile: Grape Seed Extract

Manufacturer	**Bluebonnet Nutrition Corporation (Indena S.p.A., Italy)**
U.S. distributor	**Bluebonnet Nutrition Corporation**
Botanical ingredient	**Grape seed extract**
Extract name	**LeucoSelect®**
Quantity	100 mg
Processing	Plant to extract ratio: 100:1
Standardization	Standardized to contain 80-85% oligomeric proanthocyanidins
Formulation	Capsule

Recommended dose: Take one capsule daily or as directed.

Other ingredients: Calcium phosphate, cellulose, silica, magnesium stearate.

Source(s) of information: Product label; information from Indena USA, Inc.

Product Profile: O.P.C.-100

Manufacturer	**Thorne Research (Indena S.p.A., Italy)**
U.S. distributor	**Thorne Research**
Botanical ingredient	**Grape seed extract**
Extract name	**LeucoSelect™**
Quantity	100 mg
Processing	Plant to extract ratio: 100:1
Standardization	95% oligomeric proanthocyanidins
Formulation	Capsule

Cautions: If pregnant, consult a health care practitioner before using this, or any other product.

Other ingredients: Cellulose capsule. May contain one or more of the following hypoallergenic ingredients to fill space: magnesium citrate, leucine, silicon dioxide.

Comments: This product is available only through pharmacies and health care practitioners. Also available in a 30 mg capsule (O.P.C.-30).

Source(s) of information: Product label; information from Indena USA, Inc.

Clinical Study: Endotelon®

Extract name	LeucoSelect™
Manufacturer	Sanofi Pharmaceuticals, France (Indena S.p.A., Italy)

Indication	**Chronic venous insufficiency**
Level of evidence	**II**
Therapeutic benefit	**Yes**

Bibliographic reference
Henriet JP (1988). Endotélon® dans les manifestations fonctionnelles de l'insuffisance veineuse périphérique: Etude EIVE [Endotelon® in the functional disorders caused by peripheral vascular insufficiency]. *Actualité Médicales Internationales—Angiologie* 5 (74): n.p.

Trial design
Parallel. Pretrial run-in with placebo lasting one month.

Study duration	3 months
Dose	3 (50 mg) pills twice daily
Route of administration	Oral
Randomized	Yes
Randomization adequate	Yes
Blinding	Double-blind
Blinding adequate	Yes
Placebo	Yes
Drug comparison	No
Site description	65 centers
No. of subjects enrolled	364
No. of subjects completed	357
Sex	Male and female
Age	18-63 years (mean: 37)

Inclusion criteria
Subjects between 18 and 60 years old with functional difficulties in their lower extremities, including a sensation of heaviness, tension, or pain diagnosable

as vascular symptoms which have been present for at least the last six months.

Exclusion criteria
Complications such as deep or superficial thrombosis, or vascular treatments during the six months before the study. Subjects with postphlebitis diseases, lymphatic anomalies, and evolving nutritional problems. Patients who resorted to analgesics or anti-inflammatories during the study were also excluded.

End points
Functional vascular symptoms were assessed at inclusion, at the beginning of therapy, and after one, two, and three months. These symptoms included heaviness or sensation of weight, tension, fatigue; paresthesia or prickling, itching, burning sensation, tingling; nocturnal leg cramps; leg agitation; and subjective edema. Edema was also measured quantitatively by water displacement.

Results
Improvement was observed in the clinical score of symptoms in the Endotelon group compared to placebo after 56 days of treatment, and the difference between the two groups increased after 84 days. The efficacy of Endotelon was more significant for those with initially higher symptom scores. Leg volumes did not change for either group.

Side effects
Gastric problems, nausea, headaches, and dizziness were reported in both groups.

Author's comments
The efficacy of Endotelon compared to placebo confirmed the usefulness of this drug therapy at the dosage of 300 mg per day against functional vascular-lymphatic insufficiency.

Reviewer's comments
Overall this was a good trial, with adequate blinding and randomization. The trial was large, had a long placebo washout period, and attempts were made to control circumstances for outcome measurement. The statistical methods were not adequately described or applied, however, and the data was not sufficiently summarized to allow for alternative analyses. (Translation reviewed) (5, 4)

Clinical Study: Endotelon®

Extract name	LeucoSelect™
Manufacturer	Sanofi Pharmaceuticals, France (Indena S.p.A., Italy)
Indication	**Chronic venous insufficiency; varicose veins**
Level of evidence	**II**
Therapeutic benefit	**Yes**

Bibliographic reference
Delacroix P (1981). Double-blind trial of Endotelon in chronic venous insufficiency. *Revue de Medecine* 27/28: 1793-1802.

Trial design
Parallel. Pretrial placebo period of one month followed by the treatment period of one month. Half of the subjects received Endotelon, and the other half received semisynthetic Diosmine (450 mg daily).

Study duration	1 month
Dose	3 (50 mg) gel caps daily
Route of administration	Oral
Randomized	Yes
Randomization adequate	Yes
Blinding	Double-blind
Blinding adequate	Yes
Placebo	No
Drug comparison	Yes
Drug name	Diosmine
Site description	Gynecology-obstetrics outpatient clinic
No. of subjects enrolled	50
No. of subjects completed	50
Sex	Female
Age	Mean: 34 ± 6 years

Inclusion criteria
Subjects between 20 and 60 years of age with functional symptoms of chronic venous insufficiency, or varicose veins due to pregnancy or oral contraceptives.

Exclusion criteria
Women in the first two months of pregnancy; with venous pathology in the lower limbs including arteriopathy, lymphadenitis, and painless varicose

veins; on low salt diets; or those taking diuretics, anti-inflammatories, or other therapies that might interfere with the trial. Also excluded were unstable, undisciplined, or neurotic patients.

End points
Patients were evaluated after the pretrial placebo period and after one month of treatment according to both functional and objective criteria. Functional criteria included pain typical of venous insufficiency including heaviness sensation in the legs, other pain, and swelling. Objective criteria included measurement of swelling via leg circumference and hypodermal lesions, including varicose veins and skin lesions due to hemorrhage.

Results
Both drugs were effective in treating peripheral venous insufficiency. Endotelon appeared more effective in treating functional parameters, since 65 percent of patients improved compared to 45 percent with Diosmine. Improvement was seen after nine days of treatment with Endotelon and after 14 days treatment with Diosmine. The therapeutic effect of Endotelon persisted 15 days after termination of treatment, whereas the effect persisted for only 10 days with Diosmine.

Side effects
Side effect were uncommon and never serious. Endotelon produced transient epigastric discomfort in some patients, and one case of nausea.

Author's comments
Compared with Diosmine, the therapeutic effect of Endotelon is more intense, more constant, and longer lasting, and can therefore be more readily utilized in the treatment of chronic venous insufficiency.

Reviewer's comments
This trial was well reported and conducted, except for the small number of subjects. The randomization and blinding were adequate and well described. (Translation reviewed) (5, 5)

Clinical Study: Endotelon®

Extract name	LeucoSelect™
Manufacturer	Laboratoires Labaz, France (Indena S.p.A., Italy)
Indication	**Chronic venous insufficiency**
Level of evidence	**II**
Therapeutic benefit	**Trend**

Bibliographic reference
Paitel D (1981). Rheographic and thermographic study of the effects on peripheral hemodynamics of an endotheoliotrophic, double blind versus placebo study. *Vie Medicale* 11: 776-783.

Trial design
Parallel.

Study duration	45 days
Dose	1 (50 mg) tablet 3 times daily
Route of administration	Oral
Randomized	Yes
Randomization adequate	Yes
Blinding	Double-blind
Blinding adequate	Yes
Placebo	Yes
Drug comparison	No
Site description	Single center
No. of subjects enrolled	50
No. of subjects completed	50
Sex	Male and female
Age	31-69 years (mean: 47)

Inclusion criteria
Patients with mild venous insufficiency, without significant reflux at the level of saphenous internal arch, or dilatation of the same vein. For patients affected by vascular sclerosis, the tests were performed on veins not previously treated.

Exclusion criteria
Younger than 20 or older than 70 years, use of vasculomotor therapies during the trials, or serious venous insufficiencies associated with important ostial insufficiency.

End points
Arterial and venous tone were measured using rheography (impedance plethysmography). Circulation was measured using thermography. Patients were examined before treatment and after 15, 30, and 45 days of treatment.

Results
Clinical, rheographic, and thermographic results all show a statistically significant difference in favor of Endotelon over placebo after one month of treatment. Of 25 patients treated with Endotelon, results are excellent in

seven cases, very good in 14 cases, good in two cases and acceptable in two cases. Of the 25 patients that received placebo, there were no excellent results, one very good result, two good results, seven acceptable results, and 15 cases of no results.

Side effects
None mentioned.

Author's comments
This study showed that Endotelon is effective in the treatment of peripheral vascular insufficiency.

Reviewer's comments
The end points of thermography/rheography measurements are not well validated in clinical literature. This trial was both double-blinded and randomized, but the data were not presented in sufficient detail to permit alternative analyses. (Translation reviewed) (5, 5)

Clinical Study: Endotelon®

Extract name	LeucoSelect®
Manufacturer	Laboratoires Labaz, France (Indena S.p.A., Italy)
Indication	**Capillary fragility** in hypertensive and diabetic patients
Level of evidence	**III**
Therapeutic benefit	**Trend**

Bibliographic reference
Lagrue G, Olivier-Martin F, Grillot A (1981). A study of the effect of procyanidolic oligomers on capillary resistance in the hypertension and certain nephropathies. *La Semaine des Hopitaux Paris* 57 (33-36): 1399-1401.

Trial design
Parallel. Two-phase study: first an open trial and second a comparative double-blind trial. The latter is reported here.

Study duration	1 to 3 months
Dose	3 (50 mg) tablets daily
Route of administration	Oral
Randomized	Yes
Randomization adequate	No

Blinding	Double-blind
Blinding adequate	Yes
Placebo	Yes
Drug comparison	No
Site description	Single center
No. of subjects enrolled	25
No. of subjects completed	25
Sex	Male and female
Age	18-68 years (mean: 46.5)

Inclusion criteria
Hypertensive and diabetic patients with capillary resistance decidedly less than normal.

Exclusion criteria
Subjects receiving other vascular therapies.

End points
Capillary resistance was measured using a Lavollay's capillarodynamo-meter. Capillary resistance, renal functions, arterial pressure and drug tolerance were monitored before and after treatment.

Results
Capillary resistance increased significantly after treatment with Endotelon, from 14.6 cmHg to 18.0 cmHg ($p < 0.0005$). No significant change was observed in the placebo group. Endotelon was significantly more effective compared to placebo ($p < 0.01$).

Side effects
In the open trial segment, treatment was interrupted in four out of 28 cases because of secondary effects (pruriginous eruption, palpitations, elation, and insomnia).

Authors' comments
Considering the increase in capillary resistance caused by Endotelon compared to placebo, it appears to be an interesting drug for microcirculation disorders associated with capillary fragility.

Reviewer's comments
The end point of capillary fragility/resistance is not well connected to a clinical condition, i.e., capillary fragility/resistance is a secondary end point or intermediate end point, and the exact relationship to other diseases is not established. Although the study was double-blind and randomized, the randomization process was not adequately described, the study was too small, and the

statistical methods were not adequately described or applied. (Translation reviewed) (3, 2)

Clinical Study: Endotelon®

Extract name	LeucoSelect™
Manufacturer	Laboratoires Labaz, France (Indena S.p.A., Italy)
Indication	**Capillary fragility**
Level of evidence	**III**
Therapeutic benefit	**Undetermined**

Bibliographic reference
Dartenuc JY, Marache P, Choussat H (1980). Capillary resistance in geriatrics: Study of a microangioprotector = Endotelon. *Bordeaux Medical* 13: 903-907.

Trial design
Parallel. Two-part trial: open trial and a double-blind placebo-controlled trial. The second is reported here.

Study duration	15 days
Dose	2 (50 mg) tablets daily
Route of administration	Oral
Randomized	No
Randomization adequate	No
Blinding	Double-blind
Blinding adequate	Yes
Placebo	Yes
Drug comparison	No
Site description	Single center
No. of subjects enrolled	37
No. of subjects completed	Not given
Sex	Male and female
Age	42-92 years (mean: 74.7)

Inclusion criteria
Hospitalized patients with capillary fragility with abnormal angiosterrometry (except eight patients that did not show more than five to ten petechias at −30 cmHg). Nine patients showed capillary fragility in the form of ecchymosis or petechias.

Exclusion criteria
Subjects taking therapies that were not related to the circulatory system.

End points
Capillary resistance was recorded using an angiosterrometer before treatment and at the end of the first and second treatments.

Results
Although cases of improvement were fewer than cases of no improvement, it is important to keep in mind that six patients had normal capillary resistance before treatment. Endotelon showed effectiveness in ten cases out of 21, whereas the placebo produced improvement in three patients out of 12. It appears that Endotelon is more effective against capillary fragility compared to placebo.

Side effects
None mentioned.

Authors' comments
The study showed that Endotelon is suitable in all clinical peripheral micro-angiopathy, all capillary permeability troubles, and in cases of capillary fragility revealed by angiosterrometric measures.

Reviewer's comments
It is not clear that the outcome measure used is clinically relevant. The variable dosage and variable length of trials (comparing both parts of trial) confound results. Variable tests were also performed on members of treatment groups. Although the study was double-blind, it was not randomized, the data were not summarized in sufficient detail, and the statistical methods were not adequately described or applied. (Translation reviewed) (2, 3)

Clinical Study: Endotelon®

Extract name	LeucoSelect™
Manufacturer	Laboratoires Labaz, France (Indena S.p.A., Italy)
Indication	**Capillary fragility** in patients with venous insufficiency and induced in healthy volunteers
Level of evidence	**III**
Therapeutic benefit	**Undetermined**

Bibliographic reference
Dubos G, Durst G, Hugonot R (1980). Capillary resistance evolution, spontaneously or artificially lessened by action of a capillaro-toxic substance in aged people. *Extrait de Geriatrie* September: 302-305.

Trial design
Parallel. Two-part study: open and double-blind controlled. The second part is described here. Each part of the study included two different groups of subjects: one group had low initial low capillary resistance, and another group who initially had normal levels but took 1 g aspirin for 15 days before treatment to reduce capillary resistance.

Study duration	1 month
Dose	150 mg daily
Route of administration	Oral
Randomized	Yes
Randomization adequate	Yes
Blinding	Double-blind
Blinding adequate	No
Placebo	Yes
Drug comparison	No
Site description	Single center
No. of subjects enrolled	30
No. of subjects completed	30
Sex	Male and female
Age	Mean: 74 years

Inclusion criteria
Two groups of subjects: some with venous insufficiency and others who were healthy. Those with capillary fragility had an initial mean capillary resistance of 13.32 cmHg. Those with normal capillary resistance had an initial mean level of 25.21 cmHg.

Exclusion criteria
None mentioned.

End points
Capillary resistance was evaluated using Parrot's angiosterrometer before taking the product and at the end of each week during the month of treatment.

Results
The subjects with initially low capillary resistance improved significantly af-

ter 15 and 30 days of treatment ($p < 0.02$ and $p < 0.01$, respectively). No significant change was observed with placebo. Similarly, the group with aspirin-induced capillary fragility improved after 15 and 30 days (both $p < 0.001$), whereas no significant change occurred with placebo.

Side effects
Endotelon did not cause any clinical or biological tolerance problems.

Authors' comments
Administered at a dose of 150 mg per day, Endotelon was capable of restoring normal values in subjects affected by capillary fragility caused by multiple pathologies and was able to oppose the decrease in capillary resistance produced by aspirin.

Reviewer's comments
This is a very complicated trial for such small numbers, and I am not convinced of the direct clinical relevance of this outcome and of the process of artificially lessening capillary resistance with aspirin. This study was adequately randomized, although the blinding was not described in enough detail. The sample size was also small, and the statistical methods and data were not adequately described. (Translation reviewed) (3, 3)

Clinical Study: Endotelon®

Extract name	LeucoSelect™
Manufacturer	Laboratoires Labaz, France (Indena S.p.A., Italy)

Indication	**Postoperative edema**
Level of evidence	**III**
Therapeutic benefit	**Trend**

Bibliographic reference
Baruch J (1984). The effects of Endotelon on postoperative edema: Results of a double-blind study vs. placebo in thirty-two patients. *Annales de Chirurgie Plastique et Esthetique* 29 (4): 393-395.

Trial design
Parallel. Treatment was given five days before surgery and from the second day until the sixth day after surgery (a second five-day treatment period).

Study duration	10 days
Dose	2 (50 mg) tablets 3 times daily

Route of administration	Oral
Randomized	Yes
Randomization adequate	No
Blinding	Double-blind
Blinding adequate	No
Placebo	Yes
Drug comparison	No
Site description	Cosmetic surgery practice
No. of subjects enrolled	33
No. of subjects completed	32
Sex	Female
Age	44-65 years (mean: 56.5)

Inclusion criteria
Women undergoing facelift surgery.

Exclusion criteria
Concurrent therapy.

End points
Three criteria were used to assess efficacy: the speed of edema disappearance expressed in days, the volume of edema assessed by the clinician, and a global clinical assessment. Patients were assessed on the second, fifth, and twelfth day postoperatively.

Results
The time until disappearance of edema after operation was 11.4 days for the treatment group and 15.8 days for the placebo group. This difference is statistically significant ($p = 0.01$). No significant difference in edema volume was observed between the two groups. However, global clinical evaluation on day 12 was in favor of the treatment group ($p = 0.04$).

Side effects
None observed.

Author's comments
The preventive effect of Endotelon on postoperative edema in face-lift surgery was demonstrated in this homogeneous group of patients.

Reviewer's comments
The primary outcome measure was not very objective, and this lack of an "objective" outcome limits the usefulness of this trial. Although the study was both

randomized and double-blind, neither process was adequately described. The length of the trial was also very short. (Translation reviewed) (1, 3)

Clinical Study: Endotelon®

Extract name	LeucoSelect™
Manufacturer	Sanofi Pharmaceuticals, France (Indena S.p.A., Italy)
Indication	**Vision**
Level of evidence	**II**
Therapeutic benefit	**Yes**

Bibliographic reference
Corbe C, Boissin JP, Siou A (1988). Chromatic sense and chorioretinal circulation: Study of the effect of O.P.C (Endotelon). *Journal Français d'Ophtalmologie* 11 (5): 453-460.

Trial design
Parallel. Half of the subjects received Endotelon treatment and the other half received no treatment. Evaluators were blind.

Study duration	5 weeks
Dose	2 (50 mg procyanidolic oligomers) tablets twice daily
Route of administration	Oral
Randomized	Yes
Randomization adequate	Yes
Blinding	Single-Blind
Blinding adequate	No
Placebo	No
Drug comparison	No
Site description	2 centers
No. of subjects enrolled	100
No. of subjects completed	95
Sex	Male and female
Age	Mean: 37 years

Inclusion criteria
Adults whose work in front of video displays subjected them to frequent bright stimuli of long duration, and drivers subject to bright lights and repeated glare from headlights.

Exclusion criteria
Any major retinal or ophthalmological pathology. This included patients with retinal pathology from diabetes and hypertension, retinopathy and retinal detachment, glaucoma, myopia over six dioptric units, astigmatism over three units, and nystagmus.

End points
The evaluations included visual recovery after glare as a function of time (Comberg's nycometer), night morphoscopic vision threshold (Beyne's scoptometer), and ergovision tests. Examinations were completed before treatment and after five weeks.

Results
For subjects treated with Endotelon, the improvement in the visual performances after glare, as well as the rapidity of recovery from glare, was very significant compared to the results obtained by the control group. Visual adaptation to low luminance also improved under treatment. The ergovision tests support the above results.

Side effects
Gastric symptoms in one subject and dizziness in another with known hypertension.

Authors' comments
The efficacy of Endotelon and the observed good tolerance in the study allows the endorsement of this therapy for subjects having increased sensitivity to glare and a decrease in nocturnal vision, especially a lesser distinguishing ability in a weak luminance environment.

Reviewer's comments
This trial demonstrated a benefit for sensitivity to glare, but no conclusion can be made regarding any other ophthalmologic conditions. The study was not double-blind, and the data was not summarized in sufficient detail to permit replication. (Translation reviewed) (3, 5)

Product Profile: LeucoSelect™-phytosome®

Manufacturer	**Indena S.p.A., Italy**
U.S. distributor	**Indena USA, Inc.**
Botanical ingredient	**Grape seed phytosome**
Extract name	**LeucoSelect-phytosome**
Quantity	150 mg

Processing	1 part LeucoSelect® (extract of grape seeds) to 2 parts phosphatidylcholine. LeucoSelect plant/extract ratio 100:1
Standardization	No information
Formulation	Capsule

Other ingredients: Phosphatidylcholine from soybean

Source(s) of information: Nuttall et al., 1998; information provided by the distributor.

Clinical Study: LeucoSelect™-phytosome®

Extract name	LeucoSelect-phytosome
Manufacturer	Indena S.p.A, Italy
Indication	**Antioxidant activity** in healthy volunteers
Level of evidence	**III**
Therapeutic benefit	**MOA**

Bibliographic reference
Nuttall SL, Kendall MJ, Bombardelli E, Morazzoni P (1998). An evaluation of the antioxidant activity of a standardized grape seed extract, Leucoselect. *Journal of Clinical Pharmacy and Therapeutics* 23 (5): 385-389.

Trial design
Crossover study. Levels of antioxidant activity were measured after one dose and after five days of treatment. The experiment was repeated following at least a two-week washout period.

Study duration	5 days
Dose	2 (150 mg) capsules daily
Route of administration	Oral
Randomized	Yes
Randomization adequate	No
Blinding	Single-blind
Blinding adequate	No
Placebo	Yes
Drug comparison	No
Site description	Single center
No. of subjects enrolled	20

No. of subjects completed	Not given
Sex	Male and female
Age	19-31 years (mean: 23)

Inclusion criteria

Healthy young students. All volunteers were nonsmokers, maintained a standardized dietary pattern throughout the study period, and did not take vitamin supplements.

Exclusion criteria

Major medical or surgical illness in the previous five years, hospital admissions, or current medications.

End points

A series of blood samples were taken before breakfast and following breakfast plus either placebo or active treatment over a period of six hours on days 1 and 5 of each treatment arm. Blood samples were assayed for antioxidant activity and levels of vitamins C and E.

Results

LeucoSelect had no effect on serum vitamins C and E levels, but increased serum total antioxidant activity (TAC). On day 1, TAC was significantly increased 30 minutes after drug treatment compared with baseline values, $p < 0.05$. TAC was further increased at 60 minutes postdose, and remained elevated more than three hours postdose ($p < 0.01$). On day 5, results showed similar increases in TAC at 30 and 60 minutes postdose compared with baseline levels ($p < 0.05$ and $p < 0.01$). No significant difference was observed between days 1 and 5. There was no significant change in serum TAC following administration of placebo on either test day.

Side effects

Not mentioned.

Authors' comments

LeucoSelect capsules increase serum antioxidant activity, but the longer-term clinical implications need to be assessed in further randomized clinical trials.

Reviewer's comments

Antioxidant activity is an intermediate outcome, not a clinical end point (for example, heart disease). This study was single-blind and not randomized, and the sample size was too small. (0, 5)

Product Profile: Procianidol

Manufacturer	**Bruschettini s.r.l., Italy**
U.S. distributor	None
Botanical ingredient	**Grape seed fermented product**
Extract name	N/A
Quantity	100 mg
Processing	No information
Standardization	No information
Formulation	Capsule

Source(s) of information: Fusi et al., 1990.

Clinical Study: Procianidol

Extract name	N/A
Manufacturer	Bruschettini s.r.l., Italy
Indication	**Vision**
Level of evidence	**II**
Therapeutic benefit	**Trend**

Bibliographic reference
Fusi L, Czimeg F, Pesce F, Germogli R, Boero A, Vanzetti M, and Gandiglio G (1990). Effects of procyanidolic olygomers from *Vitis vinifera* in subjects working at video-display units. *Annali di Ottalmologia e Clinica Oculistica* 116: 575-584.

Trial design
Parallel. Three-arm treatment: Group 1 included 50 subjects treated with procyanidolic oligomers; group 2 included ten subjects treated with bilberry anthocyanosides at a dose of 1 × 100 mg capsule three times daily; and group 3 included 15 subjects treated with placebo.

Study duration	2 months
Dose	1 (100 mg) capsule 3 times daily procyanidolic oligomers
Route of administration	Oral
Randomized	Yes
Randomization adequate	No

Blinding	Double-blind
Blinding adequate	Yes
Placebo	Yes
Drug comparison	Yes
Drug name	Bilberry anthocyanosides
Site description	Not described
No. of subjects enrolled	75
No. of subjects completed	75
Sex	Male and female
Age	20-60 years (mean: 37.9)

Inclusion criteria
Employees using video displays for at least six hours daily, some with various ophthalmological abnormalities.

Exclusion criteria
None mentioned.

End points
A complete ophthalmological examination, orthotic, chromatic sense, determination of contrast sensitivity curve, and a computerized examination of visual field were conducted before and after treatment.

Results
At baseline, the mean curve of contrast sensitivity was below the normal range at most contrast values. After treatment, a statistically significant increase was observed at all ten points of the curve in the group treated with procyanidolic olygomers, at six points of the curve for the bilberry anthocyanoside group, and two points of the curve for the placebo group. The visual acuity and chromatic sense data showed no treatment related changes. An examination of the kinetic visual field did not reveal pathological alterations in any patient. Comparison of overall therapeutic efficacy ratings shows that favorable results were obtained significantly more frequently in both groups treated with active compounds than in the placebo-treated group.

Side effects
Gastric complaints, which did not differ between the 3 groups, were reported.

Authors' comments
Procyanidolic oligomers and bilberry anthocyanosides significantly improved contrast sensitivity and angular resolution power, which are both re-

duced as a result of the visual stress induced by working with video-display units.

Reviewer's comments
This study is adequately double-blinded, and although it is also randomized, the randomization process is not well described. The statistical methods are not adequately described or applied. An unequal division of groups is present, with no statistical difference between them. (Translation reviewed) (3, 4)

Grass Pollen

Rye pollen (*Secale cereale* L.) [Poaceae]
Timothy pollen (*Phleum pratense* L.) [Poaceae]
Corn pollen (*Zea mays* L.) [Poaceae]

PREPARATION USED
IN REVIEWED CLINICAL STUDIES

Pollen is the male fertilizing element of flowering plants. It consists of fine yellow grains that are dispersed by the wind and also by insects such as honeybees. A mechanical method of harvesting pollen by puncturing the pollen husk and extracting the nutrients has produced a product that has been tested in numerous studies (Schulz, Hänsel, and Tyler, 2001).

Cernilton® is a standardized product prepared from a proprietary blend of selected pollens, identified by the company literature only as flower pollen. However, it is suggested by Schulz, Hänsel, and Tyler (2001) that Cernilton complies with the German Commission E monograph description of an extract of pollens from grass flowers, consisting of rye pollen (*Secale cereale* L.), timothy pollen (*Phleum pratense* L.), and corn pollen (*Zea mays* L.) (family Poaceae, formally Graminae). Cernilton contains two extracts: Cernitin™ T60™, a water-soluble pollen extract fraction; and Cernitin™ GBX™, a fat-soluble pollen extract fraction. Each capsule/tablet contains 60 mg T60 and 3 mg GBX. Cernilton is manufactured and distributed by A.B. Cernelle, Sweden, and Graminex LLC.

SUMMARY OF REVIEWED CLINICAL STUDIES

Cernilton was tested in clinical studies for treatment of symptomatic benign prostatic hyperplasia (BPH), also known as benign prostatic hypertrophy and prostatic adenoma. BPH is a nonmalignant en-

773

GRASS POLLEN SUMMARY TABLE

Product Name	Manufacturer/ U.S. Distributor	Product Characteristics	Dose in Trials	Indication	No. of Trials	Benefit (Evidence Level-Trial No.)
Cernilton®	A.B. Cernelle, Sweden (Graminex LLC)/Graminex LLC	Cernitin™ T60™ (water-soluble pollen extract fraction); Cernitin™ GBX™ (acetone-soluble pollen extract fraction)	3 to 6 capsules or tablets (containing 60 mg T60 and 3 mg GBX) daily	Benign prostatic hyperplasia	3	Yes (II-1) Trend (II-1) Undetermined (III-1)

largement of the prostate that is common in men over 40 years of age. Symptoms include hesitancy in initiating the urinary stream, a weak or intermittent stream, terminal dribbling of urine, increased urinary urgency and frequency (diuresis: increased formation and release of urine; and nocturia: frequent and/or excessive urination at night), and sensation of incomplete voiding.

The progressive symptoms of BPH have been categorized by Vahlensieck, Alken, and others. The Vahlensieck classification has four stages of symptoms. Stage I is characterized by no voiding difficulties, no residual urine, and a urine flow of more than 15 ml per second. Stage II is characterized by transient voiding difficulties and urine flow between 10 and 15 ml per second. Stage III is characterized by constant voiding dysfunction, urine flow less than 10 ml per second, residual urine greater than 50 ml, and a trabeculated (ridged) bladder. Stage IV is characterized by residual urine volume greater than 100 ml and bladder dilatation (Schulz, Hänsel, and Tyler, 2001). The Alken classification has three stages. Stages I to III are similar to Vahlensieck stages II through IV. Stage I is characterized by an increase in the frequency of urination, pollakiuria (abnormally frequent urination), nocturia, delayed onset of urination, and weak urinary stream. Stage II is characterized by the beginning of the decomposition of the bladder function accompanied by formation of residual urine and urge to urinate. Stage III is characterized by decomposition of the bladder, vesicular overflowing, continuous drip incontinence, and damage to the urinary system and kidneys due to regressive obstruction (Löbelenz, 1992).

Cernilton

Benign Prostatic Hyperplasia

We reviewed three studies, two of which were double-blind and placebo-controlled. The larger study included 96 men with Vahlensieck stage II or III, who were treated Cernilton (two capsules three times daily) or placebo for three months. Observations at 6 and 12 weeks revealed that symptoms of nocturia, diuresis, and sensation of residual urine were significantly improved compared to placebo. No difference in hesitancy, urgency, intermittency, terminal dribbling, dysuria, peak urine flow, or voided volume was reported (Becker and Ebeling, 1988).

The second study included 53 men awaiting an operation to relieve urinary obstruction, who were given either two capsules twice daily or placebo for six months. The study reported a significant decrease in residual urine and a decrease in the diameter of the prostate with treatment compared to placebo. As with the previous study, flow rate and voided volume were not changed (Buck et al., 1990).

The third study, which included 89 men with BPH stages I and II (classification system not given), compared Cernilton to Tadenan (a product containing a *Pygeum africanum* extract that is also covered in this book). The Cernilton group received one to two tablets of Cernilton three times daily, and the Tadenan group received two tablets twice daily. After four months of treatment, a positive therapeutic response was reported for both treatments, with improved peak flow rate, decreased residual urine volume, decreased prostate volume, and improved obstructive and irritative symptom scores. Scores for the Cernilton group showed more improvement than scores for the Tadenan group, although statistical analysis was not conducted (Dutkiewicz, 1996). The lack of a placebo group limited the usefulness of this study.

According to our reviewer, Dr. Elliot Fagelman, the studies range from fair to good in quality and provide evidence that Cernilton may be beneficial in patients with BPH. However, no studies compared Cernilton with an alpha-adrenergic receptor blocker (e.g., prazosin, terazosin) or a five-alpha reductase inhibitor (e.g., finasteride), the two classes of drugs used in standard clinical practice.

SYSTEMATIC REVIEWS

Four controlled trials, published between 1981 and 1996 with a minimum of one month's duration, were included in a systematic review of Cernilton for the treatment of benign prostatic hyperplasia. The trials' durations were from three to six months, and included 444 men (163 in placebo-controlled trials and 281 in the comparison trials). The subjects received dosages ranging from three to six capsules daily. Three of these trials were reviewed previously (Becker and Ebeling, 1988; Buck et al., 1990; Dutkiewicz, 1996). The forth trial is a double-blind study that compared Cernilton with Paraprost (a mixture of amino acids). In all studies, Cernilton performed better than the controls (placebo, Paraprost, and Tadenan) in terms of the self-reported improvement of symptoms. The frequency of urination was reduced by Cernilton compared with controls, whereas urinary flow measures were not significantly different. Postvoid residual urine volume was reduced modestly by Cernilton compared to placebo, and was similarly reduced by the other control agents. Cernilton's performance was similar to Paraprost and Tadenan with obstructive and irritative symptoms. Only one placebo-controlled study reported a significant reduction in prostate size with Cernilton. The authors of the review conclude, however, that because of the methodological shortcomings of the studies (such as short duration, small sample sizes, and unclear concealment of treatment allocation), Cernilton's efficacy in preventing complications of BPH is undetermined. The trials could not be combined in a meta-analysis due to the differences in reporting methods and control agents (MacDonald et al., 1999).

ADVERSE REACTIONS OR SIDE EFFECTS

Nausea was noted in one study we reviewed (Becker and Ebeling, 1988). A systematic review reported that Cernilton was well tolerated with no serious side effects (MacDonald et al., 1999). In an unpublished report including 1,798 patients treated with Cernilton N, 15 patients (0.8 percent) reported adverse effects, which included mostly gastrointestinal symptoms (indigestion, stomach pain, nausea, pressure sensation, and diarrhea) (Bach and Ebeling, n.d.).

INFORMATION FROM PHARMACOPOEIAL MONOGRAPHS

Source of Published Therapeutic Monographs

German Commission E

Indications

In 1994, the German Commission E recommended a grass pollen preparation for the treatment of benign prostatic hyperplasia (micturition difficulties associated with Alken stage I-II benign prostatic enlargement). The preparation is described as containing a complex extract of 92 percent rye pollen (*Secale cereale* L.), 5 percent timothy pollen (*Phleum pratense* L.), and 3 percent corn pollen (*Zea mays* L.). The herbs are extracted with a water and acetone mixture, yielding a product with an herb to extract ratio of 2.5:1 (Schulz, Hänsel, and Tyler, 2001).

Doses

Extract: 80 to 120 mg daily in two or three divided doses (Schulz, Hänsel, and Tyler, 2001).

Treatment Period

Treatment should last at least three months (Schulz, Hänsel, and Tyler, 2001).

Contraindications

None (Schulz, Hänsel, and Tyler, 2001)

Adverse Reactions

Adverse reactions include rare instances of gastrointestinal complaints or allergic skin reactions (Schulz, Hänsel, and Tyler, 2001).

REFERENCES

Bach D, Ebeling L (n.d.). Possibilities and limitations of phytotherapy for benign prostatic hyperplasia (BPH): Results of treatment with Cernilton®N for stages 1-3 according to Alken (or II-IV according to Vahlensieck). Available at <http://www.cerniltonamerica.com/study12. html> and <http://www.graminex.com/clinical_studies/study12.php>.

Becker H, Ebeling L (1988). Conservative therapy of benign prostate hyperplasia (BPH) with Cernilton: Results of a placebo-controlled, double blind study. *Urologe [B]* 28: 301-306.

Buck AC, Cox R, Rees R, Ebeling L, John A (1990). Treatment of outflow tract obstruction due to benign prostatic hyperplasia with the pollen extract, Cernilton. *British Journal of Urology* 66 (4): 398-404.

Dutkiewicz S (1996). Usefulness of Cernilton in the treatment of benign prostatic hyperplasia. *International Urology and Nephrology* 28 (1): 49-53.

Löbelenz J (1992). *Extractum sabal fructus* in the therapy of benign prostatic hyperplasia (BPH). *Tpk Therapeutikon* 6 (1/2): 34-37.

MacDonald R, Ishani A, Rutks I, Wilt TJ (1999). A systematic review of Cernilton for the treatment of benign prostatic hyperplasia. *BJU International* 85 (7): 836-841.

Schulz V, Hänsel R, Tyler VE (2001). *Rational Phytotherapy: A Physicians' Guide to Herbal Medicine,* Fourth Edition. Trans. TC Telgar. Berlin: Springer-Verlag.

DETAILS ON GRASS POLLEN PRODUCTS
AND CLINICAL STUDIES

Product and clinical study information is grouped in the same order as in the Summary Table. A profile on an individual product is followed by details of the clinical studies associated with that product. In some instances, a clinical study, or studies, supports several products that contain the same principal ingredient(s). In these instances, those products are grouped together.

Clinical studies that follow each product, or group of products, are grouped by therapeutic indication, in accordance with the order in the Summary Table.

Product Profile: Cernilton®

Manufacturer	**AB Cernelle, Sweden**
U.S. distributor	**Graminex L.L.C.**
Botanical ingredient	**Flower pollen extract**
Extract name	**Cernitin™ T60™; Cernitin™ GBX™**
Quantity	60 mg Cernitin T60, 3 mg Cernitin GBX in one tablet
Processing	Cernitin T60 (water-soluble pollen extract concentrate) and Cernitin GBX (fat-soluble pollen extract concentrate), ratio of 20:1
Standardization	No information
Formulation	Tablet

Recommended dose: Four tablets daily as a dietary supplement with meals or a glass of water.

DSHEA-Structure/Function: Promotes a healthy prostate. Supplies vital nutrients to the body and cells (including all essential amino acids, unsaturated fatty acids, and enzymes). Improves absorption of vitamins, minerals, and trace elements from the food we eat. Enables better adaptation to stress, enhancing physical and mental capacity. Helps bioregulate organism functions such as immune system, lipid metabolism, blood cholesterol level, and function of prostate.

Other ingredients: Microcrystalline cellulose, silicon dioxide colloidal, and magnesium stearate.

Source(s) of information: Product label; product information pamphlet.

Clinical Study: Cernilton® N

Extract name	T60™; GBX™
Manufacturer	AB Cernelle, Sweden
Indication	**Benign prostatic hyperplasia**
Level of evidence	**II**
Therapeutic benefit	**Yes**

Bibliographic reference
Becker H, Ebeling L (1988). Conservative therapy of benign prostate hyperplasia (BPH) with Cernilton: Results of a placebo-controlled, double blind study. *Urologe [B]* 28: 301-306.

Trial design
Parallel. Study was preceded by a washout phase.

Study duration	3 months
Dose	2 capsules 3 times daily
Route of administration	Oral
Randomized	Yes
Randomization adequate	No
Blinding	Double-blind
Blinding adequate	Yes
Placebo	Yes
Drug comparison	No
Site description	6 urology clinics
No. of subjects enrolled	103
No. of subjects completed	96
Sex	Male
Age	42-85 years

Inclusion criteria
Patients with benign prostatic hyperplasia (BPH) in stages II and III according to Vahlensieck.

Exclusion criteria
Suspicion of a prostate carcinoma; urinary retention of >150 ml; neuro-

genous bladder-emptying difficulties; acute and/or chronic prostatitis/pro-statovesiculities; deformity or postoperative condition in the urogenital area with obstruction of the urethra; bladder calculus.

End points
The controlled parameters were micturition problems, urinary retention, palpation result, uroflow, and overall assessment of therapy by patient and doctor. Patients were examined before the trial and after 6 and 12 weeks.

Results
Observations at 6 and 12 weeks showed that all individual symptoms had higher improvement rates and/or positive responses under Cernilton compared to placebo. These differences were especially evident for nocturia, diuresis, and sensation of residual urine. Nocturia improved significantly in 68.8 percent of Cernilton patients and in 37.2 percent of placebo group (comparison $p < 0.005$). The average decrease in urinary retention during treatment was significantly different ($p = 0.006$). No difference was seen between the groups in terms of dysuria, urge, and discomfort. Patients and doctors rated the results of the treatment as very good and good with statistical significance, corresponding to the efficacy of treatment.

Side effects
Slight nausea in one patient taking Cernilton.

Authors' comments
The results of this study demonstrate the effectiveness of the pollen extract preparation for clinical symptoms, urodynamics, and overall opinion of BPH patients stages II and III. The pollen extract is salubrious, and makes long-term treatment with little risk of side effects possible. The use of Cernilton for the symptomatic treatment of BPH stages II and III is recommended.

Reviewer's comments
Overall this is a good study showing symptomatic improvement in those treated with Cernilton. However, 12 weeks is a relatively short duration of treatment. (Translation reviewed) (3, 6)

Clinical Study: Cernilton®

Extract name	T60™, GBX™
Manufacturer	AB Cernelle, Sweden
Indication	**Benign prostatic hyperplasia**
Level of evidence	**II**
Therapeutic benefit	**Trend**

Bibliographic reference
Buck AC, Cox R, Rees R, Ebeling L, John A (1990). Treatment of outflow tract obstruction due to benign prostatic hyperplasia with the pollen extract, Cernilton. *British Journal of Urology* 66 (4): 398-404.

Trial design
Parallel.

Study duration	6 months
Dose	2 capsules twice daily
Route of administration	Oral
Randomized	No
Randomization adequate	No
Blinding	Double-blind
Blinding adequate	Yes
Placebo	Yes
Drug comparison	No
Site description	Not described
No. of subjects enrolled	60
No. of subjects completed	53
Sex	Male
Age	56-89 years (mean: 68.6)

Inclusion criteria
Patients awaiting operative treatment for outflow obstruction due to benign enlargement of the prostate.

Exclusion criteria
None mentioned.

End points
Objective criteria for the evaluation of outflow obstruction were urine flow rate, voided volume, residual urine, and prostate size. Subjective assessment was based on a modified Boyarsky scoring scale for symptoms of frequency, hesitancy, urgency, intermittency, incomplete emptying, terminal dribbling, and dysuria. Investigations were performed before the patients entered treatment, at three months, and at six months.

Results
A statically significant subjective improvement with Cernilton (69 percent of patients) was observed compared with placebo (30 percent) ($p < 0.009$). Residual urine volume decreased significantly in the patients receiving Cernilton compared with the placebo group, in whom it increased ($p <$

0.025). No statistical difference in the symptoms of diurnal frequency was observed between the two groups ($p = 0.66$). Sixty percent of patients on Cernilton were improved or symptom free of nocturia compared with 30 percent of patients on placebo ($p < 0.063$). On Cernilton, 57 percent of patients showed improvement in bladder emptying, compared to 10 percent on placebo ($p < 0.004$). No significant differences between the two groups were found in hesitancy, urgency, intermittency, terminal dribbling, dysuria, peak urine flow rate, or voided volume.

Side effects
No adverse side effects.

Authors' comments
The precise mode of action of Cernilton in benign prostatic hyperplasia is not known. However, this study has shown distinct subjective and objective improvement with a positive response in the Cernilton group. Cernilton may prove to be a useful agent in alleviating the early symptoms of outflow tract obstruction due to BPH.

Reviewer's comments
This study is limited by the small number of patients and lack of randomization (however, the groups were similar at baseline). Overall a symptomatic benefit was seen in those on Cernilton. A decrease in residual urine was statistically significant, but may not be clinically significant. (3, 4)

Clinical Study: Cernilton®

Extract name	T60™; GBX™
Manufacturer	AB Cernelle, Sweden
Indication	**Benign prostatic hyperplasia**
Level of evidence	**III**
Therapeutic benefit	**Undetermined**

Bibliographic reference
Dutkiewicz S (1996). Usefulness of Cernilton in the treatment of benign prostatic hyperplasia. *International Urology and Nephrology* 28 (1): 49-53.

Trial design
Parallel. For the first two weeks of the trial, the Cernilton group received two tablets three times daily; for the remainder of the trial, patients received one tablet three times daily. Patients in the control (Tadenan) group received two tablets twice daily.

Study duration	4 months
Dose	1 to 2 tablets 3 times daily
Route of administration	Oral
Randomized	No
Randomization adequate	No
Blinding	Open
Blinding adequate	No
Placebo	No
Drug comparison	Yes
Drug name	Tadenan
Site description	Not described
No. of subjects enrolled	89
No. of subjects completed	89
Sex	Male
Age	50-68 years

Inclusion criteria
Patients with clinical stages I and II benign prostate hyperplasia, with a short history of symptoms no longer than a few weeks in duration (classification system not given).

Exclusion criteria
Patients with complete urine retention.

End points
Subjective assessment was made using a symptom score system and objective evaluation by physical examination, uroflowmetry, and ultrasound examination of residual urine and prostate size.

Results
The therapeutic response was positive in 40 (78 percent) and 21 (55 percent) patients in the Cernilton and Tadenan groups, respectively. Peak flow rate improved by 19.5 percent in the Cernilton group, and by 10.8 percent in the Tadenan group. Residual urine volume improved by 47.8 percent and by 21.6 percent in the Cernilton and Tadenan groups, respectively. Prostate volume also improved by 5.15 percent (Cernilton) and by 0.45 percent (Tadenan). Obstructive symptom scores improved by 62.75 percent in the Cernilton group and by 45.8 percent in the Tadenan group. Irritative symptoms improved in the Cernilton group by 68.4 percent and by 40 percent in the Tadenan group.

Side effects
No adverse reactions were seen.

Author's comments

In BPH, the decongestive effect of Cernilton leads to a lasting improvement of voiding difficulties. The residual urine volume decreases significantly. In comparison to *Pygeum africanum* extract (Tadenan), Cernilton proved much more effective.

Reviewer's comments

This study compares Cernilton with Tadenan. Although a benefit was observed in the patients treated with Cernilton, a poor study design and lack of a placebo group limit the usefulness of the study. The treatment was also given for a short duration. (1, 3)

Green Tea

Latin name: *Camellia sinensis* (**L.**) **Kuntze** [Theaceae]
Latin synonyms: *Thea sinensis* **L.**
Plant part: **Leaf**

PREPARATIONS USED IN REVIEWED CLINICAL STUDIES

Chinese legend has it that tea was discovered in 2700 B.C. when a gust of wind blew some tea leaves into a kettle of boiling water. A competing legend advanced by the British East India Company claims tea originated in India and not China (Gutman and Ryu, 1996).

Green tea and black tea are both derived from the young shoots (the first two or three leaves plus the growing bud) of *Camellia sinensis* (L.) Kuntze. The teas are differentiated by their method of processing. Heating the freshly picked leaves shortly after harvest produces green tea. This process inactivates enzymes (polyphenol oxidases) that form the dark pigments associated with black tea. The heated leaves are then rolled to squeeze the juices to the surface of the leaf and dried using hot air. Black teas are produced by a natural enzymatic fermentation of the leaves that occurs after harvest (Gutman and Ryu, 1996).

A cup of green tea usually contains 300 to 400 mg polyphenols. Polyphenols are a large class of mildly acidic compounds with antioxidant properties. Polyphenols can be divided into many subclasses, including catechins, an example of which is epigallocatechin gallate (EGCG) (Gutman and Ryu, 1996).

Two studies were conducted on a product defined as US Tea Associations regular tea freeze-dried solids and called "Lipton® Research Blend." The tea was prepared by Thomas J. Lipton Co., of Englewood Cliffs, New Jersey, which is now part of Unilever Bestfoods, North America. The rest of the studies were conducted on extracts of tea leaves with concentrated amounts of polyphenols.

GREEN TEA SUMMARY TABLE

Product Name	Manufacturer/ U.S. Distributor	Product Characteristics	Dose in Trials	Indication	No. of Trials	Benefit (Evidence Level-Trial No.)
Exolise™	Arktopharma Laboratoires Pharmaceutiques, France/Health from the Sun/ Arkopharma	Aqueous ethanolic dry extract standardized to 25% catechins, expressed as EGCG	1 capsule 3 times daily (375 mg catechins, 150 mg caffeine)	Weight loss	1	MOA (III-1)
Lipton® Research Blend	Thomas J Lipton Co. (Unilever Bestfoods, North America)/none	Tea solids	3 g tea solids (900 ml/day)	Cardio-vascular risk factors	1	MOA (III-1)
			2 g tea solids (300 ml/day)	Antioxidant activity	1	MOA (III-1)
Tegreen 97® (US), Xin Nao Jian (China)	Pharmanex LLC/Pharmanex Natural Healthcare	Extract containing 97% polyphenols	600 mg extract per day	Hemato-poietic effects of cancer therapy	1	Undetermined (III-1)
				Renal insuf-ficiency	1	Undetermined (III-1)
Polyphenon E®	Mitsui Nohrin Co., Ltd., Japan/None	Polyphenol extract	600 mg extract per day	Cardio-vascular risk factors	1	Undetermined (III-1)

Editor's note: Exolise was taken off the market while this book was in press.

Exolise™, which is manufactured by Arktopharma Laboratoires Pharmaceutiques in France and distributed by Health from the Sun/ Arkopharma, Stamford, Connecticut, contains an 80 percent ethanolic dry extract standardized to 25 percent catechins, expressed as EGCG. The amount used in the weight-loss study was specifically characterized as three capsules per day containing a total of 375 mg catechin (270 mg of which as epigallocatechin) and 150 mg caffeine.

Tegreen®, produced by Pharmanex LLC, a wholly owned subsidiary of Nu Skin Enterprises, Inc., Provo, Utah, is characterized as containing 97 percent polyphenols.

Polyphenon E®, produced by Mitsui Nohrin Co. Ltd., Tokyo, Japan, is characterized simply as a polyphenol extract. This product is not available commercially in the United States.

SUMMARY OF REVIEWED CLINICAL STUDIES

Studies of green tea as tea solids or extracts have been conducted exploring its use in weight loss and as an antioxidant useful in reducing cardiovascular risk factors, in alleviating the adverse effects of renal insufficiency, and in reducing the negative effects of cancer therapy on blood cells. On balance, green tea extracts and green tea have positive effects on metabolism and antioxidant activity. However, the impact of these effects on health outcomes remains to be determined.

Exolise

Weight Loss

A study exploring green tea's effect on weight loss was conducted using Exolise, one capsule three times daily. This mechanistic study showed an increase in energy expenditure over a 24-hour period with Exolise compared to placebo. The energy expenditure was 4 percent above the stimulatory effects produced by equivalent amounts of caffeine found in Exolise (Dulloo et al., 1999). Although this carefully controlled study demonstrated thermogenic activity and promotion of the oxidation of fat, the results were of questionable significance for clinical weight management. A follow-up study with moderately obese subjects did report weight loss as a result of treatment. However that study did not include a control group, and thus did not qualify for review in this book (Chantre and Lairon, 2002).

Lipton Green Tea, Research Blend

Cardiovascular Risk Factors/Antioxidant Activity

Potential antioxidant activity was explored in two studies comparing green and black teas. In a study with 45 participants, the daily consumption of six cups of green or black tea (Lipton tea solids, 0.5 g in 150 ml water) over a four-week period did not lead to any effect on serum lipid concentrations, resistance of low-density-lipoprotein-cholesterol (LDL) to oxidation, or to markers of oxidative damage to lipids. However, consumption of green tea led to a slight increase in total antioxidant activity in plasma (van het Hof et al., 1997). The other study included 21 adults who received six different treatments on six different days with at least two days in between treatments. The administration of a single dose of 2 g of green or black tea solids (Lipton) in 300 ml water led to a significant increase in plasma catechin levels and in plasma antioxidant activity one hour later. The rise in total catechins was greater with green tea than black tea, as expected based on the higher content of catechins in green tea compared to black tea. The addition of milk to either green or black tea did not affect results (Leenen et al., 2000). These studies were both rated as low in quality due to a lack of blinding and poor descriptions of the randomization process.

Tegreen

Hematopoietic Effects of Cancer Therapy

A study examined the potential protective effect of a green tea polyphenol extract (Xin Nao Jian) on the damage to the development and formation of blood cells due to cancer radiation therapy or chemotherapy. Sixty cancer inpatients with a normal blood cell profile undergoing their first treatment were included in the study. They were given 200 mg of extract three times daily, another herbal formula for improving blood quality (Sha Gan Chun), or no additional treatment for one month. Total white blood cell counts improved in the green tea group but declined in the Sha Gan Chun group after five weeks and in the control group after three weeks. No significant changes were observed in hemoglobin levels or platelet counts in any group (Walsh, 1997a). Our reviewer, Dr. David Heber, commented that the effects of green tea on lymphocyte stabilization and immune function deserve further study. This study was limited by inadequately described statistical methods and a small sample size.

Renal Insufficiency

In another study, Tegreen was given in the same dose (200 mg three times daily) to patients with chronic renal insufficiency for three months. Renal function (as measured by blood urea nitrogen) was improved, erythrocyte superoxide dismutase activity was significantly increased, and plasma lipid peroxide levels were significantly decreased. The author of the study commented that the benefits of Tegreen to this population were due to its antioxidant activity and free radical scavenging activity (Walsh, 1997b). Although it had some serious methodological flaws, this study remains a good guide for future studies.

Polyphenon E

Cardiovascular Risk Factors

A small study using a green tea concentrate, Polyphenon E, measured the effect of 300 mg extract twice daily, the equivalent of seven to eight cups of tea, on markers of antioxidant activity in the blood compared to untreated controls. After one week, plasma catechin levels were measurable, whereas they were not detectable at baseline. No effect was reported on the concentration of plasma lipids or on lipid peroxides compared to baseline. However, an increase in resistance to oxidation of LDL-cholesterol was measured ex vivo (Miura et al., 2000). The study was weak due to the small sample size and the lack of blinding and randomization of patient populations.

EPIDEMIOLOGICAL STUDIES

Many of the studies on green tea are epidemiological: population studies and statistical comparisons of the health status and subsequent disease history of large groups of people who customarily drink several cups of green tea daily in comparison with other groups who do not.

A meta-analysis of 17 epidemiological studies explored the possible relationship between black and green tea consumption and cardiovascular disease. Although the study-specific effect estimates for heart attack and coronary heart disease were too heterogeneous to summarize, the relative risk for heart attack was estimated to decrease by 11 percent with consumption of three cups of tea per day (Peters, Poole, and Arab, 2001). The study did not distinguish, however, between the various types of tea, methods of preparation, or the strength of the tea.

A recent study with 13,916 healthy Japanese workers concluded that consumption of green tea was associated with lower serum total cholesterol. There appeared to be an inverse dose relationship with increasing quantities of green tea consumption correlating with decreasing levels of total cholesterol. This inverse relationship appeared to level off with consumption of more than ten cups per day. Consumption of green tea was unrelated to serum levels of high-density lipoprotein cholesterol or serum triglycerides. (Tokunaga et al., 2002).

The authors of a review of epidemiological studies on tea drinking and cancer concluded that there was no evidence of a protective role against cancer in general. However, when the studies were broken down to specific body sites, the authors reported that the results suggest a protective effect from green tea consumption on the development of colon cancer. The authors indicated that benefits are likely restricted to high consumption of tea in high-risk populations. The range and crude categorization of tea consumption, as well as the choice of control groups and inadequate control for confounding variables, limited this review (Kohlmeier et al., 1997).

A population-based, case-controlled study was conducted in China with 1,324 women, wherein women diagnosed with lung cancer were matched by age with women in the general population. Information was obtained from both groups regarding their tea drinking habits. The researchers found that consumption of green tea was associated with a reduced risk of lung cancer. Among nonsmoking women, regular consumption of green tea (501 to 1,500 grams per year) over a five-year period was associated with a reduced risk of lung cancer (odds ratio 0.65). The risks decreased with increasing consumption of green tea (over 1,500 grams per year; odds ratio 0.46). However, there was no reduced risk in women who smoked (Zhong et al., 2001).

A hospital-based, epidemiological research program in Japan that followed a total of 1,160 new surgical cases of female invasive breast cancer reported a decreased risk for recurrence with consumption of three or more cups of green tea per day (odds ratio 0.69). The decreased risk was significant for those with stage I cancer (odds ratio 0.43), and strongest for those who consumed three to five cups per day (odds ratio 0.37). Those with stage II cancer exhibited a nonsignificant trend toward reduced cancer recurrence, whereas no benefit was observed for those with more advanced stages of cancer (Inoue et al., 2001).

A population-based, case-controlled study conducted in China, with 133 patients with stomach cancer, 166 with chronic gastritis, and 433 healthy controls, reported an inverse association between green tea drinking and risk of both stomach cancer and chronic gastritis (odds ratios 0.52 and 0.49, respectively, with more than 21 cups per week). The possible benefit increased with larger amounts of tea and additional years of tea drinking (Setiawan et al., 2001). In contrast, a prospective study that followed 38,540 Japanese men and women in Hiroshima and Nagasaki for 13 to 14 years found no correlation between green tea consumption and the incidence of an array of solid cancers or hematopoietic cancers (lymphoma, multiple myeloma, and leukemia) (Nagano et al., 2001).

ADVERSE REACTIONS OR SIDE EFFECTS

No side effects were reported in the individual trials discussed earlier. The caffeine contained in green tea may have a stimulant effect, especially for those who choose to drink large quantities.

REFERENCES

Chantre P, Lairon D (2002). Recent findings of green tea extract AR25 (Exolise) and its activity for the treatment of obesity. *Phytomedicine* 9 (1): 3-8.

Dulloo AG, Duret C, Rohrer D, Girardier L, Mensi N, Fathi M, Chantre P, Vandermander J (1999). Efficacy of a green tea extract rich in catechin polyphenols and caffeine in increasing 24-h energy expenditure and fat oxidation in humans. *American Journal of Clinical Nutrition* 70 (6): 1040-1045.

Gutman RL, Ryu BH (1996). Rediscovering tea. *HerbalGram* 37: 33-48.

Inoue M, Tajima K, Mizutani M, Iwata H, Iwase T, Miura S, Hirose K, Hamajima N (2001). Regular consumption of green tea and the risk of breast cancer recurrence: Follow-up study from the Hospital-Based Epidemiologic Research Program at Aichi Cancer Center. *Cancer Letters* 167 (2): 175-182.

Kohlmeier L, Weterings KG, Steck S, Kok FJ. (1997). Tea and cancer prevention: An evaluation of the epidemiological literature. *Nutrition and Cancer—An International Journal* 27 (1): 1-13.

Leenen R, Roodenburg AJC, Tijburg LBM, Wiseman SA (2000). A single dose of tea with or without milk increases plasma antioxidant activity in humans. *European Journal of Clinical Nutrition* 54 (1): 87-92.

Miura Y, Chiba T, Miura S, Tomita I, Umegaki K, Ikeda M, Tomita T (2000). Green tea polyphenols (flavan 3-ols) prevent oxidative modification of low density lipoproteins: An ex vivo study in humans. *Journal of Nutritional Biochemistry* 11 (4): 216-222.

Nagano J, Kono S, Preston DL, Mabuchi K (2001). A prospective study of green tea consumption and cancer incidence, Hiroshima and Nagasaki (Japan). *Cancer Causes and Control* 12 (6): 501-508.

Peters U, Poole C, Arab L (2001). Does tea affect cardiovascular disease? A meta-analysis. *American Journal of Epidemiology* 154 (6): 495-503.

Setiawan VW, Zhang ZF, Yu GP, Li YL, Lu ML, Wang MR, Guo CH, Yu SZ, Kurtz RC, Hsieh CC (2001). Protective effect of green tea on the risks of chronic gastritis and stomach cancer. *International Journal of Cancer* 92 (4): 600-604.

Tokunaga S, White IR, Frost C, Tanaka K, Kono S, Tokudome S, Akamatsu T, Moriyama T, Zakouji H (2002). Green tea consumption and serum lipids and lipoproteins in a population of healthy workers in Japan. *Annals of Epidemiology* 12 (3): 157-165.

van het Hof KH, de Boer HSM, Wiseman SA, Lien N, Westrate JA, Tijburg LBM (1997). Consumption of green or black tea does not increase resistance of low-density lipoprotein to oxidation in humans. *American Journal of Clinical Nutrition* 66 (5): 1125-1132.

Walsh B (1997a). Scientific report: Observation of the anti-free-radical effect in the treatment of chronic renal insufficiency using tea polyphenol. Pharmanex Inc. Confidential Report # PN0409.

Walsh B (1997b). Scientific report: The protective effect of "Xin Nao Jian" capsule on the hemogram of cancer patients undergoing radiotherapy and chemotherapy. Pharmanex Inc. Confidential Report #PN0411.

Zhong L, Goldberg MS, Gao YT, Hanley JA, Parent ME, Jin F (2001). A population-based case-control study of lung cancer and green tea consumption among women living in Shanghai, China. *Epidemiology* 12 (6): 695-700.

DETAILS ON GREEN TEA PRODUCTS
AND CLINICAL STUDIES

Product and clinical study information is grouped in the same order as in the Summary Table. A profile on an individual product is followed by details of the clinical studies associated with that product. In some instances, a clinical study, or studies, supports several products that contain the same principal ingredient(s). In these instances, those products are grouped together.

Clinical studies that follow each product, or group of products, are grouped by therapeutic indication, in accordance with the order in the Summary Table.

Index to Green Tea Products

Product Profile: Exolise™

Manufacturer	**Arkopharma Laboratoires Pharmaceutiques, France**
U.S. distributor	**Health from the Sun/Arkopharma**
Botanical ingredient	**Green tea leaf extract**
Extract name	**AR25**
Quantity	375 mg
Processing	Alcohol extraction from dry leaves of unfermented *Camellia sinensis*
Standardization	Standardized to 25% catechins
Formulation	Capsule

Recommended dose: Take two capsules with breakfast and two capsules with lunch with a glass of water.

DSHEA structure/function: Helps maintain a healthy body weight.

Other ingredients: Cellulose derivative (capsule shell), vegetal magnesium stearate, silicon dioxide.

Source(s) of information: Product package; Dulloo et al., 1999.

Clinical Study: Exolise™

Extract name	AR25
Manufacturer	Arkopharma Laboratoires Pharmaceutiques, France
Indication	**Weight loss; thermogenic effect** (energy expenditure)
Level of evidence	**III**
Therapeutic benefit	**MOA**

Bibliographic reference
Dulloo AG, Duret C, Rohrer D, Girardier L, Mensi N, Fathi M, Chantre P, Vandermander J (1999). Efficacy of a green tea extract rich in catechin polyphenols and caffeine in increasing 24-h energy expenditure and fat oxidation in humans. *American Journal of Clinical Nutrition* 70 (6): 1040-1045.

Trial design
Parallel. Each subject spent 24 hours in the respiratory chamber on three separate occasions (each separated by five to ten days) and was randomly assigned to receive one of the following three treatments at breakfast, lunch, and dinner: green tea extract (containing 50 mg caffeine and 90 mg epigallocatechin), 50 mg caffeine, or placebo.

Study duration	3 days
Dose	2 capsules green tea extract (50 mg caffeine and 90 mg epigallocatechin per dose) 3 times daily
Route of administration	Oral
Randomized	Yes
Randomization adequate	No
Blinding	Double-blind
Blinding adequate	No
Placebo	Yes
Drug comparison	Yes
Drug name	Caffeine
Site description	Single center

No. of subjects enrolled   10
No. of subjects completed 10
Sex   Male
Age   Mean: 25 ± 1 years

Inclusion criteria

Healthy young men with body composition ranging from lean to mildly obese (8 to 30 percent body fat), consumption of a typical Western diet with fat contributing 35 to 40 percent of dietary energy intake, and estimated intake of methylxanthines (mostly caffeine-containing beverages) ranging from 100 to 200 mg/day.

Exclusion criteria

Smokers, competitive athletes, and persons who engaged in intense physical activities or who had a history of weight loss.

End points

Energy expenditure (EE), respiratory quotient (RQ), and urinary excretion of nitrogen and catecholamines were measured for each 24-hour stay in the respiratory chamber.

Results

Relative to placebo, treatment with the green tea extract resulted in a significant increase in 24-hour EE (4 percent, $p < 0.01$) and a significant decrease in 24-hour RQ (from 0.88 to 0.85, $p < .001$) without any change in urinary nitrogen. Twenty-four-hour urinary norepinephrine excretion was higher during treatment with green tea extract than with the placebo (40 percent, $p < 0.05$). Treatment with caffeine in amounts equivalent to those found in the green tea extract had no effect on EE and RQ nor on urinary nitrogen or catecholamines. With green tea extract, fat oxidation was significantly higher ($p < 0.001$) and carbohydrate oxidation was significantly lower ($p < 0.01$) than with placebo.

Side effects

None reported.

Authors' comments

Green tea has thermogenic properties, and promotes fat oxidation beyond that explained by its caffeine content per se. The green tea extract may play a role in the control of body composition via sympathetic activation of thermogenesis.

Reviewer's comments

This was a mechanistic study showing green tea to have thermogenic and fat-oxidation-promoting activity; however, its role in weight loss is undetermined. Neither the randomization nor the double-blinding were adequately described. (1, 6)

Product Profile: Lipton Research Blend

Manufacturer	**Thomas J. Lipton Co.** (now Unilever Bestfoods, North America)
U.S. distributor	None
Botanical ingredient	**Green tea leaf extract**
Extract name	None given
Quantity	No information
Processing	Lyophilized (freeze-dried) tea solids
Standardization	No information
Formulation	Tea solids

Source(s) of information: Leenen et al., 2000.

Clinical Study: Lipton Research Blend

Extract name	None given
Manufacturer	Thomas J. Lipton Co.
Indication	**Cardiovascular risk factors** in healthy volunteers
Level of evidence	**III**
Therapeutic benefit	**MOA**

Bibliographic reference
van het Hof KH, de Boer HSM, Wiseman SA, Lien N, Westrate JA, Tijburg LBM (1997). Consumption of green or black tea does not increase resistance of low-density lipoprotein to oxidation in humans. *American Journal of Clinical Nutrition* 66 (5): 1125-1132.

Trial design
Parallel. After a two-week pretrial period in which all subjects consumed 900 ml (6 cups) of water per day, they were divided into three groups and given 900 ml (6 cups) of either water, green tea, or black tea (0.5 g black tea extract per cup) daily.

Study duration	1 month
Dose	6 (0.5 g tea extract in 150 ml) cups daily

Route of administration	Oral
Randomized	No
Randomization adequate	No
Blinding	Open
Blinding adequate	No
Placebo	No
Drug comparison	No
Site description	Single center
No. of subjects enrolled	48
No. of subjects completed	45
Sex	Male and female
Age	20-61 years

Inclusion criteria
Ages 18 to 65 years, healthy, nonsmoking, not using vitamin C, vitamin E, carotenoid, selenium, or zinc supplements or consuming a medically pre-scribed or weight-loss diet, and a stable weight for at least one month before the start of the study.

Exclusion criteria
Pregnant or lactating women.

End points
Blood samples were obtained before and after experimental period. Serum lipid concentrations, plasma and low-density lipoprotein (LDL) antioxidant status, resistance of LDL to oxidation, and plasma malondialdehyde and LDL-hydroperoxide concentrations were measured.

Results
Consumption of green or black tea did not affect serum lipid concentrations, resistance of LDL to oxidation ex vivo, or markers of oxidative damage to lipids in vivo. However, consumption of green tea slightly increased total an-tioxidant activity of plasma.

Side effects
None mentioned.

Authors' comments
Daily consumption of 900 ml (six cups) green or black tea per day for four weeks had no effect on serum lipid concentrations or resistance of LDL to oxidation ex vivo. Future research should focus on mechanisms by which tea flavonoids may reduce the risk of cardiovascular disease other than by increasing the intrinsic antioxidant status of LDL.

Reviewer's comments
Although this study gave negative results, the sample size was small, and the subjects were not randomized or blinded. (1, 5)

Clinical Study: Lipton® Research Blend

Extract name	None given
Manufacturer	Thomas J. Lipton Co.
Indication	**Antioxidant activity** in healthy volunteers
Level of evidence	**III**
Therapeutic benefit	**MOA**

Bibliographic reference
Leenen R, Roodenburg AJC, Tijburg LBM, Wiseman SA (2000). A single dose of tea with or without milk increases plasma antioxidant activity in humans. *European Journal of Clinical Nutrition* 54 (1): 87-92.

Trial design
Crossover. Each subject received six treatments on six different days with at least two days in between. After an overnight fast, volunteers were given a single dose of black tea, green tea, or water, with or without milk.

Study duration	1 day
Dose	2 g tea solids in 300 ml water (equivalent to 3 cups of tea)
Route of administration	Oral
Randomized	Yes
Randomization adequate	No
Blinding	Open
Blinding adequate	No
Placebo	Yes
Drug comparison	Yes
Drug name	Black tea
Site description	Single center
No. of subjects enrolled	24
No. of subjects completed	21
Sex	Male and female
Age	18-65 years

Inclusion criteria
Between 18 and 70 years old, healthy, nonsmokers. Subjects did not use any medicines, a medically prescribed diet, a weight-loss regime, or supplements containing vitamin C, vitamin E, carotenoids, calcium, or iron, and had a stable body weight for at least one month before the start of the study.

Exclusion criteria
Pregnant or lactating women.

End points
Blood samples were obtained at baseline and at 30, 60, 90, and 120 minutes after tea drinking. Plasma was analyzed for total catechins and antioxidant activity, using the ferric reducing ability of plasma (FRAP) assay.

Results
Consumption of black tea resulted in a significant increase in plasma antioxidant activity, which reached maximal levels at about 60 minutes ($p < 0.001$ tea versus water). A larger increase was observed after consumption of green tea ($p < 0.05$ green versus black). As anticipated from the higher catechin concentration in green tea, the rise in plasma total catechins was significantly higher after consumption of green tea when compared to black tea ($p < 0.001$). Addition of milk to black or green tea did not affect the observed increases in plasma antioxidant activity.

Side effects
None mentioned.

Authors' comments
Consumption of a single dose of black or green tea induces a significant rise in plasma antioxidant activity in vivo. Addition of milk to tea does not abolish this increase. Whether the observed increases in plasma antioxidant activity after a single dose of tea prevent in vivo oxidative damage remains to be established.

Reviewer's comments
This study shows that a single dose of black or green tea increases antioxidant activity in plasma. The study was not blinded, and the randomization was not adequately described. (1, 6)

Product Profile: Tegreen 97®

Manufacturer	**Pharmanex LLC**
U.S. distributor	**Pharmanex Natural Healthcare**

Botanical ingredient	**Green tea leaf extract**
Extract name	**Tegreen 97**
Quantity	250 mg
Processing	Plant/extract ratio 20:1
Standardization	97% green tea polyphenols
Formulation	Capsule

Recommended dose: Take one capsule daily with food and drink. Take consistently for best results.

DSHEA structure/function: Supports the antioxidant defense system in the presence of pollution, stress, and toxins.

Cautions: If pregnant or nursing, or taking a prescription medication, consult a physician before using this product.

Other ingredients: Millet, gelatin, magnesium silicate, silicon dioxide.

Source(s) of information: Product package.

Clinical Study: Xin Nao Jian (Tegreen 97®)

Extract name	Tea polyphenol
Manufacturer	Pharmanex LLC
Indication	**Hematopoietic effects** of cancer therapy
Level of evidence	**III**
Therapeutic benefit	**Undetermined**

Bibliographic reference
Walsh B (1997). Scientific report: The protective effect of "Xin Nao Jian" capsule on the hemogram of cancer patients undergoing radiotherapy and chemotherapy. Pharmanex Inc. Confidential Report #PN0411.

Trial design
Parallel. The study began with the first day of radiotherapy or chemotherapy. Patients were divided randomly into three groups and given either Xin Nao Jian, Sha Gan Chun (a traditional Chinese medicine used to improve blood quality; 100 mg three times daily), or no additional therapy.

Study duration	1 month
Dose	200 mg tea polyphenol three times daily
Route of administration	Oral
Randomized	Yes

Randomization adequate   Yes
Blinding   Not described
Blinding adequate   No

Placebo   No
Drug comparison   Yes
Drug name   Sha Gan Chun

Site description   Multicenter

No. of subjects enrolled   60
No. of subjects completed 60
Sex   Not given
Age   Not given

Inclusion criteria
Cancer inpatients with a normal hemogram undergoing the first course of radiotherapy and chemotherapy.

Exclusion criteria
None mentioned.

End points
After the beginning of treatment, patient blood samples were taken every week. Hemoglobin content was determined, along with platelet and white blood cell levels.

Results
Total white blood cell counts improved in the Xin Nao Jian group, but significantly declined in the Sha Gan Chun group after five weeks ($p < 0.05$) and in the control group after three weeks ($p < 0.001$). No significant changes in hemoglobin or blood platelet levels were observed.

Side effects
Three cases of nausea and loss of appetite were reported in the Xin Nao Jian group. However, the other groups reported these effects as well.

Author's comments
It can be seen that Xin Nao Jian has a protective effect on the hemogram of patients undergoing radiotherapy and chemotherapy, especially a definite effect on the stabilization of the number of total leucocytes.

Reviewer's comments
This study had several flaws: inadequately described statistical methods and data, and it was nonblinded. However, the stabilization of lymphocytes and the effects on immune function deserve further study. (2, 3)

Clinical Study: Tegreen 97®

Extract name	Tea polyphenol
Manufacturer	Pharmanex LLC

Indication	**Renal insufficiency**
Level of evidence	**III**
Therapeutic benefit	**Undetermined**

Bibliographic reference

Walsh B (1997). Scientific report: Observation of the anti-free-radical effect in the treatment of chronic renal insufficiency using tea polyphenol. Pharmanex Inc. Confidential Report #PN0409.

Trial design

Parallel. Both groups adopted a low-protein, low-salt diet, and routine therapy. In addition, the treatment group was given capsules with tea polyphenols.

Study duration	3 months
Dose	2 (100 mg) capsules three times daily
Route of administration	Oral
Randomized	Yes
Randomization adequate	No
Blinding	Not described
Blinding adequate	No
Placebo	No
Drug comparison	No
Site description	Multicenter
No. of subjects enrolled	60
No. of subjects completed	60
Sex	Male and female
Age	19-59 years (mean: 36.7)

Inclusion criteria

Patients with chronic renal insufficiency.

Exclusion criteria

None mentioned.

End points

Measurement of the content of blood plasma lipid peroxide (LPO), erythrocyte superoxide dismutase (SOD) activity, blood urea nitrogen (BUN), serum creatine (SCr), and clinical symptoms.

Results
Erythrocyte SOD was significantly increased ($p < 0.05$), and the plasma LPO was significantly decreased ($p < 0.01$) in the treatment group relative to the control group. Renal function was improved in the treatment group relative to the control group as assessed by BUN ($p < 0.01$) and SCr ($p < 0.05$).

Side effects
None mentioned.

Author's comments
Tea polyphenol is able to clear free radicals and prohibit lipid peroxidation. It can also mobilize and activate the endogenous antioxidant system of the body, raise the activity of SOD and other enzymes, cause the reduction of blood plasma LPO levels, and therefore produce body-protecting effects.

Reviewer's comments
Although serious flaws are present in the study design and description of results, this heterogeneous group of renal failure patients claimed to have improvement in renal function: BUN decreased from 21 to 11 in treatment group; serum creatinine decreased from 405 to 275; and positive effects on plasma SOD and lipid peroxide were observed. This is a good guide for future study. (0, 0)

Product Profile: Polyphenon E®

Manufacturer	**Mitsui Nohrin Co., Ltd., Japan**
U.S. distributor	None
Botanical ingredient	**Green tea leaf extract**
Extract name	None given
Quantity	No information
Processing	No information
Standardization	No information

Source(s) of information: Miura et al., 2000.

Clinical Study: Polyphenon E®

Extract name	Not given
Manufacturer	Mitsui Nohrin Co., Ltd., Japan

Indication	**Cardiovascular risk factors** in normal volunteers
Level of evidence	**III**
Therapeutic benefit	**Undetermined**

Bibliographic reference

Miura Y, Chiba T, Miura S, Tomita I, Umegaki K, Ikeda M, Tomita T (2000). Green tea polyphenols (flavan 3-ols) prevent oxidative modification of low density lipoproteins: An ex vivo study in humans. *Journal of Nutritional Biochemistry* 11 (4): 216-222.

Trial design

Parallel. All subjects had a strict dietary regimen, including drinks. After a one-week baseline period, they were divided into control and tea groups.

Study duration	1 week
Dose	300 mg tea extract twice daily
Route of administration	Oral
Randomized	No
Randomization adequate	No
Blinding	Not described
Blinding adequate	No
Placebo	No
Drug comparison	No
Site description	Single center
No. of subjects enrolled	22
No. of subjects completed	22
Sex	Male
Age	22-32 years (mean: 24.5)

Inclusion criteria

Normolipidemic, smokers or nonsmokers, who did not take any medications or special dietary additives.

Exclusion criteria

Medication, vitamin supplements, or special dietary additives. Additional consumption of green or black teas, fruit juice, or vegetable juice was not allowed during the pretrial and trial periods.

End points

Fasting blood samples were drawn before the pretrial baseline period, after the pretrial period, and after one week of treatment. Plasma catechin levels were measured as well as plasma lipids, antioxidative vitamins, and thio-barbituric acid-reactive substances.

Results
Plasma catechin (epigallocatchin-gallate) concentration at the end of the experiment was 56 nmol/l on average (56 percent in free form) after one week ingestion of tea, whereas none was detected beforehand. Plasma concentration of lipids, ascorbate, alpha-tocopherol, and lipid peroxides did not change before and after the experiment in either group, but beta-carotene was higher in the tea group ($p < 0.01$ by paired Student's t-test). Low-density lipoprotein (LDL) oxidation lag time was prolonged by 13.7 minutes in the tea group, whereas such a change was not observed in the control group ($p < 0.05$).

Side effects
None mentioned.

Authors' comments
These results suggest that daily consumption of seven to eight cups (approximately 100 ml each cup) of green tea may increase resistance of LDL to in vivo oxidation, leading to a reduction in the risk of cardiovascular diseases.

Reviewer's comments
This is a carefully controlled and well-reported study. However, it was not randomized and the blinding was not described. (0, 6)

Hawthorn

Other common names: **English hawthorn; May tree; white thorn**
Latin name: *Crataegus laevigata* **(Poir.) DC.** and *C. monogyna* **Jacq.** as well as other species [Rosaceae]
Latin synonyms: *Crataegus oxyacantha* **L.** = *C. laevigata*
Plant parts: **Leaf, flower**

PREPARATIONS USED IN REVIEWED CLINICAL STUDIES

Hawthorn, a tall shrub that grows throughout Europe, was first documented as having medical use in the first century A.D., but the plant's use as a heart medicine can only be traced back to the 1600s. The two primary species are *Crataegus laevigata* (Poir.) DC. and *C. monogyna* Jacq. However, other species have been used medicinally, and to make matters more complex, the two primary species are known to hybridize (Upton, Graff, Williamson, et al., 1999). Therapeutic efficacy has been documented most reliably for the leaves and flowers. The dried, berrylike fruits have also been used, either alone or in combination with the leaves and flowers. The main constituents of hawthorn are identified as procyanidins, flavonoids, triterpenoids, catechins, aromatic carboxylic acids, and amino and purine derivatives. For quality control purposes, the flavonoid content and/or the oligomeric procyanidin content are determined. The leaves and flowers contain approximately 1 percent flavonoids and 1 to 3 percent oligomeric procyanidins (Schulz, Hänsel, and Tyler, 2001).

HeartCare™ contains 80 mg WS 1442, a hydroalcoholic extract of hawthorn leaves and flowers (5:1) standardized to 18.75 percent oligomeric procyanidins. This product is made by Dr. Willmar Schwabe GmbH & Co. in Germany, and is distributed in the United States by Nature's Way Products, Inc. WS 1442 is sold in Europe in a product named Crataegutt®.

HAWTHORN SUMMARY TABLE

Product Name	Manufacturer/ U.S. Distributor	Product Characteristics	Dose in Trials	Indication	No. of Trials	Benefit (Evidence Level-Trial No.)
HeartCare™ (US); Crataegutt® (EU)	Dr. Willmar Schwabe GmbH & Co., Germany/ Nature's Way Products, Inc.	Hydroalcoholic extract of leaves and flowers (WS 1442)	160 or 180 mg daily	Chronic heart failure	6	Yes (II-1, III-1) Trend (I-1) Undetermined (III-3)
Faros® 300 (EU)	Lichtwer Pharma AG, Germany/ None	Hydroalcoholic extract of leaves and flowers (LI 132)	300, 600, or 900 mg daily	Chronic heart failure	4	Yes (II-1) Trend (I-1, II-2)

Faros® 300 is manufactured by Lichtwer Pharma AG in Germany and contains a hydroalcoholic extract of leaves and flowers (LI 132). Tablets or capsules containing 50, 200, and 300 mg hawthorn extract have been used in clinical studies. Faros 300 is not sold in the United States.

SUMMARY OF REVIEWED CLINICAL STUDIES

Hawthorn has been studied for its clinical use in the treatment of early stage heart failure, which is also called cardiac insufficiency. Heart failure is defined as the inadequate supply of oxygen and nutrients to the body as the result of heart disease. Animal studies indicate that hawthorn preparations increase the contraction of the heart muscle, increase the integrity of the blood vessel wall, and improve the flow of blood to the heart without changing heart rate or aggregation of red blood cells (Loew, 1997).

The New York Heart Association (NYHA) has classified heart failure in four stages. Patients with Class I heart failure have cardiac disease but are able to conduct ordinary physical activity without limitation. Class II is defined as a slight limitation of ordinary physical activity due to fatigue, palpitation, dyspnea, or anginal pain. Class III is defined as marked limitation of physical activity even on light exertion. Patients with Class IV heart failure are unable to carry on any physical activity without discomfort—they may experience symptoms of congestive heart failure even at rest (Cochran Foundation, 1997). Many of the clinical studies using hawthorn have been conducted on patients with Class II disease.

HeartCare

Chronic Heart Failure

Five placebo-controlled studies evaluated the effectiveness of WS 1442 in the treatment of stable chronic heart failure classified as NYHA Class II. An additional study evaluated patients with NYHA Class III.

Two of the studies with patients classified as NYHA Class II were rated as good quality. The largest good-quality study included 129 patients treated with either 160 mg extract or placebo daily for two months. As a result of treatment, there was a statistically significant increase in cardiac performance compared to placebo, as measured by blood pressure and heart rate at rest and after exercise. Clinical symptoms such as restricted physical performance, shortness of breath, and edema around the ankles were improved (Weikl et al., 1996). Another good-quality, but smaller, study with only 39 subjects showed a trend toward improvement in exercise tolerance following three months of treatment with 80 mg three times daily. A decrease in a measurement combining heart rate and blood pressure was observed in the hawthorn group but not in the placebo group (Zapfe, 2001). According to our reviewer, Dr. Mary Hardy, an increase in the study size may have strengthened the results.

Three other studies, with small groups of patients (30 to 58) classified as having NYHA Class II, were rated poorly due to methodological flaws. A crossover study that used a dose of 180 mg per day for six weeks reported that the patients' exercise-induced rise in systolic blood pressure and heart rate was reduced compared to placebo. In addition, a decrease in blood pressure at the end of the recovery period was observed compared to baseline and placebo (O'Conolly et al., 1986). An eight-week parallel study found that a measure of blood pressure and heart rate during exercise decreased continuously after four and eight weeks of treatment compared to baseline. This measure was also statistically below that from the placebo group. In addition, a greater decrease in subjective complaints was observed in the treatment group compared to the placebo group (Leuchtgens, 1993). Another study reported a significant increase in exercise tolerance compared to the placebo group following treatment with 180 mg per day for three weeks. The treatment group's ischemic reaction to exercise also decreased as measured by electrocardiogram. This study found no difference in blood pressure or heart rate (Hanack and Brückel, 1983).

A three-arm trial with 197 subjects with NYHA Class III heart failure assessed the ability of WS 1442 to increase exercise capacity and decrease symptoms. Either 900 or 1,800 mg WS 1442 daily, or placebo, was given in addition to preexisting diuretic therapy (50 mg triamterene and 25 mg hydrochlorothiazide). After four months of treatment, maximum tolerated workload during exercise with the 1,800 mg dose increased significantly compared to the 900 mg dose and to placebo. Subjective heart failure symptoms were significantly reduced by both doses compared to placebo (Tauchert, 2002).

Faros 300

Chronic Heart Failure

Four trials were reviewed that evaluate the use of Litchwer's extract LI 132 for patients with NYHA Class II heart failure. The trials used a dose ranging from 100 to 300 mg three times daily for a period of one to two months. The largest trial, which was rated as being of good quality, included 124 subjects, and compared the effectiveness of LI 132 (300 mg three times daily) with captopril (12.5 mg three times daily). Captopril is an ACE (angiotension converting enzyme) inhibitor that lowers blood pressure in hypertensive individuals and reduces peripheral resistance of blood vessels. In this trial, both LI 132 and captropril equally improved exercise capacity and decreased a measured product of heart rate and blood pressure after two months of treatment (Tauchert, Ploch, and Hübner, 1994).

Three smaller trials, with about 70 subjects each, were placebo-controlled. One of them, using a dose of 200 mg three times daily for two months, reported a statistical improvement in exercise capacity and a decrease in the measured product of heart rate and blood pressure compared to placebo (Schmidt et al., 1994). Another trial, using a dose of 300 mg three times daily, showed only a trend toward an increase in exercise capacity, but reported a significant increase both in exercise time taken to reach anaerobic metabolism and in oxygen absorbed by the lungs both during exercise and afterward (Forster et al., 1994). The final study used a smaller dose (100 mg three times daily) for short period of time (only one month) and showed statistically insignificant increases in exercise capacity compared with placebo (Bodigheimer and Chase, 1994).

POSTMARKETING SURVEILLANCE STUDIES

A study including 940 medical practioners and 3,664 patients diagnosed with cardiac insufficiency NYHA Class I or Class II documented a therapeutic benefit in 1,476 patients given hawthorn and no other medication to treat their disease. Patients were evaluated after four and eight weeks of treatment, consisting of Faros 300 in a dose of 300 mg three times daily. At the end of the surveillance period, the average cardiac insufficiency symptom score was reduced from 6.9 to 1.7 points out of nine total. Work tolerance, as measured using bike ergometry, was increased, and a measurement of heart rate and blood pressure associated with exercise was reduced. In a subset of patients with borderline hypertension, reductions were observed in systolic and diastolic blood pressure. In patients with tachycardia, a reduction in heart rate and incidence of arrhythmias was reported (Schmidt et al., 1998).

ADVERSE REACTIONS OR SIDE EFFECTS

No significant side effects were reported in the trials reviewed in this section. In a surveillance study with 3,664 patients diagnosed with NYHA Class I or Class II heart failure, 48 of the patients (1.3 percent) reported 72 adverse reactions. The majority of these reactions were gastrointestinal complaints (24 cases), palpitations (10), vertigo (7), headache (7), and flushing (3). The treatment was Faros 300 taken in a dose of 300 mg three times daily (Schmidt et al., 1998).

INFORMATION FROM PHARMACOPOEIAL MONOGRAPHS

Sources of Published Therapeutic Monographs

American Herbal Pharmacopoeia
European Scientific Cooperative on Phytotherapy
German Commission E

Indications

The German Commission E has approved the dried flowering twig tips (leaf with flower) for decreasing cardiac output as described in functional Stage II of heart disease as described by the New York Heart Association (Blumenthal et al., 1998). The European Scientific

Cooperative on Phytotherapy (ESCOP) also lists this treatment, but specifies that the preparation used be a hydroalcoholic extract. ESCOP also suggests hawthorn leaf and flowers for nervous heart complaints and support of cardiac and circulatory functions when prepared as tea or other preparations (not as a hydroalcoholic extract) (ESCOP, 1999).

The *American Herbal Pharmacopoeia (AHP)* lists hawthorn leaf and flowers for the treatment of Class I and II cardiac insufficiency, hypertonic heart with and without signs of coronary insufficiencies, myocardial insufficiencies, arrhythmia, cerebral insufficiency, mild hypertension, and patients with a history of myocardial infarction. It is also distinguished as having the ability to potentiate the effects of cardiac glycosides. The actions listed by the *AHP* include: increases coronary and myocardial perfusion, lowers peripheral resistance, and has economizing action with respect to oxygen and energy consumption; it is positively inotropic, positively dromotropic, negatively chronotropic, and negatively bathmotropic; and hawthorn is considered to be an antiarrhythmic, an antioxidant, a diuretic, a hypocholesterolemic, a hypotensive, and a sedative (Upton, Graff, Williamson, et al., 1999). The *AHP* has also published a monograph on hawthorn berry with similar indications (Upton, Graff, Bencie, et al., 1999).

Doses

> Powder: 200 to 500 mg (Upton, Graff, Williamson, et al., 1999); 2 to 5 g daily (ESCOP, 1999)
>
> Infusion: one cup morning and evening; at beginning of therapy, three cups daily (Upton, Graff, Williamson et al., 1999); 1 to 1.5 g of comminuted drug as an infusion three to four times daily (ESCOP, 1999)
>
> Tincture: 20 drops two to three times daily (Upton, Graff, Williamson, et al., 1999; ESCOP, 1999)
>
> Extract: 160 to 900 mg , extract (ethanol 45 percent v/v or methanol 70 percent v/v with a drug-extract ratio of 4 to 7:1), corresponding to 30 to 168.7 mg procyanidins, calculated as epicatechin, or 3.5 to 19.8 mg flavonoids, calculated in accordance with the *German Pharmacopoeia (DAB 10),* in two or three individual doses (Blumenthal et al., 1998; ESCOP, 1999; Upton, Graff, Williamson et al., 1999)

Fluid extract (as defined by the *French Codex IX*): 0.5 to 2.0 g daily, 60 to 120 drops three times daily (ESCOP, 1999)
Dry extract (as defined by *Belgium Farm V*): 50 to 300 mg dry extract three times daily (ESCOP, 1999)
Glycerol macerate: 50 drops three times daily (ESCOP, 1999)

Treatment Period

The Commission E suggests a treatment period of six weeks minimum, whereas ESCOP gives no restrictions (Blumenthal et al., 1998; ESCOP, 1999).

Contraindications

None of the pharmacopoeias list any contraindications (Blumenthal et al., 1998; ESCOP, 1999; Upton, Graff, Williamson, et al., 1999).

Adverse Reactions

The Commission E and ESCOP list no known adverse reactions (Blumenthal et al., 1998; ESCOP, 1999). The *AHP*, however, mentions that adverse reactions are minimal, but that some patients have reported gastrointestinal disorders, palpitations, headaches, and dizziness (Upton, Graff, Williamson, et al., 1999).

Precautions

The Commission E and ESCOP suggest that a physician must be consulted in cases where symptoms continue unchanged for longer than six weeks or in case of swelling of the legs. Medical diagnosis is necessary when pains occur in the region of the heart, spreading out to the arms, upper abdomen or the area around the neck, or in cases of respiratory distress (dyspnea) (Blumenthal et al., 1998; ESCOP, 1999). The *AHP* also advises that patients with cardiovascular disease should inform their primary health care provider if they are using hawthorn preparations (Upton, Graff, Williamson, et al., 1999).

Drug Interactions

Both the Commission E and ESCOP list no known drug interactions (Blumenthal et al., 1998; ESCOP, 1999). However, the *AHP* states that hawthorn potentiates the effects of cardiac glycosides as well as barbiturate-induced sleeping times. One particular hawthorn product, Esbericard® (Schaper & Brümmer GmbH & Co., KG, Germany), has reportedly augmented the coronary artery dilating effect brought on by caffeine, adenosine, epinephrine, theophylline, sodium nitrate, and papaverine. Hawthorn has also been found to work synergistically with garlic to protect against enzymatic changes caused by isoprenaline-induced myocardial necroses in rats (Upton, Graff, Williamson, et al., 1999).

REFERENCES

Blumenthal M, Busse W, Hall T, Goldberg A, Grünwald J, Riggins C, Rister S, eds. (1998). *The Complete German Commission E Monographs: Therapeutic Guide to Herbal Medicines.* Trans. S Klein. Austin: American Botanical Council.

Bödigheimer K, Chase D (1994). Efficacy of hawthorn extract in a daily dose of 3 x 100 mg: Multicenter double-blind study in 85 patients with NYHA stage II heart failure. *Münchener Medizinische Wochenschrift* 136 (Suppl. 1): 7-11.

Cochran Foundation (1997). Cardiovascular Disease Classification Chart. <http://www.cochranfoundation.com/main/cardiovascular.htm>. Accessed May 29, 2003.

European Scientific Cooperative on Phytotherapy (ESCOP) (1999). Crataegi folium cum flore: Hawthorn leaf and flower. In *Monographs on the Medicinal Uses of Plant Drugs.* Exeter, UK: European Scientific Cooperative on Phytotherapy.

Forster A, Forster K, Buhring M, Wolfstadter HD (1994). *Crataegus* for moderately reduced left ventricular ejection fraction: Ergospirometric monitoring study on 72 patients in a double-blind comparison with placebo. *Münchener Medizinische Wochenschrift* 136 (Suppl. 1): 21-26.

Hanack T, Brückel MH (1983). The treatment of mild stable forms of angina pectoris using Crataegutt novo. *Therapiewoche* 33: 4331-4333.

Leuchtgens H (1993). *Crataegus* special extract WS 1442 in cardiac insufficiency NYHA II. *Fortschritte der Medizin* 111 (20-21): 352-354.

Loew D (1997). Phytotherapy in heart failure. *Phytomedicine* 4 (3): 267-271.

O'Conolly VM, Jansen W, Bernhöft G, Bartsch G (1986). Treatment of decreasing cardiac performance (NYHA stages I to II) in advanced age with standardized *Crataegus* extract. *Fortschritte der Medizin* 104 (42): 805-808.

Schmidt U, Albrecht M, Podzuweit H, Ploch M, Maisenbacher J (1998). High dosage therapy with *Crataegus* extract in patients suffering from heart failure NYHA class I and II. *Zeitschrift für Phytotherapie* 19: 22-30.

Schmidt U, Kuhn U, Ploch M, Hübner WD (1994). Efficacy of the hawthorn *(Crataegus)* preparation LI 132 in 78 patients with chronic congestive heart failure defined as NYHA functional class II. *Phytomedicine* 1 (1): 17-24.

Schulz V, Hänsel R, Tyler VE (2001). *Rational Phytotherapy: A Physicians' Guide to Herbal Medicine,* Fourth Edition. Trans. TC Telgar. Berlin: Springer-Verlag.

Tauchert M (2002). Efficacy and safety of *Crataegus* extract WS 1442 in comparison with placebo in patients with chronic stable New York Heart Association class-III heart failure. *American Heart Journal* 143 (5): 910-915.

Tauchert M, Ploch M, Hübner WD (1994). Efficacy of hawthorn extract LI 132 in comparison with captopril: Multicenter double-blind study on 132 patients with cardiac insufficiency of NYHA grade II. *Münchener Medizinische Wochenschrift* 136 (Suppl. 1): 27-33.

Upton R, Graff A, Bencie R, Williamson E, Länger R, Hartung T, Rehwald A, Flachsmann E, Reich E, Martinez M, et al. (1999). *Hawthorn Berry, Crataegus spp. Analytical, Quality Control, and Therapeutic Monograph.* Eds. R Upton, C Petrone. Santa Cruz: American Herbal Pharmacopoeia.

Upton R, Graff A, Williamson E, Länger R, Hartung T, Rehwald A, Flachsmann E, Reich E, Martinez M, Chandra A et al. (1999). *Hawthorn Leaf with Flower, Crataegus spp. Analytical, Quality Control, and Therapeutic Monograph.* Eds. R Upton, C Petrone. Santa Cruz: American Herbal Pharmacopoeia.

Weikl A, Assmus KD, Neukum-Schmidt A, Schmitz J, Zapfe G, Noh HS, Siegrist J (1996). *Crataegus* special extract WS 1442: Objective proof of efficacy in patients with cardiac insufficiency (NYHA II). *Fortscritte der Medizin* 114 (24): 291-296. (Reported in *The Quarterly Review of Natural Medicine* Fall 1997: 201-209.)

Zapfe G (2001). Clinical efficacy of *Crataegus* extract WS 1442 in congestive heart failure NYHA class II. *Phytomedicine* 8 (4): 262-266.

DETAILS ON HAWTHORN PRODUCTS
AND CLINICAL STUDIES

Product and clinical study information is grouped in the same order as in the Summary Table. A profile on an individual product is followed by details of the clinical studies associated with that product. In some instances, a clinical study, or studies, supports several products that contain the same principal ingredient(s). In these instances, those products are grouped together.

Clinical studies that follow each product, or group of products, are grouped by therapeutic indication, in accordance with the order in the Summary Table.

Index to Hawthorn Products

Product Profile: HeartCare™

Manufacturer	**Dr. Willmar Schwabe GmbH & Co., Germany**
U.S. distributor	**Nature's Way Products, Inc.**
Botanical ingredient	**Hawthorn leaves and flowers extract**
Extract name	**WS 1442**
Quantity	80 mg
Processing (m/m)	Plant to extract ratio 5:1, 45% ethanol
Standardization	18.75% oligomeric procyanidins
Formulation	Tablet

Recommended dose: One tablet twice daily with water. For intensive use take up to two tablets three times daily. Best results are obtained with continual use.

DSHEA structure/function: Improves blood and nutrient flow to the heart muscle. Supports efficient heart muscle metabolism by improving its oxygen and energy utilization.

Other ingredients: Cellulose, maltodextrin, modified cellulose gum, stearic acid, modified cellulose, silica, titanium dioxide, riboflavin, glycerine, carmine.

Comments: WS 1442 has been sold in Europe as Crataegutt®, Crataegutt® forte, and Crataegutt® novo.

Source(s) of information: Product label (©2000 R/O Nature's Way Products, Inc.); Weikl et al., 1996; information provided by distributor.

Clinical Study: Crataegutt®

Extract name	WS 1442
Manufacturer	Dr. Willmar Schwabe GmbH & Co., Germany
Indication	**Chronic heart failure (NYHA II)**
Level of evidence	**II**
Therapeutic benefit	**Yes**

Bibliographic reference
Weikl A, Assmus KD, Neukum-Schmidt A, Schmitz J, Zapfe G, Noh HS, Siegrist J (1996). *Crataegus* special extract WS 1442: Objective proof of efficacy in patients with cardiac insufficiency (NYHA II). *Fortscritte der Medizin* 114 (24): 291-296. (Reported in *The Quarterly Review of Natural Medicine* Fall 1997: 201-209.)

Trial design
Parallel. Pretrial placebo run-in phase of two weeks.

Study duration	2 months
Dose	1 (80 mg extract) capsule twice daily
Route of administration	Oral
Randomized	Yes
Randomization adequate	No
Blinding	Double-blind
Blinding adequate	Yes
Placebo	Yes
Drug comparison	No
Site description	5 centers
No. of subjects enrolled	136
No. of subjects completed	129

Sex   Male and female
Age   Mean: 65.4 years

Inclusion criteria
Cardiac insufficiency Stage II according to the NYHA; ages 40 to 80 years; at least two symptoms of "cardiac findings" (nocturia, ankle edema, congestion of the cervical veins, incipient enlargement of the left ventricle, dyspnea under exertion and restricted "loadability"); change in blood pressure x rate, product (PRP) difference (50 watt [W] exertion versus rest) at the end of the run-in phase <15 percent. All nonpermissible concomitant medication was stopped at the start of the placebo run-in phase.

Exclusion criteria
Severe cerebral degeneration, severe organic or mental disease, decompensated cardiac insufficiency, arterial hypertension, ventricular arrhythmias, myocardial infarction during the preceding six months, unstable angina pectoris, stenosis of the aortal valves, hypertrophic obstructive cardiomyopathia, pregnancy/lactation, degenerative changes in the joints, insufficient cooperation during the run-in phase, participation in another clinical trial at the same time or during the preceding four weeks. Cardiac glycosides were not allowed, and concomitant medications, specifically calcium antagonists and ACE inhibitors, were only maintained at an unchanged doses for long-term therapy lasting at least six months.

End points
The change in pressure rate/product difference (systolic blood pressure times heart rate divided by 100 (PRP), exercise exertion of 50 W versus rest) between the beginning and the end of therapy was the primary target parameter. The secondary parameter was "life quality" as assessed by patients.

Results
From the pressure rate/product differences recorded, a clear improvement in cardiac performance was demonstrated in the Hawthorn group ($p = 0.018$), whereas a progressive aggravation occurred in the placebo group. The difference between therapy groups was significant statistically. The positive results were confirmed by a statistically clear improvement in major symptoms such as restricted physical performance, shortness of breath (dyspnea), and edema around the ankles. Active treatment in comparison with placebo resulted in an improvement in the quality of life for the patients, including a better sense of mental well-being.

Side effects
Nine adverse events were reported (six in placebo and three in the Hawthorn group) that were transitory, mild or medium in intensity, and not attributed to the treatment.

Authors' comments
This clinical trial confirmed the results of preceding studies, which have shown the *Crataegus* special extract WS 1442 to be an effective and low-risk treatment for patients with cardiac insufficiency NYHA Stage II.

Reviewer's comments
This evaluation is based on a published translation, therefore, some details may not be accurate. The trial was fairly well-designed and reported. However, the randomization method is not described adequately enough to assess. Further, no statistics were performed on the groups at the onset of the study. (Translation reviewed) (3, 6)

Clinical Study: WS 1442

Extract name	WS 1442
Manufacturer	Dr. Willmar Schwabe GmbH & Co., Germany
Indication	**Chronic heart failure (NYHA II)**
Level of evidence	**I**
Therapeutic benefit	**Trend**

Bibliographic reference
Zapfe G (2001). Clinical efficacy of *Crataegus* extract WS 1442 in congestive heart failure NYHA class II. *Phytomedicine 8* (4): 262-266.

Trial design
Parallel. Pretrial washout period of up to seven days.

Study duration	3 months
Dose	1 (80 mg) capsule 3 times daily
Route of administration	Oral
Randomized	Yes
Randomization adequate	Yes
Blinding	Double-blind
Blinding adequate	Yes
Placebo	Yes
Drug comparison	No
Site description	Not described
No. of subjects enrolled	40
No. of subjects completed	39

Sex   Male and female
Age   Mean: 62 ± 11 years

Inclusion criteria
Patients ages 40 to 80 years with congestive heart failure NYHA II.

Exclusion criteria
Patients were excluded if they had severe cerebral deterioration, severe organic or mental disease (e.g., addiction), decompensated heart disease, pregnancy or lactation, severe blood pressure elevation (diastolic >120 mmHg), ventricular arrhythmia (greater than Lown Class III), cardiac infarction within the last six months, unstable angina pectoris, participation in other clinical trials simultaneously or within the last four weeks, degenerative joint disease or other disorder that limits ergometric investigation from the outset.

End points
The primary outcome variable was exercise tolerance (watts times minutes) calculated from the results of bicycle tests carried out at the start and end of the treatment. The secondary outcome was the double product (pressure-rate product: heart rate x systolic blood pressure times 10–2) calculated at rest and after two minutes of 50 watt (W) workload in the bicycle test.

Results
After treatment with WS 1442, patients experienced an improvement in exercise tolerance of an average of 66.3 W times minutes, whereas the placebo group experienced a decrease of 105.3 W times minutes. The difference between the groups is borderline significant ($p = 0.06$). In the hawthorn group, the double product declined by 26.8 percent (14.4 mmHg/s). In the placebo group, this parameter did not change markedly.

Side effects
None observed.

Author's comments
Crataegus extract WS 1442 is a safe and effective alternative for the treatment of patients suffering from mild heart failure corresponding to NYNA Class II.

Reviewer's comments
This is a well-done study with adequately described randomization and blinding. The outcome measures were clearly defined, the data were summarized in sufficient detail, and the statistical methods were adequately described and applied (intention-to-treat analysis). Unfortunately, the results were not clinically significant. A larger sample size would possibly strengthen the results. (5, 6)

Clinical Study: Crataegutt® novo

Extract name	WS 1442
Manufacturer	Dr. Willmar Schwabe GmbH & Co., Germany

Indication	**Chronic heart failure (NYHA I and II)**
Level of evidence	**III**
Therapeutic benefit	**Undetermined**

Bibliographic reference
O'Conolly VM, Jansen W, Bernhöft G, Bartsch G (1986). Treatment of decreasing cardiac performance (NYHA Stages I to II) in advanced age with standardized *Crataegus* extract. *Fortschritte der Medizin* 104 (42): 805-808.

Trial design
Crossover. A two-week washout phase preceded the study composed of alternating six-week periods.

Study duration	6 weeks
Dose	1 (60 mg extract) tablet 3 times daily
Route of administration	Oral
Randomized	No
Randomization adequate	No
Blinding	Double-blind
Blinding adequate	No
Placebo	Yes
Drug comparison	No
Site description	Geriatric hospital
No. of subjects enrolled	34
No. of subjects completed	32
Sex	Male and female
Age	62-84 years

Inclusion criteria
Patients in a geriatric hospital diagnosed with decreasing cardiac performance associated with heart failure of NYHA Classes I to II, present for at least two years. Cardioactive medication and psychopharmaceutical drugs (including neuroleptics) were discontinued at the start of the washout phase.

Exclusion criteria
Patients with an electrocardiogram ST wave segment depression below 0.1 mV, cor pulmonale, cardiac rhythm disturbances, arthritic alterations pre-

venting the performance of an exercise-tolerance test, and cerebrovascular insufficiency with distinct loss of mental performance (IQ < 90).

End points
Patients were assessed at baseline, 6 weeks, and 12 weeks. Patients were evaluated before and after exercise (two minutes at 25 W, and if possible at 50 W). Treatment effect was evaluated by the doctor on the basis of general state of health. Patients also assessed the changes in their general well-being. Two scales were also used to ascertain the psychologically relevant symptoms that accompany the onset of heart failure: Nurses' Observation Scale for Inpatient Evaluation (NOSIE) and Brief Psychiatric Rating Scale.

Results
Following treatment with hawthorn, patients' exercise-induced rise in systolic blood pressure and heart rate was reduced. There was a significant difference from placebo ($p < 0.0001$ for both). Hawthorn treatment also caused a decrease in blood pressure at the end of the recovery period compared to baseline and placebo. A decrease in the number of prematurely terminated exercise sessions served as evidence of an increased tolerance to loading. The success of the medication was associated with an improvement in the patients' well-being, including psychological parameters.

Side effects
None observed.

Authors' comments
The results of this study confirm that Crataegutt novo is therapeutically effective in incipient loss of cardiac performance (NYHA Grades I to II). The therapeutic efficacy, combined with its absence of contraindications and its good tolerability, all serve to justify the use of Crataegutt novo in elderly patients.

Reviewer's comments
This study was not randomized, and the blinding process was not described. The study lacked documentation for study designs and methods, but it was evaluated in translation, which may not be complete or accurate. (Translation reviewed) (1, 3)

Clinical study: Crataegutt® forte

Extract name	WS 1442
Manufacturer	Dr. Willmar Schwabe GmbH & Co., Germany

Indication   **Chronic heart failure (NYHA II)**
Level of evidence   **III**
Therapeutic benefit   **Undetermined**

Bibliographic reference
Leuchtgens H (1993). *Crataegus* special extract WS 1442 in cardiac insufficiency NYHA II. *Fortschritte der Medizin* 111 (20-21): 352-354.

Trial design
Parallel.

Study duration	2 months
Dose	1 (80 mg) capsule twice daily
Route of administration	Oral
Randomized	Yes
Randomization adequate	No
Blinding	Double-blind
Blinding adequate	No
Placebo	Yes
Drug comparison	No
Site description	Not described
No. of subjects enrolled	30
No. of subjects completed	30
Sex	Male and female
Age	Mean: 65.5 ± 6 years

Inclusion criteria
Patients with cardiac insufficiency in Class II according to the NYHA, age between 50 and 70 years, with no complaints at rest and under mild physical exercise, but dyspnea and tiredness under increasing physical exertion.

Exclusion criteria
Exclusion criteria were cardiac arrhythmia greater than Lown Class III, electrocardiogram (ECG)-recorded ST segment depression at rest > 0.1 mV, degenerative conditions of the joints or other disease that would restrict exercise on an ergometric bicycle, and decompensated cardiac insufficiency or myocardial infarction up to six months previously.

End points
The major parameters were the change in the pressure times rate product (PRP = product of systolic blood pressure and heart rate divided by 100) under standardized exercise on a bicycle ergometer, as well as a questionnaire on subjective improvement of complaints (B-L-Total Score). Exercise toler-

ance, change in heart rate and change in arterial blood pressure were accepted as secondary parameters. Patients were examined prior to therapy and then after four and eight weeks.

Results
In both of the principal target variables, the differences in favor of the WS 1442 group were statistically significant after eight weeks of therapy. The PRP with exercise decreased continuously after four and eight weeks of treatment compared to baseline, and was statistically below that of the placebo group. Individual progression confirmed improvement in 13/15 WS 1442 patients, and in 3/15 placebo patients. In the hawthorn group, the B-L-Total Score decreased more than with placebo. In the secondary variables, the heart rate decreased in the hawthorn group whereas the increased values remained approximately the same in the placebo group. The systolic and diastolic blood pressures dropped slightly to about the same extent in both groups.

Side effects
Adverse events were not recorded.

Author's comments
The increase in well-being and the reduction of complaints could be demonstrated in the WS 1442-treated group of patients. This study confirms the therapeutic efficacy and good tolerance of Crataegutt forte, and justifies its application in patients suffering from NYHA Class II cardiac insufficiency.

Reviewer's comments
Significant methodological flaws as well as a poor description of methods make it hard to evaluate these results. Neither the randomization nor the blinding processs are well described, and the sample size is small. (1, 4)

Clinical Study: Crataegutt® novo

Extract name	WS 1442
Manufacturer	Dr. Willmar Schwabe GmbH & Co., Germany
Indication	**Chronic heart failure (NYHA I and II)**
Level of evidence	**III**
Therapeutic benefit	**Undetermined**

Bibliographic reference
Hanack T, Brückel MH (1983). The treatment of mild stable forms of angina pectoris using Crataegutt novo. *Therapiewoche* 33: 4331-4333.

Trial design
Parallel. Pretrial placebo washout period of eight days.

Study duration	3 weeks
Dose	1 (60 mg) tablet 3 times daily
Route of administration	Oral
Randomized	Yes
Randomization adequate	No
Blinding	Double-blind
Blinding adequate	No
Placebo	Yes
Drug comparison	No
Site description	Not described
No. of subjects enrolled	60
No. of subjects completed	58
Sex	Male and female
Age	Mean: 55 years

Inclusion criteria
Patients suffering from coronary disease New York Health Association (NYHA) Class I and II. Additional medication for circulatory and cardiac complaints was not allowed.

Exclusion criteria
Patients were excluded if they had instable angina pectoris, hypopotassemia, manifest cardiac insufficiency, essential hypertension according to WHO Grades II and III, and hyperlipoproteinemia (> 400 mg% cholesterol). Patients were also excluded if, after the first ergometric exertion after the washout period, they had an increase in pectoralgia, dysrhythmia, dyspnoea, or attainment of the submaximum heart rate.

End points
Patients' tolerance to ergometric loading was assessed using the bicycle ergometer before and after the trial. Typical changes in ECG under exertion were also evaluated to objectivize myocardial ischemia and to assess Crataegutt novo's therapeutic efficacy. Clinical and chemical parameters (blood count, blood sugar level, cholesterol, triglycerides, uric acid, serum creatinine, iron [including total iron-binding capacity], potassium, and magnesium) were also measured at the start and end of the trial.

Results
After treatment with Crataegutt novo, patients were able to increase (by 25 percent) tolerance to ergometric load by 100 watt times minute, whereas patients treated with placebo could not increase their tolerance. This difference

was statistically significant ($p < 0.08$). After 21 days of treatment, 18 patients in the hawthorn group had a marked reverse in their ischemic reaction in ECG under load, but only six patients in the placebo had the same reaction. No significant difference was found between the two groups in terms of the pulse rate, blood pressure, or the clinical and chemical parameters.

Side effects
None mentioned.

Authors' comments
Our examinations have confirmed that Crataegutt novo is suitable for the effective and side-effect-free treatment of stable forms of angina pectoris in NYHA Classes I and II.

Reviewer's comments
Workload was increased, but other parameters were unchanged. The lack of evidence of therapeutic efficacy may be due to the short trial length. The randomization and blinding were not adequately described. However, the outcome measures were clearly defined, the sample size was appropriate, and the data were summarized in sufficient detail. (Translation reviewed) (1, 5)

Clinical Study: WS 1442

Extract name	WS 1442
Manufacturer	Dr. Willmar Schwabe GmbH & Co., Germany
Indication	**Chronic heart failure (NYHA III)**
Level of evidence	**III**
Therapeutic benefit	**Yes**

Bibliographic reference
Tauchert M (2002). Efficacy and safety of *Crataegus* extract WS 1442 in comparison with placebo in patients with chronic stable New York Heart Association class-III heart failure. *American Heart Journal* 143 (5): 910-915.

Trial design
Parallel. Patients underwent a four-week, single-blind, placebo washout period before being randomized to receive either 900 or 1,800 mg WS 1442, or placebo, daily. Throughout the washout and trial period, all patients were also taking their preexisting diuretic therapy daily: triamterene (50 mg) and hydrochlorothiazide (25 mg).

Study duration	4 months
Dose	900 or 1,800 mg daily
Route of administration	Oral
Randomized	Yes
Randomization adequate	No
Blinding	Double-blind
Blinding adequate	No
Placebo	Yes
Drug comparison	No
Site description	Multicenter
No. of subjects enrolled	232
No. of subjects completed	197
Sex	Male and female
Age	Mean: 67.6 ± 9.4 years

Inclusion criteria

Patients at least 40 years old with chronic congestive heart failure (NYHA Class III) known for at least six months, who had not been treated with a diuretic and/or a low dose of an angiotensin-converting enzyme (ACE) inhibitor, and with an exercise capacity of ≤ 75 watts (W) as assessed by seated bicycle ergometry.

Exclusion criteria

Major exclusion criteria consisted of: NYHA Classes I, II, or IV; treatment with digitalis within the previous six months; exercise capacity of > 75 W for two minutes at the test during run-in; unstable angina or myocardial infarction within the previous six months; atrial fibrillation or ventricular arrhythmia ≥ Lown Class III; cardiac valvular disease or hypertrophic cardiomyopathy; significant hypertension or hypotension (< 60 mmHg or ≥ 105 mmHg diastolic or < 90 mmHg or > 175 mmHg systolic); electrolyte disturbances, hyperuricemia, hypovolemia; impaired renal function (creatinine > 1.8 mg/dl) or hepatic function; obstructive airways disease; hypersensitivity to study drug; pregnancy, unreliable contraception, or breast-feeding mothers; and participation in another clinical trial within the previous six weeks. The following medications were prohibited during the study: ACE inhibitors, digitalis, antiarrhythmics, sympathomimetics, vasodilators, and diuretics other than triamterene/hydrochlorothiazide.

End points

The maximal workload tolerated was tested by symptom-limited bicycle exercise tests. The tests were carried out in a sitting position at the same time of day. The initial workload was 25 W, with the workload increasing by 25 W every two minutes. This test, as well as safety laboratory tests, was carried out at the beginning and end of the washout period, and after 8 and 16 weeks of treatment. Also measured at these tests were: blood pressure after each exercise stage, intensity of effort-induced dyspnea, and any ST-segment depression and arrhythmia. Subjective symptoms were also recorded every four weeks during the treatment phase.

Results
The increase in maximal workload tolerated at the end of the study in subjects in the 1,800 mg WS 1442 group was statistically significant compared with the placebo group. The high-dose group also improved more than the lower dose group (900 mg WS 1442). The subjective symptoms scores for the typical heart failure symptoms for those taking active treatment were lower than the scores for the placebo group, and these differences were statistically significant.

Side effects
Significantly fewer side effects occurred in the groups taking hawthorn compared with placebo. Overall, the group taking 1,800 mg WS 1442 experienced fewer side effects, particularly with respect to vertigo and dizziness. Tolerability was rated best by both the patients and the investigators for the 1,800 mg group.

Author's comments
The study confirms that treatment with WS 1442 is capable of improving the exercise capacity of patients with heart failure, including patients with an advanced state of the disease (NYHA Class III). This was demonstrated not only by the statistically significant improvement in the maximal workload tolerated by the 1,800 mg dose of WS 1442 versus placebo, but also by the fact that the efficacy of WS 1442 was dose dependent.

Reviewer's comments
The low score on the Jadad scale likely reflects problems with the report rather than problems with the conducted trial. Again, it is unfortunate that an objective medical measure was not included. (1, 6)

Product Profile: Faros® 300

Manufacturer	**Lichtwer Pharma AG, Germany**
U.S. distributor	None
Botanical ingredient	**Hawthorn leaf and flower extract**
Extract name	**LI 132**
Quantity	No information
Processing	No information
Standardization	No information
Formulation	Tablet

Source(s) of information: Bödigheimer and Chase, 1994; Hawthorn Leaf with Flower, *American Herbal Pharmacopoeia*, February 1999.

Clinical Study: Faros® 300

Extract name	LI 132
Manufacturer	Lichtwer Pharma AG, Germany
Indication	**Chronic heart failure (NYHA II)**
Level of evidence	**II**
Therapeutic benefit	**Yes**

Bibliographic reference
Tauchert M, Ploch M, Hübner WD (1994). Efficacy of hawthorn extract LI 132 in comparison with captopril: Multicenter double-blind study on 132 patients with cardiac insufficiency of NYHA grade II. *Münchener Medizinische Wochenschrift* 136 (Suppl. 1): 27-33.

Trial design
Parallel. Pretrial placebo run-in phase of one week. The dosages for the trial were as follows: patients took either one 300 mg hawthorn extract or one 6.25 mg captopril on day 0; two 300 mg hawthorn or two 6.25 mg captopril from days 1 through 3; three 300 mg hawthorn or three 6.25 mg captopril from days 4 through 6; and then took three 300 mg hawthorn or three 12.5 mg captopril for the rest of the trial.

Study duration	2 months
Dose	1 (300 mg extract) capsule 3 times daily
Route of administration	Oral
Randomized	Yes
Randomization adequate	Yes
Blinding	Double-blind
Blinding adequate	Yes
Placebo	No
Drug comparison	Yes
Drug name	Captopril
Site description	14 test centers
No. of subjects enrolled	132
No. of subjects completed	124

Sex   Male and female
Age   Mean: 62.5 ± 6 years

Inclusion criteria
Patients from 50 to 70 years of age with stable cardiac insufficiency of NYHA Class II, with work tolerance in standardized bicycle ergometry less than 100 W.

Exclusion criteria
Patients with cardiac insufficiency of NYHA Class III and IV, unstable angina pectoris, myocardial infarction during the previous six months, atrial fibrillation, ventricular extrasystoles of Lown Class IV, second-degree and third-degree AV block, bundle-branch block, hyperthyroidism, hypothyroidism, anemia, hypertension with blood pressures of more than 165/95 mmHg, more than 25 percent overweight, obstructive ventilation disorders, and physical infirmities such that exhaustive exercise in bicycle ergometry would have been ruled out. Further contraindications were hypersensitivity to captopril, angioneurotic edema, and severe kidney and liver disease. Medication with cardioprotective preparations before or during the trial were not generally permitted, except for diuretics that had been taken at a constant dose for at least four weeks before and were continued throughout the trial.

End points
Patients were monitored at inclusion and after 14, 28, and 56 days. The primary end point was symptom-limited ergometric exercise. Secondary criteria for the study were blood pressure, heart rate, and pressure-rate product (each measured both at rest and under maximum exertion), analysis of the resting ECG, assessment of the decrease in physical performance, exhaustion, susceptibility to fatigue, exertional dyspnea and edema, and general final judgments of efficacy and tolerance by the doctor and the patient.

Results
Both treatment groups showed statistically significant increases in work tolerance over the course of treatment. The pressure-rate product decreased in both groups, and the frequency and severity of symptoms decreased by about 50 percent in both groups. No significant differences were found for any of the target parameters between the two treatments. Judgment of efficacy by doctors slightly favored the captopril group at day 28, but reported better efficacy for the *Crataegus* group on day 56.

Side effects
No serious side effects were reported in the hawthorn group (two patients reported gastrointestinal symptoms and one reported cardiac pains).

Authors' comments
Apart from termination of treatment because of an adverse effect in one

case during treatment with captopril, the study gave substantially equivalent results for the principal and secondary criteria under treatment with both hawthorn and captopril.

Reviewer's comments
This was a very well-conducted study with a pharmaceutical comparison. The study was adequately powered to show moderate difference in efficacy, and both the randomization and blinding processes were well described. However, a sufficient description of data was lacking, as means and standard deviations were not reported. (Translation reviewed) (5, 5)

Clinical Study: Faros® 300

Extract name	LI 132
Manufacturer	Lichtwer Pharma AG, Germany
Indication	**Chronic heart failure (NYHA II)**
Level of evidence	**I**
Therapeutic benefit	**Trend**

Bibliographic reference
Schmidt U, Kuhn U, Ploch M, Hübner WD (1994). Efficacy of the hawthorn *(Crataegus)* preparation LI 132 in 78 patients with chronic congestive heart failure defined as NYHA functional class II. *Phytomedicine* 1 (1): 17-24.

Trial design
Parallel. Pretrial washout period of one week.

Study duration	2 months
Dose	200 mg 3 times daily
Route of administration	Oral
Randomized	Yes
Randomization adequate	Yes
Blinding	Double-blind
Blinding adequate	Yes
Placebo	Yes
Drug comparison	No
Site description	10 centers
No. of subjects enrolled	78
No. of subjects completed	70
Sex	Male and female
Age	Mean: 60 ± 6.9 years

Inclusion criteria

Patients with stable chronic heart failure defined as NYHA Class II, between the ages of 45 and 73, and initial maximum cardiac capacity measured by way of bicycle ergometry below 100 watts.

Exclusion criteria

Patients affected by chronic heart failure defined as NYHA Class III and IV, with cardiac angina at rest, cardiac infarction in the preceding three months, atrial fibrillation, ventricular extrasystoles of Class IV according to Lown, second- and third-degree atrioventricular block, more than 20 percent over-weight, obstructive respiratory tract diseases, bodily defects that did not al-low for the patients to be tested on the ergometer bicycle, pregnant or nurs-ing women, and those addicted to alcohol or medical drugs.

End points

The primary target was the maximum working capacity measured using a bicycle ergometer (three minutes in 25 W increments). As secondary target criteria, the clinical symptoms, patients' subjective feelings of health, blood pressure, heart rate, and pressure/rate product at rest and under load were used.

Results

After 56 days of treatment, the median values obtained for the working ca-pacity of the patients treated with hawthorn increased by 28 W, whereas the increase in the placebo group was as little as 5 watts. The difference was statistically significant ($p < 0.001$). A significant reduction of the systolic blood pressure, of the heart rate, and of the pressure/rate product was ob-served for the patients treated with hawthorn compared to the patients treated with the placebo preparation. The clinical symptoms were also found to have improved significantly.

Side effects

None observed.

Authors' comments

No improvement was observed in the working capacity of subjects with exer-cise levels below 75 W, whereas a distinct improvement was observed for those with exercise levels of 100 and 125 W. From this we can conclude that patients who are exposed to physical load corresponding to 100 to 125 W will benefit from hawthorn, if the drug is administered in adequate doses.

Reviewer's comments

This is a well-conducted trial. Unfortunately, the primary end point was work capacity, and I am unsure of the clinical significance regarding the progno-sis. Obviously, some of the secondary end points are not inappropriate, but I wish the authors had looked at anginal episodes, episodes of excitational angina, or another clinically relevant end point. (5, 5)

Clinical Study: Faros® 300

Extract name	LI 132
Manufacturer	Lichtwer Pharma AG, Germany
Indication	**Chronic heart failure (NYHA II)**
Level of evidence	**II**
Therapeutic benefit	**Trend**

Bibliographic reference
Forster A, Forster K, Buhring M, Wolfstadter HD (1994). *Crataegus* for moderately reduced left ventricular ejection fraction: Ergospirometric monitoring study on 72 patients in a double-blind comparison with placebo. *Münchener Medizinische Wochenschrift* 136 (Suppl. 1): 21-26.

Trial design
Parallel. Pretrial washout period of seven days.

Study duration	2 months
Dose	1 (300 mg) tablet 3 times daily
Route of administration	Oral
Randomized	Yes
Randomization adequate	Yes
Blinding	Double-blind
Blinding adequate	Yes
Placebo	Yes
Drug comparison	No
Site description	Cardiology outpatient center
No. of subjects enrolled	72
No. of subjects completed	69
Sex	Male and female
Age	31-79 years (mean: 51)

Inclusion criteria
Cardiology outpatients with diagnoses of cardiac insufficiency NYHA Class II with earlier diagnosis of postmyocarditic state, coronary heart disease, hypertensive heart disease, or other similar diagnosis.

Exclusion criteria

Cardiac insufficiency of NYHA Classes III and IV, myocardial infarction during the previous three months, arrhythmias such as atrial fibrillation, ventricular extrasystoles of Lown Class IV, and second-degree and third-degree AV block, more than 20 percent overweight, obstructive ventilation disorders, and physical infirmities such that a meaningful ergospirometric test would have been impossible. Patients could not use cardioactive preparations (except stabilized diuretic therapy) for eight days before the trial start and during the trial itself.

End points

Clinical examination and ergospirometric tests were carried out at the beginning of the study and after eight weeks of treatment. Running averages of the following parameters were obtained under resting conditions, under maximum efforts, and at the time of reaching the anaerobic threshold: maximum oxygen uptake, oxygen uptake at the time of reaching the anaerobic threshold, output achieved, heart rate, time taken to reach anaerobic threshold, oxygen pulse, respiratory equivalent for oxygen, and continuous effort endurance time. Patients were also questioned about their well-being after four and eight weeks of treatment.

Results

After treatment for eight weeks, statistically different improvements in subjective well-being were reported by 86 percent of patients in the hawthorn group and by 47 percent in the placebo group ($p < 0.01$). Exercise capacity increased more in the hawthorn group than in the placebo group, but not significantly. The quantity of oxygen absorbed by the lungs increased in the treated group compared to placebo, both at the exercise peak and afterward ($p < 0.05$ for both). For significantly more patients in the hawthorn group, the exercise time taken to reach the point of anaerobic metabolism increased ($p < 0.05$). An average increase of 30 seconds was observed for patients of the *Crataegus* group, whereas the time for the placebo group did not change. No significant differences were found between the two groups in terms of the control parameters of blood pressure, heart rate, oxygen pulse, and respiratory equivalent.

Side effects

No significant side effects were observed.

Authors' comments

A cardiac effect of hawthorn extract was demonstrated both in the ergospirometric parameters and in a distinct improvement of subjective symptoms. In view of its positive effects, hawthorn extract LI 132 can be recommended for the treatment of milder disturbances of cardiac function.

Reviewer's comments
This was a fairly well-designed and well-run study, with the randomization and double-blinding processes described adequately. It is not clear, however, that a 30 second increase in exercise time represents a clinically significant outcome. The changes in symptoms were reported as categorical. In addition, the subjective variable of well-being is not as reliable a measure, and the sample size was too small for a mild to moderate effect. (Translation reviewed) (5, 5)

Clinical Study: Faros® 300

Extract name	LI 132
Manufacturer	Lichtwer Pharma AG, Germany
Indication	**Chronic heart failure (NYHA II)**
Level of evidence	**II**
Therapeutic benefit	**Trend**

Bibliographic reference
Bödigheimer K, Chase D (1994). Efficacy of hawthorn extract in a daily dose of 3 x 100 mg: Multicenter double-blind study in 85 patients with NYHA stage II heart failure. *Münchener Medizinische Wochenschrift* 136 (Suppl. 1): 7-11.

Trial design
Parallel. Pretrial washout period of seven days.

Study duration	1 month
Dose	2 (50 mg) tablets 3 times daily
Route of administration	Oral
Randomized	Yes
Randomization adequate	Yes
Blinding	Double-blind
Blinding adequate	Yes
Placebo	Yes
Drug comparison	No
Site description	Multicenter
No. of subjects enrolled	85
No. of subjects completed	73
Sex	Male and female
Age	40-80 years (mean 61.5)

Inclusion criteria
Patients ages 40 to 80 years with stable NYHA Class II heart failure.

Exclusion criteria
Patients with NYHA Classes III and IV heart failure, coronary heart disease with angina pectoris, myocardial infarction less than three months before the start of the study, atrial fibrillation, ventricular extrasystoles (Lown Class IV), AV block Grade 2 or 3, hypertension requiring treatment, more than 20 percent overweight, pregnancy, obstructive airways diseases and physical infirmities that prevented the patient from being fully tested by bicycle ergometry. The use of cardiac substances, especially cardiac glycosides, ACE inhibitors, sympathicomimetics, antiarrhythmics, vasodilators, beta-blockers, calcium-channel blockers, and long-acting nitrates was not permitted during the study. The use of diuretics was allowed if they had been given in a constant dose for at least four weeks before the start of the study and this dosage was continued throughout the study.

End points
Exercise tolerance during bicycle ergometric testing was measured to a maximum watt level that a patient could sustain for at least two minutes, applied in 25 W increments. Heart rate, blood pressure, ECG course, and clinical symptoms were recorded. In addition, clinical findings (neck-vein distension, third/fourth heart sounds, rales and edema, blood pressure, and heart rate at rest) were recorded, as well as the global assessment by the doctor and the patient. Patients were assessed at inclusion, after the seven-day washout period, and after 14 and 28 days of treatment.

Results
Exercise tolerance in the active treatment group increased by 13 W, whereas the placebo group had an increase of 3 W. Heart rate, systolic blood pressure, and the two multiplied together decreased more markedly in the hawthorn group than in the placebo group—at rest and at maximal loading. However, none of the differences between the groups were statistically significant. In the final evaluation of the treatment outcome by the doctor and patient, hawthorn formulation received a more favorable assessment than the placebo treatment.

Side effects
Two cases of nonspecific side effects, including migraine, gastrointestinal complaints and palpitations, occurred in each group.

Authors' comments
Other studies using larger doses and longer durations reported significant effects of hawthorn on cardiac function. The fact that merely trends toward improvements were observed in the present study therefore suggests that neither the dose used here nor the treatment period was sufficient. It may be

that a dose of almost 1 g of extract should be recommended for *Crataegus* preparations, with minimum treatment periods of six to eight weeks.

Reviewer's comments

This was a well-done trial that was double-blind and randomized, but the results were not clinically significant. Also, no means or standard deviations were reported. The trial length was minimal, but adequate. (5, 6)

Horse Chestnut

Latin name: *Aesculus hippocastanum* **L.** [Hippocastanaceae]
Plant part: **Seed**

PREPARATIONS USED
IN REVIEWED CLINICAL STUDIES

Native to the Near East, the horse chestnut tree was brought to northern Europe in the sixteenth century. As early as the 1800s, horse chestnut seed extracts were used therapeutically in France. Although preparations of other parts of the tree have been used medicinally, only the efficacy of the dried seeds has been proven. Powdered dried seeds contain 3 to 5 percent saponins, and powdered hydroalcoholic extracts of the seeds contain 16 to 20 percent triterpene glycosides (a class of saponins), calculated as aescin (escin). Aescin, itself a mixture of several glycosides derived from two triterpenoid aglycones, is believed to be the main active constituent of horse chestnut seed extract (Schulz, Hänsel, and Tyler, 2001).

Venastat™ contains the horse chestnut seed extract HCE 50 and is manufactured by Pharmaton S.A., in Switzerland and distributed in the United States by Pharmaton Natural Health Products. HCE 50 is characterized as containing 16 percent triterpene glycosides calculated as aescin. Each 300 mg capsule contains 50 mg aescin. Venastat is sold in Europe as Venostasin® retard.

Venaforce™ is manufactured in Switzerland by Bioforce AG, and is distributed in the United States by Bioforce USA. Venaforce contains horse chestnut seed extract (5 to 6.1:1, 60 percent ethanol m/m), and 76.5 mg tablets are standardized to contain 20 mg aescin. Venaforce is sold as Aesculaforce in Europe.

One trial used a generic horse chestnut seed extract with a plant/extract ratio of 5:1. Each capsule contained 369 to 412 mg standardized extract containing 75 mg triterpene glycosides calculated as aescin.

HORSE CHESTNUT SUMMARY TABLE

Product Name	Manufacturer/ U.S. Distributor	Product Characteristics	Dose in Trials	Indication	No. of Trials	Benefit (Evidence Level-Trial No.)
Venastat™ (US); Venostasin® retard (EU)	Pharmaton, S.A., Switzerland/ Pharmaton Natural Health Products	Extract (HCE 50) contains 16% aescin	2 (300 mg ex-tract) capsules daily (100 mg aescin)	Chronic venous insufficiency	12	Yes (II-4, III-3) Trend (II-1) No (II-1) Undetermined (III-1) MOA (II-1, III-1)
Venaforce™ (US); Aesculaforce (EU)	Bioforce AG, Switzerland/ Bioforce USA	Hydro-alcoholic extract	378-540 mg (120 mg aescin) daily	Chronic venous insufficiency	1	Yes (II-1)
Generic	None	Extract ratio of 5:1	2 capsules (150 mg aescin) daily	Chronic venous insufficiency	1	Yes (II-1)
Escin gel	Madaus AG, Germany/None	2% aescin	10 g gel	Hematoma	1	Undetermined (II-1)

Escin gel is a topical formulation of horse chestnut seed extract standardized to contain 2 percent aescin that is manufactured by Madaus AG of Germany. Escin gel, which is not available in the United States, is available in Europe as Reparil gel.

SUMMARY OF REVIEWED CLINICAL STUDIES

Horse chestnut has been used traditionally as an herbal remedy for chronic venous insufficiency, and numerous clinical trials support that use. Chronic venous insufficiency (CVI) is characterized by chronic inadequate drainage of venous blood and venous hypertension, which results in leg edema, dermatosclerosis (hardening of the skin), and feelings of pain, fatigue, and tenseness in the lower extremities. As a result, patients often require hospitalization and surgery, for instance, for symptomatic varicose veins. Pharmacological therapies and/or leg compression with specialized stockings or surgery are the treatment options (Pittler and Ernst, 2002).

CVI is divided into three stages according to the degree of severity. The symptoms of Grade I, according to Widmer and Marshall, are dilation of the veins of the feet and a tendency for edema. Grade II is defined by additional symptoms, including pigmentation of the skin, hypertrophy of the skin corneal layer, and hardening of the skin. Grade III is characterized by leg ulcers, either healed (IIIa) or unhealed (IIIb). In the early stages of CVI (Grade I), the veins have not suffered any permanent damage, and pharmacological therapy may reduce the leakage of fluid from the veins. At the later stages of CVI (Grades II and III), the disease process involves the larger veins, and ultimately the damage to the veins is irreversible (Ottillinger and Greeske, 2001). Studies reviewed here included patients with CVI Grades I or II. One study, on a generic product, included patients with CVI Grade II according to Hach. Although we found no information on this scale the description of symptoms were similar to Grade II according to Widmer and Marshall. They were obstructive edema, possible tropic skin changes, and venous capacity and/or venous return outside normal limits (Diehm et al, 1992).

Venastat

Chronic Venous Insufficiency

Twelve reviewed trials conducted with Venastat (Venostasin) measured symptoms related to CVI. All trials reported some benefit in clinical symptoms with a dose of 600 mg extract (100 mg aescin) per day, although the quality of some trials was better than others.

Three small, well-conducted, placebo-controlled studies reported significant decreases in leg/foot volume, circumference, edema, and pain in patients with CVI given 300 mg extract twice daily compared to placebo. The first study included 39 subjects with CVI Grades I or II who were treated for one month. The volume of the foot and the distal shank, and the circumference of the ankle and calf, all significantly decreased with horse chestnut compared to placebo. Neither group had a change in venous capacity (Rudofsky et al., 1986). In the second study, 28 outpatients with CVI (grade not given) were treated for 20 days, and a reduction in leg circumference compared to placebo was noted (Pilz, 1990). In the third study, 30 subjects (CVI grade not given) were treated for two months. After both one and two months, a reduction in edema, pain, and symptoms such as heaviness, pins and needles, restlessness, and nocturnal cramps was observed compared to placebo. After two months, significant differences in the circumferences of the ankle and leg in the Venostasin group were observed compared to placebo (Cloarec, 1993).

Another trial, including 74 subjects with CVI, measured the effect of treatment for two months with either 600 mg extract or placebo on edema provoked by sitting on an exercise bicycle with legs dangling in the air. As a result of treatment, provoked increases in leg volume and leg circumference were significantly reduced (Lohr et al., 1986). A group of 20 women with pregnancy-related edema or CVI Grade I were treated with 600 mg per day or placebo in a crossover study of two weeks duration for each treatment phase. Treatment with Venastat led to a significant reduction in leg volume and circumference (Steiner and Hillemanns, 1986).

A large, good-quality trial included 240 subjects (CVI Grade I) and compared Venastat (600 mg per day) with compression stockings and placebo. Following three months of treatment there was a significant decrease in leg volume and edema with both treatments compared to placebo (Diehm et al., 1996). Another study of similar design included 355 patients with advanced CVI of Grades II or IIIa. In this study, both active therapies produced a reduction in lower leg volume, but the decrease was much larger for the group with compression stockings. Compression treatment was the only treatment that performed significantly better than placebo. A subgroup analysis determined that Venostasin was more effective in subjects with CVI Grade II than those with Grade IIIa. Compression, on the other hand, was more effective for those with the higher grade (Diehm and Schmidt, 2000). Ottillinger and Greeske (2001) compared these two trials and concluded that the lower CVI grades were suitable for therapy with horse chestnut, but that those with higher grades were better off with compression therapy.

A good-quality study with 30 subjects with CVI compared Venostasin to another edema-protective agent. Venostasin, 600 mg per day for one month, reduced an increase in ankle circumference caused by standing for 15 minutes when compared to baseline. The effectiveness of Venostasin was greater than the control agent (Erdlen, 1989). Although the control agent was not identified in the translation we reviewed, Pittler and Ernst (2002) identified the agent as rutoside (oxerutin) in their review. Oxerutin (*O*-beta-hydroxyethyl-rutosides) is a semisynthetic derivative of plant constituents that has been used as an alternative to horse chestnut preparations. It is used as a comparative agent in the following three studies.

A study included 137 postmenopausal women with CVI Grade II who were given one of three treatments for three months. The study compared a horse chestnut extract (thought to be Venostasin, 600 mg per day) to oxerutin (1,000 mg per day) and to oxerutin (1,000 mg per day for four weeks followed by 500 mg per day). Oxerutin at 1,000 mg per day was significantly more effective at reducing leg volume than horse chestnut extract. The constant 1,000 mg dose was better than the 1,000 to 500 mg stepped treatment (Rehn et al., 1996). Two other studies compared Venostasin to oxerutin, but are not reviewed in detail due to a lack of translation into English. They found the effectiveness of Venostasin (50 mg or 150 mg aescin per day, respectively) greater than or equal to oxerutin (500 or 2000 mg per day, respectively) (Kalbfleisch and Pfalzgraf, 1989; Erler, 1991).

A study using 19 normal volunteers explored the effectiveness of Venostasin in preventing the edema caused by a 14-hour airline flight. Participants took 600 mg or placebo daily for ten days prior to the flight. The control group showed a steady and significant increase in the circumference of the ankle and foot. This swelling was significantly reduced by treatment with Venostasin (Marshall and Dormady, 1987).

A crossover mechanistic study explored the effect of Venostasin on the development of edema through measuring the quantity of fluid flowing from blood capillaries into the surrounding tissue (transcapillary filtration coefficient). The study included 22 women with CVI grades I to III who were given a single dose of 600 mg or placebo on test days. Measurements before and after dosing revealed a reduction in the transcapillary filtration coefficient of 22 percent in the Venostasin group compared to baseline (Pauschinger, 1987).

Another mechanistic study explored the effect of Venostasin on levels of serum proteoglycan hydrolases. Proteoglycan hydrolases cause the degradation of proteoglycans, a part of the capillary endothelium and a main component of the extravascular matrix. This matrix is thought to play a role in capillary permeability and fragility. Treatment of 15 patients with varicose veins with 900 mg Venostasin per day for 12 days resulted in a significant reduction in the activities of three glycosaminoglycan hydrolases. Thus, treatment with Venostasin may shift the equilibrium of degradation and synthesis of proteoglycans toward synthesis, thereby preventing vascular leakage (Kreysel, Nissen, and Enghofer, 1983).

Venaforce

Chronic Venous Insufficiency

Venaforce was reported to statistically reduce ankle edema, but not subjective symptoms of heaviness, pain, burning, itching, or pins and needles in the legs. This placebo-controlled study included 52 subjects with CVI Grades I or II. Treatment consisted of six tablets, containing 120 mg aescin, per day for six weeks (Shah, Bommer, and Degenring, 1997).

Generic

Chronic Venous Insufficiency

A well-conducted, placebo-controlled trial with 39 patients with CVI (Stage II according to Hach) reported a statistical reduction in mean leg volume after six weeks of treatment, both before and after edema provocation, compared to placebo. Treatment was an un-branded extract delivering 150 mg aescin per day (Diehm et al., 1992).

Escin Gel

Hematoma

Escin gel containing 2 percent aescin was compared to placebo in an experimentally induced hematoma model. Hematomas are swellings filled with blood that can form as the result of physical trauma to the body, causing damage to blood vessels beneath the skin. In this study, hematomas were induced in 70 healthy volunteers by subcutaneous injection of 2 ml of the subjects' own blood. Treatment with 10 g of gel or placebo followed within five minutes. Sensitivity measurements were taken from one to nine hours after treatment. As a result, the Escin gel statistically reduced pain at all time points compared to placebo (Calabrese and Preston, 1993). Our reviewer, Dr. Mary Hardy, criticized the model because the subcutaneous injection of blood does not produce all of the parameters as a bruise or hematoma acquired through trauma. Thus, she rated the possible benefit as undetermined.

SYSTEMATIC REVIEWS

A systematic review of double-blind, randomized, controlled trials was conducted on oral horse chestnut seed extract preparations for symptomatic treatment of CVI. Thirteen studies fulfilled the inclusion criteria, of which eight were placebo-controlled and five were controlled with a reference substance (oxerutin) or compression. The authors found that the use of horse chestnut was associated with a decrease in lower leg volume and a reduction in leg circumference at the calf and ankle. Symptoms such as leg pain, pruritus, and a feeling of fatigue and tenseness were reduced. The authors concluded that horse chestnut seed extract is superior to placebo and as effective as reference medications in alleviating the objective signs and symptoms of CVI (Pittler and Ernst, 1998). In a subsequent review conducted by the same authors, using the "Cochrane Library" format, several placebo-controlled trials were considered adequate to enter into meta-analysis. Leg pain, as assessed in six placebo-controlled trials using visual analog scales and four-point scales, was significantly reduced in comparison to placebo. An analysis of four trials ($n = 239$) that used water displacement to measure leg volume determined a significant reduction in favor of horse chestnut extract compared with placebo (weighted mean difference 58.6 ml [95 percent CI 24.9-92.2]). A meta-analysis of three trials found that treatment reduced the circumference at the ankle (weighted mean difference 4.7 mm [95 percent CI 1.13-8.28]) as well as at the calf (weighted mean difference 3.5 mm [95 percent CI 0.58-6.45]) compared to placebo (Pittler and Ernst, 2002).

ADVERSE REACTIONS OR SIDE EFFECTS

The trials reviewed in this section rarely reported minimal adverse events that did not differ significantly from placebo. Eight of the 13 studies included in a systematic review reported symptoms of adverse reactions, including gastrointestinal tract symptoms, dizziness, nausea, headache, and pruritus. The frequency of adverse event reports ranged from 0.9 percent to 3.0 percent. In three studies the adverse events were not different from those reported by the placebo group (Pittler and Ernst, 1998). An observational study involving more than 5,000 patients with CVI receiving various therapies reported the incidence of adverse reaction with horse chestnut to be 0.6 percent. Gastrointestinal symptoms and calf spasm were reported most frequently (Greeske and Pohlmann, 1996).

INFORMATION FROM PHARMACOPOEIAL MONOGRAPHS

Sources of Published Therapeutic Monographs

German Commission E
European Scientific Cooperative on Phytotherapy

Indications

The German Commission E recommends a dry extract manufactured from horse chestnut seed for the treatment of complaints found in pathological conditions of the veins of the legs (chronic venous insufficiency), for example, pains and a sensation of heaviness in the legs, nocturnal systremma (cramps in the calves), pruritus, and swelling of the legs (Blumenthal et al., 1998). The European Scientific Cooperative on Phytotherapy (ESCOP) also suggests horse chestnut for the treatment of chronic venous insufficiency, as well as for varicosis (ESCOP, 1999).

Doses

Dry extract of the seed adjusted to 16 to 20 percent triterpene glycosides (calculated as aescin [escin]): 100 mg aescin corresponding to 250 to 312.5 mg extract two times per day in a delayed release form (Blumenthal et al., 1998)
Hydroalcoholic extract containing 50 to 150 mg of triterpene glycosides (calculated as aescin) usually in divided doses (ESCOP, 1999)

Treatment Period

ESCOP lists no restriction for treatment period length (ESCOP, 1999).

Contraindications

The Commission E and ESCOP list no known contraindications (Blumenthal et al., 1998; ESCOP, 1999).

Adverse Reactions

The Commission E and ESCOP state that pruritis, nausea, and gastric complaints may occur in isolated cases after oral intake (Blumenthal et al., 1998; ESCOP, 1999).

Precautions

The Commission E lists no precautions; however, ESCOP does not recommend horse chestnut for children (Blumenthal et al., 1998; ESCOP, 1999).

Drug Interactions

The Commission E and ESCOP list no known drug interactions (Blumenthal et al., 1998; ESCOP, 1999).

REFERENCES

Blumenthal M, Busse W, Hall T, Goldberg A, Grünwald J, Riggins C, Rister S, eds. (1998). *The Complete German Commission E Monographs: Therapeutic Guide to Herbal Medicines*. Trans. S Klein. Austin: American Botanical Council.

Calabrese C, Preston P (1993). Report of the results of a double-blind, randomized, single-dose trial of a topical 2 percent escin gel versus placebo in the acute treatment of experimentally induced hematoma in volunteers. *Planta Medica* 59 (5): 394-397.

Cloarec M (1993). Study on the effect of a new vasoprotective Venostasin administered over a period of 2 months in chronic venous insufficiency of the lower limbs. Controlled double blind study in randomized parallel groups versus placebo. Unpublished report.

Diehm C, Schmidt C (2000). Venostasin retard gegen Plazebo und Kompression bei Patienten mit CVI II/IIIA. Final Study Report. Klinge Pharma GmbH, Munich, Germany. (Reported in Ottillinger B, Greeske K [2001]. Rational therapy of chronic venous insufficiency—Changes and limits of the therapeutic use of horse-chestnut seeds extract. *BioMed Central Cardiovascular Disorders* I: 5, <http://www.biomedcentral.com/1471-2261/1/5>.)

Diehm C, Trampisch HJ, Lange S, Schmidt C (1996). Comparison of leg compression stocking and oral horse-chestnut seed extract therapy in patients with chronic venous insufficiency. *The Lancet* 347 (8997): 292-294.

Diehm C, Vollbrecht D, Amendt K, Comberg HU (1992). Medical edema protection—clinical benefit in patients with chronic deep vein incompetence. *VASA* 21 (2): 188-192.

Erdlen F (1989). Clinical efficacy of Venostasin retard demonstrated in a double-blind trial. *Die Medizinische Welt* 40: 994-996.

Erler M (1991). Horse chestnut extract therapy for peripheral vascular edema. *Die Medizinische Welt* 42: 593-596.

European Scientific Cooperative on Phytotherapy (ESCOP) (1999). Hippocastani semen: Horse-chestnut seed. In *Monographs on the Medicinal Uses of Plant Drugs* (Fascicle 6: p. 12). Exeter, UK: European Scientific Cooperative on Phytotherapy.

Greeske K, Pohlmann BK (1996). Horse chestnut extract—An effective therapeutic concept in the doctor's office: Conservative treatment of chronic venous insufficiency. *Fortschritte der Medizin* 114 (15): 196-200. (Reported in Pittler MH, Ernst E [1998]. Horse-chestnut seed extract for chronic venous insufficiency. *Archives of Dermatology* 134 [11]: 1356-1360.)

Kalbfleisch W, Pfalzgraf H (1989). Odemprotektiva: Aquipotente dosierung—Rosskastaniensamenextrakt und o-beata-hydroxyethylrutoside im Vergleich. *Therapiewoche* 39: 3703-3707.

Kreysel HW, Nissen HP, Enghofer E (1983). A possible role of lysosomal enzymes in the pathogenesis of varicosis and the reduction in their serum activity by Venostasin. *VASA* 12 (4): 377-382.

Lohr E, Garanin G, Jesau P, Fischer H (1986). Anti-oedema treatment in chronic venous insufficiency with tendency to oedema. *Münchener Medizinische Wochenschrift* 128 (34): 579-581.

Marshall M, Dormady JA (1987). Oedema of long distant flights. *Phlebology* 2: 123-124.

Ottillinger B, Greeske K (2001). Rational therapy of chronic venous insufficiency—Changes and limits of the therapeutic use of horse-chestnut seeds extract. *BioMed Central Cardiovascular Disorders* I: 5, <http://www.biomedcentral.com/1471-2261/1/5>.

Pauschinger K (1987). Clinico-experimental investigations of the effect of horse-chestnut extract on the transcapillary filtration and the intravasal volume in patients with chronic venous insufficiency. *Phlebology and*

Proctology 2: 57-61. (Published previously in Bisler H, Pfeifer R, Kluken N, Pauschinger P |1986]. *Deutsche Medizinische Wochenschrift* 111: 1321-1329.)

Pilz E (1990). Edema associated with venous illness. *Die Medizinische Welt* 41: 1143-1144.

Pittler MH, Ernst E (1998). Horse-chestnut seed extract for chronic venous insufficiency. *Archives of Dermatology* 134 (11): 1356-1360.

Pittler MH, Ernst E (2002). Horse chestnut seed extract for chronic venous insufficiency (Cochrane Review). In *The Cochrane Library* 2: 1-17. Oxford: Update Software.

Rehn D, Unkauf M, Klein P, Jost V, Lücker PW (1996). Comparative clinical efficacy and tolerability of oxerutins and horse chestnut extract in patients with chronic venous insufficiency. *Arzneimittel-Forschung/Drug Research* 46 (5): 483-487.

Rudofsky G, Neiss A, Otto K, Seibel K (1986). Demonstration of the antioedematous effect and the clinical efficacy of horse-chestnut extract in a double-blind study. *Phelebologie und Proktologie* 15: 47-54.

Schulz V, Hänsel R, Tyler VE (2001). *Rational Phytotherapy: A Physicians' Guide to Herbal Medicine,* Fourth Edition. Trans. TC Telgar. Berlin: Springer-Verlag.

Shah D, Bommer S, Degenring FH (1997). Aesculaforce in chronic venous insufficiency. *Schweizerische Zeitschrift für GanzheitsMedizin* 9 (2): 86-91.

Steiner M, Hillemanns HG (1986). Investigation of the oedema-protective action of a venous therapeutic agent. *Münchener Medizinische Wochenscrift* 31: 551-552.

DETAILS ON HORSE CHESTNUT PRODUCTS AND CLINICAL STUDIES

Product and clinical study information is grouped in the same order as in the Summary Table. A profile on an individual product is followed by details of the clinical studies associated with that product. In some instances a clinical study, or studies, supports several products that contain the same principal ingredient(s). In these instances, those products are grouped together.

Clinical studies that follow each product, or group of products, are grouped by therapeutic indication, in accordance with the order in the Summary Table.

Index to Horse Chestnut Products

Product Profile: Venastat™

Manufacturer	**Pharmaton S.A., Switzerland**
U.S. distributor	**Pharmaton Natural Health Products**
Botanical ingredient	**Horse chestnut seed extract**
Extract name	**HCE 50**
Quantity	300 mg
Processing	No information
Standardization	16% triterpene glycosides calculated as aescin
Formulation	Capsule, sustained release

Recommended dose: Adults: one capsule every 12 hours, or two a day, swallowed whole with water. Effectiveness is reached after four to six weeks of continuous use.

DSHEA structure/function: Helps maintain leg vein circulation. Helps protect against leg swelling. Clinically shown to be a safe and beneficial way to supplement your diet for optimal leg vein health.

Cautions: Consult a health care professional if you are taking a prescription medicine, are pregnant or nursing a baby. Discontinue use and see a physician if gastric irritation, nausea, or rapid heartbeat occurs. In case of accidental ingestion/overdose, seek the advice of a health care professional immediately.

Other ingredients: Dextrin, gelatin, copolyvidone, talc, polymethacrylic acid deratives, titanium dioxide, dibutyl phthalate, synthetic iron oxides.

Comments: Sold in Europe as Venostasin® retard (Klinge Pharma GmbH, Munich, Germany)

Source(s) of information: Product package (© Boehringer Ingelheim Pharmaceuticals, Inc., 1999).

Clinical Study: Venostasin® retard

Extract name	HCE 50
Manufacturer	Klinge Pharma GmbH, Germany
	(Pharmaton S.A., Switzerland)
Indication	**Chronic venous insufficiency**
Level of evidence	**II**
Therapeutic benefit	**Yes**

Bibliographic reference
Rudofsky G, Neiss A, Otto K, Seibel K (1986). Demonstration of the antioedematous effect and the clinical efficacy of horse-chestnut extract in a double-blind study. *Phelebologie und Proktologie* 15: 47-54.

Trial design
Parallel.

Study duration	1 month
Dose	1 (300 mg extract, 50 mg of triterpene glycosides) capsule twice daily
Route of administration	Oral
Randomized	Yes
Randomization adequate	No
Blinding	Double-blind
Blinding adequate	Yes
Placebo	Yes

Drug comparison	No
Site description	Not described
No. of subjects enrolled	40
No. of subjects completed	39
Sex	Male and female
Age	Mean: 39.4 ± 9.2 years

Inclusion criteria

Patients with chronic venous insufficiency, Grades I or II, with at least two of the clinical signs, such as varicosis, cutaneous induration, hyperpigmentation, atrophie blanche, and two subjective symptoms such as sense of heaviness, pain, pruritus, sense of fullness and congestion in the legs and cramps in calves. Medication with vasoactive substances, diuretics, and "other venous therapeutics" was stopped four weeks before the study began.

Exclusion criteria

Patients who are pregnant, immobilized, with acute thrombophlebitis, nephritic syndrome heart failure, associated edema, and high-grade CVI.

End points

Volumetric measurements of volume of foot and distal shank using a water plethysmograph and circumference of ankle and calf were taken in the morning and evening. Venous capacity, assessment of pretibial impression and assessment of subjective symptoms were taken at the start of the study and after 14 and 28 days of therapy.

Results

The volume of the foot and distal shank decreased in the morning and evening during four weeks of treatment with horse chestnut. In contrast, an increase in both volumes at both measuring times was observed with the placebo group. The differences are statistically significant ($p < 0.001$, both measurements, 28 days). Neither Venostasin nor placebo had any influence on the venous capacity. A test for tibial edema revealed a significantly better response to treatment with Venostasin retard after 14 days ($p = 0.023$) and 28 days ($p = 0.003$) compared with placebo. Significant differences were also observed between Venostasin and placebo groups in circumference of ankle ($p < 0.01$) and in circumference of the calf ($p < 0.05$) after 28 days. For all subjective symptoms included in the evaluation, Venostasin was statistically and significantly better than placebo ($p < 0.05$), with the exception of "cramps in the calves."

Side effects

None observed.

Authors' comments
Based on the results of the study it is concluded that horse chestnut extract can exert an antiedematous effect.

Reviewer's comments
The very complete list of outcome measures makes this study more interesting and convincing clinically. The data were only reported in graphs, not in table form, making numbers difficult to determine. Also, no standard deviations were included. This trial had a well-described blinding procedure although the randomization was not adequately described. (Translation reviewed) (2, 5)

Clinical Study: Venostasin® retard

Extract name	HCE 50
Manufacturer	Klinge Pharma GmbH, Germany (Pharmaton S.A., Switzerland)
Indication	**Chronic venous insufficiency**
Level of evidence	**II**
Therapeutic benefit	**Yes**

Bibliographic reference
Pilz E (1990). Edema associated with venous illness. *Die Medizinische Welt* 41: 1143-1144.

Trial design
Parallel. Pretrial washout period of one week.

Study duration	20 days
Dose	1 (300 mg extract, 50 mg of triterpene glycosides) capsule twice daily
Route of administration	Oral
Randomized	Yes
Randomization adequate	Yes
Blinding	Double-blind
Blinding adequate	Yes
Placebo	Yes
Drug comparison	No
Site description	Single center
No. of subjects enrolled	30

No. of subjects completed 28
Sex   Male and female
Age   27-60 years (mean: 46)

Inclusion criteria

Outpatients with symptoms of chronic venous insufficiency (CVI) associated with peripheral venous edema, and subjective symptoms including heaviness and/or exhaustion, feeling of tension, burning sensations, itching, calf cramps, restless legs, swelling of the legs and/or the feet, discoloration, tissue hardening, and eczema.

Exclusion criteria

Patients younger than 20 and older than 70; with fewer than two symptoms of CVI; with ulcus cruris, cardiac, hepatic, nephrotic, and lymphatic edema; leg pains other than that listed; nerve root irritation; and inflamed or degenerated joints. Patients for whom compression was indispensable were also excluded. The following medications were not allowed during the trial: cardiac glycosides, diuretics, nonsteroidal anti-inflammatories, or corticosteroids.

End points

The main clinical variables were leg circumference measurements (smallest distance between the ankle and thigh, distance from heel to small of back, and largest circumference of the thigh) which were measured at room temperature.

Results

The Venostasin group had larger decreases in leg circumference measurements than the placebo. In particular, a statistically significant reduction was observed in the distance from the heel to the small of the back in the Venostasin group compared with the placebo group ($p < 0.05$).

Side effects

None observed.

Author's comments

Even with a relatively small number of patients, 20 days therapy with Venostasin led to significant reductions in circumferences of edematous feet compared to placebo treatment.

Reviewer's comments

This trial had an excellent description of randomization and double-blinding. It did not receive a Level I rating due to the small sample size and the lack of a detailed explanation of the results (no standard deviations were provided). (Translation reviewed) (5, 5)

Clinical Study: Venostasin®

Extract name	HCE 50
Manufacturer	Klinge Pharma GmbH, Germany
	(Pharmaton S.A., Switzerland)

Indication	**Chronic venous insufficiency**
Level of evidence	**II**
Therapeutic benefit	**Yes**

Bibliographic reference
Cloarec M (1993). Study on the effect of a new vasoprotective Venostasin administered over a period of 2 months in chronic venous insufficiency of the lower limbs. Controlled double blind study in randomized parallel groups versus placebo. Unpublished report.

Trial design
Parallel. Pretrial washout period of one month, followed by a one-month period with placebo, followed by two months treatment with drug or placebo

Study duration	2 months
Dose	1 (300 mg extract, 50 mg of triterpene glycosides) capsule twice daily
Route of administration	Oral
Randomized	Yes
Randomization adequate	No
Blinding	Double-blind
Blinding adequate	Yes
Placebo	Yes
Drug comparison	No
Site description	One hospital
No. of subjects enrolled	30
No. of subjects completed	30
Sex	Male and female
Age	23-69 years (mean: 46)

Inclusion criteria
Patients ages 20 to 70 years, ambulatory, with functional symptoms due to chronic venous insufficiency and impression edema on at least one leg, with at least two of the following symptoms exceeding Degree 5 on the visual analog scale: pain, heaviness, paresthesia or formication, restlessness, or nocturnal cramps.

Exclusion criteria
Patients with systolic pressure ankle/arm > 0.9; supporting bandage; acute or precedent (<1 month) thrombophlebitis; leg ulcer of venous origin; cardiac, renal, hepatic, or orthopedic edema; underwent sclerotherapy or surgery of the veins during the past six months; pregnant or lactating; having irregular menstrual cycle; severe hepatic, renal, or cardiovascular diseases; participating in another study; unable or unwilling to follow study instructions; or taking analgesics, diuretics or anti-inflammatory steroids.

End points
Patients were examined before pretrial placebo, before beginning treatment, and after 30 and 60 days. Measurements were taken of the circumference of the lower limb (ankle/calf), and by plethysmography. Pain and functional symptoms were evaluated by visual analog scale. Global assessments were made by patients and physicians.

Results
After 30 and 60 days of treatment there was a significant decrease in the size of edema in the Venostasin group compared to the placebo group ($p < 0.001$). After 60 days of treatment, the leg and ankle circumference in the Venostasin group decreased significantly compared to the placebo group ($p = 0.03$). A significant decrease in intensity of pain was observed after 30 and 60 days of treatment compared to placebo ($p < 0.001$). Functional symptoms of heaviness, paresthesia ("pins and needles"), and/or formication ("ants"), as well as restlessness and/or nocturnal cramps all decreased after 30 and 60 days of treatment ($p < 0.001$, 60 days compared with the placebo group). Plethysmography results showed a significant difference from placebo after 30 days ($p = 0.03$) and 60 days ($p = 0.001$) of treatment. Global judgments by both patients and physicians were positive.

Side effects
No difference in tolerance from placebo.

Author's comments
This study demonstrated that Venostasin improves in a statistically significant way the clinical symptoms and the values of occlusion plethysmography in patients with chronic venous insufficiency over a period of two months compared to placebo.

Reviewer's comments
The one-month washout followed by two-month treatment was very good. Also, an intention-to-treat analysis is a more rigorous evaluation for efficacy that eliminates bias due to poorly performing patients that are removed from therapy. Giving more attention to the reporting method of randomization would have increased the quality of this study. A significantly larger sample

size would have allowed better assessment of efficacy. (Translation reviewed) (3, 5)

Clinical Study: Venostasin® retard

Extract name	HCE 50
Manufacturer	Klinge Pharma GmbH, Germany
	(Pharmaton S.A., Switzerland)
Indication	**Chronic venous insufficiency**
Level of evidence	**III**
Therapeutic benefit	**Yes**

Bibliographic reference
Lohr E, Garanin G, Jesau P, Fischer H (1986). Anti-oedema treatment in chronic venous insufficiency with tendency to oedema. *Münchener Medizinische Wochenschrift* 128 (34): 579-581.

Trial design
Parallel. Pretrial washout period of 12 days.

Study duration	2 months
Dose	1 (300 mg extract, 50 mg of triterpene glycosides) capsule twice daily
Route of administration	Oral
Randomized	Yes
Randomization adequate	No
Blinding	Double-blind
Blinding adequate	No
Placebo	Yes
Drug comparison	No
Site description	Not described
No. of subjects enrolled	80
No. of subjects completed	74
Sex	Male and female
Age	Mean: 53.8 ± 13.1 years

Inclusion criteria
Chronic venous insufficiency. No further details were included in the translation.

Exclusion criteria
Not included in the translation.

End points
Variables included leg volume measurement and three circumference measurements (fibula circumference, ankle circumference, and heel above the instep), in each case both before and after edema provocation, as well as an evaluation of the subjective symptoms. Edema was provoked by sitting on an exercise bicycle for 20 minutes with legs hanging loose and motionless. Patients were evaluated before and after the eight-week treatment period.

Results
The increase in leg volume observed under edema provocation fell in the Venostasin group during the eight-week treatment period from 32 ml to 28 ml on average, but increased in the placebo group from 27 ml to 31 ml on average. The leg circumference measurements confirmed the leg volume results. Edema was comparatively reduced both before ($p < 0.01$) and after provocation ($p < 0.001$) when measuring the heel above the instep. Subjective symptoms, such as "feeling of tension in the legs," "itching," and "degree of impression of edema," were altered significantly by Venostasin compared to placebo.

Side effects
No statistical difference from placebo.

Authors' comments
The horse chestnut seed extract treatment was proved statistically to be effective, and is tolerated just as well as placebo.

Reviewer's comments
Provoked edema is less clinically relevant than standard measurements; thus, the edema-reducing and edema-protecting effects are not very useful measurements. This trial was both randomized and double-blind, but the processes were not well described. The trial also lacked adequate inclusion/exclusion criteria, statistical methods, and a sufficient summary of the data (no standard deviations were provided). (Translation reviewed) (1, 3)

Clinical Study: Venostasin® retard

Extract name	HCE 50
Manufacturer	Klinge Pharma GmbH, Germany
	(Pharmaton S.A., Switzerland)

Indication	**Chronic venous insufficiency**
Level of evidence	**III**
Therapeutic benefit	**Yes**

Bibliographic reference
Steiner M, Hillemanns HG (1986). Investigation of the oedema-protective action of a venous therapeutic agent. *Münchener Medizinische Wochenscrift* 31: 551-552.

Trial design
Crossover study. Five-day washout phase followed by two treatment phases of 14 days duration.

Study duration	2 weeks
Dose	1 (300 mg extract, 50 mg aescin) capsule twice daily
Route of administration	Oral
Randomized	Yes
Randomization adequate	No
Blinding	Double-blind
Blinding adequate	No
Placebo	Yes
Drug comparison	No
Site description	Not described
No. of subjects enrolled	20
No. of subjects completed	Not given
Sex	Female
Age	20-40 years

Inclusion criteria
Ambulant patients with pregnancy-related varicosis, or varicosis with chronic venous insufficiency Grade I.

Exclusion criteria
Subjects in the last three months of pregnancy, and those with Grades II and III chronic venous insufficiency.

End points
The main clinical variable was leg volume measured with a water plethysmometer. In addition, leg circumference was measured at three places: smallest ankle circumference, circumference of the heel above the instep, and circumference above the middle of the calf. Measurements were taken

before the start of the first treatment phase and at the end of the first and second treatment phases.

Results

Water plethysmometric measurements showed that treatment with horse chestnut lead to a reduction in leg volume of 114 ml in phase I and a reduction of 126.2 ml at the end of the treatment phase II. The volume values did not change under placebo treatment in treatment phase I and increased by 128.6 ml at the end of phase II after prior horse chestnut treatment in phase I. The difference between the two treatments was statistically significant ($p = 0.0009$). Circumference measurements also showed a statistically significantly reduction for all three measurement under horse chestnut therapy (heel value: $p < 0.001$, ankle value: $p < 0.001$, and calf value: $p < 0.05$).

Side effects

No difference between the two groups.

Authors' comments

In the present case, Venostasin retard was shown to have an edema-protective and edema-curative effect. It is also well tolerated.

Reviewer's comments

Although this trial was randomized and double-blind, neither process was described adequately. The data was not summarized in sufficient detail to allow for replication, and the sample size was too small. In addition, mixing pregnant and nonpregnant patients may not produce equivalent pathophysiological results. (Translation reviewed) (0, 4)

Clinical Study: Venostasin® retard

Extract name	HCE 50
Manufacturer	Klinge Pharma GmbH, Germany (Pharmaton S.A., Switzerland)
Indication	**Chronic venous insufficiency**
Level of evidence	**II**
Therapeutic benefit	**Yes**

Bibliographic reference: Diehm C, Trampisch HJ, Lange S, Schmidt C (1996). Comparison of leg compression stocking and oral horse-chestnut seed extract therapy in patients with chronic venous insufficiency. *The Lancet* 347 (8997): 292-294.

Trial desi ɪn

Parallel. P etrial run-in phase with placebo for two weeks. Patients were then randomized to receive compression, horse chestnut extract, or placebo. Those allocated to receive compression received a diuretic once daily to ensure the best possible fit with a Class II compression stocking. The trial is considered partially blinded because those with stockings knew which treatment they were receiving.

Study duration	3 months
Dose	1 (50 mg aescin) capsule twice daily
Route of administration	Oral
Randomized	Yes
Randomization adequate	No
Blinding	Partial
Blinding adequate	No
Placebo	Yes
Drug comparison	Yes
Drug name	Leg compression stockings
Site description	Single center
No. of subjects enrolled	262
No. of subjects completed	240
Sex	Male and female
Age	Mean: 52 years

Inclusion criteria

Subjects ages 18 years or older with substantial lower leg edema due to chronic venous insufficiency (confirmed by medical history, clinical findings and venous Doppler and/or duplex sonography).

Exclusion criteria

Patients who had received venotherapeutic drugs within the past six weeks before the run-in phase.

End points

Water displacement plethysmometry was used to measure the lower leg volume of the more severely affected limb at baseline and after 4, 8, and 12 weeks of therapy.

Results

Lower leg volume of the more severely affected limb decreased on average by 43.8 ml with horse chestnut seed extract (HCSE) and 46.7 ml with compression therapy, whereas it increased by 9.8 ml with placebo for the intent-to-treat group. Significant edema reductions were achieved by HCSE (p =

0.005) and compression ($p = 0.002$) compared to placebo, and the two therapies were shown to be equivalent ($p = 0.001$).

Side effects
No serious treatment related events were reported.

Authors' comments
These results indicate that compression stocking therapy and Venostasin therapy are alternate therapies for the effective treatment of patients with edema resulting from chronic venous insufficiency.

Reviewer's comments
This trial was actually relatively well constructed and conducted. Its value is probably greater than its Jadad score (the study could not be double-blinded due to the use of compression stockings, and the randomization was not described adequately). The trial had a good sample size, and used and described appropriate statistical methods (intention-to-treat analysis). (1, 6)

Clinical Study: Venostasin® retard

Extract name	HCE 50
Manufacturer	Klinge Pharma GmbH, Germany (Pharmaton S.A., Switzerland)
Indication	**Chronic venous insufficiency**
Level of evidence	**II**
Therapeutic benefit	**No**

Bibliographic reference
Diehm C, Schmidt C (2000). Venostasin retard gegen Plazebo und Kompression bei Patienten mit CVI II/IIIA. Final Study Report. Klinge Pharma GmbH, Munich, Germany. (Reported in Ottillinger B, Greeske K [2001]. Rational therapy of chronic venous insufficiency—Changes and limits of the therapeutic use of horse-chestnut seeds extract. *BioMed Central Cardiovascular Disorders* I: 5, <http://www.biomedcentral.com/1471-2261/1/5>.)

Trial design
Parallel. The trial was preceded by a two-week washout period with placebo. Subjects were randomized to receive either horse chestnut, placebo, or compression therapy. The allocation of the horse chestnut and placebo was double-blind, but the compression therapy was open. There was also a two-week follow-up period after treatment was finished.

Study duration	4 months
Dose	50 mg aescin daily
Route of administration	Oral
Randomized	Yes
Randomization adequate	Yes
Blinding	Double-blind/open
Blinding adequate	No
Placebo	Yes
Drug comparison	No
Site description	Not described
No. of subjects enrolled	355
No. of subjects completed	Not given
Sex	Not given
Age	Not given

Inclusion criteria
Patients with chronic venous insufficiency Grade II and Grade IIIa.

Exclusion criteria
Patients were excluded if they had received therapy with vein drugs during the six weeks prior to the study start, and patients with edemas of non-venous origin.

End points
The primary end point was the reduction of lower leg volume at the end of the study compared to baseline. Lower leg volume was determined by plethysmometry at baseline and at weeks 4, 8, 12, and 16, and twice during the follow-up period. Secondary end points included a subjective symptom score (including the following symptoms: heaviness, distension, distension pain, feeling of swelling, tiredness in the leg, itching, leg cramps, paresthesia, plantar burning, and unspecific subjective complaints) and a rating of quality of life (determined using the Fragebogen zur Lebensqualität bei Venenerkrankungen [FLQA]).

Results
The compression treatment was significantly better than placebo ($p <$ 0.001), but horse chestnut was not. Mean reductions in leg volume for the compression, horse chestnut, and placebo groups were 89, 18, and 2 ml, respectively. The subjective symptom score evaluation rated horse chestnut better than compression therapy, but the difference was not statistically significant. Horse chestnut also showed more favorable results compared with compression therapy in the quality of life parameters. After a subgroup analysis, subjects with CVI Grade II were found to respond better to horse

chestnut than those with Grade IIIa. Compression, in contrast, was better for the higher CVI grade.

Side effects
The incidence of side effects was similar in all groups. The horse chestnut group experienced more gastrointestinal adverse effects, and constipation and dry mouth occurred only in this group (two and three cases, respectively).

Authors' comments
In the early stages of CVI, when the veins and their wall structures have not yet suffered any permanent damage, pharmacological methods (such as horse chestnut seed extract) may be sufficient to affect the disease process. Horse chestnut seed extract may still close the endothelial gaps in the later stages of CVI and thus reduce edema to some extent. At this time, however, the disease process has already caused irreversible damage in the larger veins.

Reviewer's comments
This trial had a good experimental design comparing horse chestnut to a placebo control and conventional therapy (stocking). (2, 6)

Clinical Study: Venostasin® retard

Extract name	HCE 50
Manufacturer	Klinge Pharma GmbH, Germany (Pharmaton S.A., Switzerland)
Indication	**Chronic venous insufficiency**
Level of evidence	**II**
Therapeutic benefit	**Trend**

Bibliographic reference
Erdlen F (1989). Clinical efficacy of Venostasin retard demonstrated in a double-blind trial. *Die Medizinische Welt* 40: 994-996.

Trial design
Parallel. Pretrial run-in period with placebo for one week. Translation does not give the name of the comparison agent.

Study duration	1 month
Dose	1 (300 mg extract, 50 mg of triperpene glycosides) capsule twice daily

Route of administration   Oral

Randomized   Yes
Randomization adequate   Yes
Blinding   Double-blind
Blinding adequate   Yes

Placebo   No
Drug comparison   Yes
Drug name   Another edema-protective agent

Site description   Single center

No. of subjects enrolled   30
No. of subjects completed   Not given
Sex   Male and female
Age   Mean: 54 ± 12 years

Inclusion criteria

Outpatients, over 18 years of age, suffering from varicosis and chronic venous insufficiency combined with peripheral venous edema.

Exclusion criteria

Patients suffering from cardiogenic or hepatogenic edemas, disturbances of renal function, or hepatic disease; patients receiving vasoactive medication or requiring compression treatment during study; patients with a history of allergic reactions to any of the constituents. In addition, primary lymphatic edema, ulcus cruris or administration of cardiac glycosides, methyl xanthine preparations or nonsteroidal antirheumatic agents were not allowed.

End points

At the beginning of the treatment period, as well as after two and four weeks of therapy, leg circumference was measured before and after edema provocation (standing for 15 minutes).

Results

In both the Venostasin group and comparison drug group, the ankle circumference decreased between the beginning and end of therapy by an average of 0.4 cm. The edema protective effect was 0.2 cm for Venostasin and –0.1 cm for the comparison group. The negative value suggests a greater increase in the leg circumference.

Side effects

Both preparations were well tolerated.

Author's comments
Venostasin retard is effective as another antiedematous and edema-protective agent, and is slightly superior to the comparison preparation.

Reviewer's comments
Edema provocation was standing for 15 minutes, a clinically relevant challenge. Venostasin had activity comparable to the comparison agent, which unfortunately was not identified in the translation (the Cochrain review by Pittler and Ernst [2002] identifies the agent as rutoside [*The Cochraine Library* 2: 1-17]). There was a problem with the randomization, since one of the groups had many more women than men. The trial lacked a description of withdrawals and dropouts, the sample size was small, and the statistical methods were not adequately described or applied. (Translation reviewed) (4, 4)

Clinical Study: Venostasin®

Extract name	HCE50
Manufacturer	Pharmaton S.A., Switzerland
Indication	**Chronic venous insufficiency**
Level of evidence	**III**
Therapeutic benefit	**Undetermined**

Bibliographic reference
Rehn D, Unkauf M, Klein P, Jost V, Lücker PW (1996). Comparative clinical efficacy and tolerability of oxerutins and horse chestnut extract in patients with chronic venous insufficiency. *Arzneimittel-Forschung/Drug Research* 46 (5): 483-487.

Trial design
Parallel. Pretrial placebo run-in of one week. Patients were given one of three treatments for 12 weeks: horse chestnut extract, oxerutins (1,000 mg/day), or oxerutins (1,000 mg/day loading dose for four weeks, followed by 500 mg/day maintenance dose). A six-week follow-up period followed the trial end.

Study duration	3 months
Dose	600 mg per day
Route of administration	Oral
Randomized	Yes
Randomization adequate	No
Blinding	Double-blind

Blinding adequate   No

Placebo   No
Drug comparison   No
Drug name   Oxerutins (Venoruton®)

Site description   12 centers

No. of subjects enrolled   155
No. of subjects completed   137
Sex   Female
Age   Mean: 60.1 ± 8.6 years

Inclusion criteria
Postmenopausal females with a maximum age of 70 years; uni- or bilateral chronic venous insufficiency (CVI) Grade II; corona phlebectatica paraplantaris, clinical persistent edema, low-grade skin alterations (e.g., hypo- or hyperpigmentation athrophie blanche, but without severe dermatosclerosis); have had a doppler sonography and a phlebological status in the past six months.

Exclusion criteria
Leg edema not due to venous diseases of the legs; older than 70 years; women with childbearing potential; decompensated cardiac insufficiency; current acute phlebitis or thrombosis; renal insufficiency; liver disease; and other relevant diseases, e.g., diabetes mellitus, etc. Pretreatment that could influence the results of the study, e.g., regular compression therapy within the last 4 weeks, treatment with other venous drugs for the last six weeks, use of laxatives with influence on fluid or electrolyte balance within the last eight days, treatment with theophylline, diuretics, cardiac glycosides angiotension converting enzyme inhibitors or calcium antagonists within the last eight days, and changes in the postmenopausal hormone replacement therapy within the last two months. These treatments, including compression therapy, were not allowed as concomitant therapy. Patients who participated in other clinical trials within 30 previous days were also excluded.

End points
The volume of the more affected leg was assessed by water displacement at baseline and at weeks 4, 8, and 12. At each visit, the volume was assessed twice. Subjective symptoms (tired, heavy legs, sensations of tension, and tingling sensation) were also evaluated at each visit using a 10 cm visual analogue scale.

Results
After 12 weeks of treatment, oxyrutins (1,000 mg/day) proved to be equivalent or better at reducing leg volume compared to oxerutin (1,000 then 500 mg/day) and horse chestnut. Mean leg volume was reduced by 57.9 ml, 40.2

ml, and 28.2 ml, respectively. In addition, 74.6 percent, 64.9 percent, and 57.6 percent of the respective groups were responders to therapy (had a leg volume reduction in week 12). The difference between the oxerutins (1,000 mg/day) and the horse chestnut group was statistically significant (p = 0.0238). Mean VAS values of tired, heavy legs were also reduced from baseline for all three treatments at the end of the treatment phase.

Side effects
Nine patients taking oxerutins and two patients taking horse chestnut reported adverse reactions. The reported symptoms were gastrointestinal complaints, headaches, and dizziness of transitory nature.

Authors' comments
In general, both tested drugs are able to achieve a mean leg volume reduction of about 100 ml after 12 weeks treatment in responding patients. This is a therapeutically relevant amount of edema reduction and comparable to values reported or calculated for compression therapy.

Reviewer's comments
The lack of placebo control and the use of an active control of unknown efficacy (i.e., not a standard drug or a "proven" herbal) made the interpretation of significance difficult. (1, 6)

Clinical Study: Venostasin® retard

Extract name	HCE 50
Manufacturer	Klinge Pharma GmbH, Germany (Pharmaton S.A., Switzerland)
Indication	**Chronic venous insufficiency; Edema** due to long-distance flights
Level of evidence	**III**
Therapeutic benefit	**Yes**

Bibliographic reference
Marshall M, Dormady JA (1987). Oedema of long distant flights. *Phlebology* 2: 123-124.

Trial design
Parallel. Medication was given ten days prior to a 14-hour flight and continued until landing in destination.

Study duration	11 days
Dose	1 (300 mg extract containing 50 mg of triterpene glycosides) capsule twice daily
Route of administration	Oral
Randomized	Yes
Randomization adequate	No
Blinding	Double-blind
Blinding adequate	No
Placebo	Yes
Drug comparison	No
Site description	Flight
No. of subjects enrolled	19
No. of subjects completed	19
Sex	Not given
Age	Not given

Inclusion criteria
Phlebologists undergoing a 14-hour flight from Europe to Kyoto, with no past history of venous disease or chronic leg edema.

Exclusion criteria
None mentioned.

End points
Max circumference of the foot around the heel and the smallest circumference around the ankle were measured half an hour after departure on aircraft as well as three hours and 14 hours later.

Results
A steady and significant increase in both the ankle and heel size measurements was observed in the subjects receiving placebo over the 14-hour flight. The swelling in the lower legs was approximately equivalent to 60 ml. Subjects receiving Venostasin ($p < 0.05$) had significantly less swelling in the heel and ankles after 14 hours. There was no significant difference after only three hours of flight.

Side effects
None mentioned.

Authors' comments
Swelling in the lower legs of normal subjects exposed to a 14-hour flight was

completely prevented by Venostasin at the level of the ankle and very much reduced at the level of the heel.

Reviewer's comments

The outcome measures were appropriate to the clinical condition. The sample size was too small, but it is otherwise a generally well-conducted trial. I am concerned that the authors did not report their subjective data. The interpretation of this trial was limited by the poor methodology, since neither the blinding nor the randomization were described adequately. The treatment length was good, but it might be unrealistic—most patients will not take therapy for ten days prior to their flight. (1, 5)

Clinical Study: Venostasin® retard

Extract name	HCE 50
Manufacturer	Klinge Pharma GmbH, Germany
	(Pharmaton S.A., Germany)
Indication	**Chronic venous insufficiency**
Level of evidence	**II**
Therapeutic benefit	**MOA**

Bibliographic reference

Pauschinger K (1987). Clinico-experimental investigations of the effect of horse-chestnut extract on the transcapillary filtration and the intravasal volume in patients with chronic venous insufficiency. *Phlebology and Proctology* 2: 57-61. (Previously published in Bisler H, Pfeifer R, Kluken N, Pauschinger P [1986]. *Deutsche Medizinische Wochenschrift* 111: 1321-1329.)

Trial design

Crossover. The two test days were separated by an interval of two weeks. All venous agents that were being taken were discontinued during the preliminary phase of the study.

Study duration	1 day
Dose	2 (300 mg) capsules
Route of administration	Oral
Randomized	Yes
Randomization adequate	No
Blinding	Double-blind
Blinding adequate	Yes

Placebo   Yes
Drug comparison   No

Site description   Not described

No. of subjects enrolled   24
No. of subjects completed   22
Sex   Female
Age   Not given

Inclusion criteria
Females suffering from Grades I to III suprafascial chronic venous insufficiency of the lower extremities according to Widmer.

Exclusion criteria
The presence of occlusive arterial disease.

End points
The development of edema was monitored through measuring the quantity of fluid flowing from blood capillaries into the surrounding tissue. The transcapillary filtration coefficient and the intravasal volume on the shank was determined four times: before patients took the treatment and three times after taking the treatment at 35-minute intervals.

Results
Compared with baseline, the capillary filtration coefficient (CFC) remained constant when patients were given placebo. When given horse chestnut, the CFC was reduced by 22 percent, which was significantly lower when compared to baseline ($p = 0.006$). The intravasal volume of patients given placebo and horse chestnut decreased compared to baseline, with no significant difference found between groups ($p = 0.24$).

Side effects
None mentioned.

Author's comments
The results of the study allow one to conclude that horse chestnut extract inhibits development of edema in chronic venous insufficiency of the lower extremities.

Reviewer's comments
This is a single-dose study with an intermediate outcome (capillary filtration rate) that is not as effective in showing benefit as a clinical outcome measure. The data were not described in sufficient detail since no standard deviations were given, and no test of the effect of treatment order was conducted. The sample size was small and the randomization process was not adequately described. (Translation reviewed) (3, 4)

Clinical Study: Venostasin® retard

Extract name	HCE 50
Manufacturer	Klinge Pharma GmbH, Germany
	(Pharmaton S.A., Switzerland)
Indication	**Chronic venous insufficiency; varicosis**
	(varicose veins)
Level of evidence	**III**
Therapeutic benefit	**MOA**

Bibliographic reference
Kreysel HW, Nissen HP, Enghofer E (1983). A possible role of lysosomal enzymes in the pathogenesis of varicosis and the reduction in their serum activity by venostasin. *VASA* 12 (4): 377-382.

Trial design
Crossover. Study in four phases: pretrial run-in period of three days without any medication, followed by three days of placebo treatment, 12 days of active therapy following, and then another three days of placebo.

Study duration	12 days
Dose	1 (300 mg extract containing 50 mg of triperpene glycosides) capsule 3 times daily
Route of administration	Oral
Randomized	No
Randomization adequate	No
Blinding	Double-blind
Blinding adequate	No
Placebo	Yes
Drug comparison	No
Site description	Hospital
No. of subjects enrolled	15
No. of subjects completed	Not given
Sex	Male and female
Age	Mean: 40 years

Inclusion criteria
Patients with varicosis of the internal saphenous vein, Stages II and III, who were in hospital due to dermatological disorders.

Exclusion criteria
Patients with atherosclerosis, diabetes involving vascular complications, or hepatitis.

End points
Blood was drawn three days after entry, then on days 1 and 3 (first placebo phase), 5, 10, 15 (interval of active treatment), and again on day 18 (end of second placebo phase) for enzyme assays such as β-glucuronidase, β-N-acetylglucosaminidase and arylsulphatase.

Results
Treatment of varicose patients with an extract of horse chestnut for 12 days led to a significant reduction in the activities of three glycosaminoglycan hydrolases. At the end of treatment, serum activities were lowered by 29.1 percent ($p < 0.01$) for β-N-acetylglucosaminidase, 25.7 percent ($p < 0.01$) for β-glucuronidase, and 28.7 percent ($p < 0.01$) for arysulphatase. A further three days of control treatment caused only a slight and insignificant rise in the enzymes' activities, thus hinting at an effect that outlasts drug ingestion.

Side effects
None mentioned.

Authors' comments
Since the reductions in all three glycosaminoglycan hydrolases were of the same order of magnitude, Venostasin may act through a protective effect on the site of enzymatic release: the lysosomal membrane. The reduction in enzyme activity might be of clinical importance in reducing proteoglycan breakdown, and hence affecting capillary permeability and fragility. Long-term therapy with Venostasin could have an influence on the collagen content and architecture of the varicose vein, thus normalizing its elastic and contractile properties.

Reviewer's comments
It is not clear that the enzyme assays used as end points in this study are clinically relevant as they are not directly connected with the end points of the disease process. In addition, the trial was not randomized, and the blinding process was not described adequately. (0, 5)

Product Profile: Venaforce™

Manufacturer	**Bioforce AG, Switzerland**
U.S. distributor	**Bioforce USA**
Botanical ingredient	**Horse chestnut seed extract**

Extract name	None given
Quantity	76.5 mg
Processing	Plant to extract ratio 5.0-6.1:1, 60% (m/m) ethanol
Standardization	20 mg aescin
Formulation	Tablet (enteric coated)

Recommended dose: Adults take three tablets in morning, two tablets in evening, with meals, for the first week; thereafter, take two tablets in morning, one in evening.

DSHEA structure/function: Promotes integrity of veins, healthy circulation, stamina of legs.

Other ingredients: Microcrystalline cellulose, potato starch, silicea, polysaccharide of soy, methacrylic copolymer, colloidal silicon dioxide, triethyl citrate.

Comments: Sold as Aesculaforce in Europe.

Source(s) of information: Product package; information provided by distributor; Shah, Bommer, and Degenring, 1997.

Clinical Study: Aesculaforce

Extract name	None given
Manufacturer	Bioforce AG, Switzerland
Indication	**Chronic venous insufficiency**
Level of evidence	**II**
Therapeutic benefit	**Yes**

Bibliographic reference
Shah D, Bommer S, Degenring FH (1997). Aesculaforce in chronic venous insufficiency. *Schweizerische Zeitschrift für GanzheitsMedizin* 9 (2): 86-91.

Trial design
Parallel.

Study duration	6 weeks
Dose	2 tablets (63-90 mg extract containing 20 mg aescin) 3 times daily
Route of administration	Oral
Randomized	Yes

Randomization adequate	No
Blinding	Double-blind
Blinding adequate	Yes
Placebo	Yes
Drug comparison	No
Site description	3 centers
No. of subjects enrolled	60
No. of subjects completed	52
Sex	Male and female
Age	Mean: 55 ± 12 years

Inclusion criteria
Subjects with a minimum age of 18 years, Widmer Stages I or II chronic venous insufficiency, with an admission summed score (edema, skin pigmentation, and eczema) and a symptoms summed score (sensation of heaviness or tension, pain, burning sensation, itching, and paresthesias affecting the legs) of at least 6.

Exclusion criteria
None mentioned.

End points
Patients were examined upon admission and after two and six weeks of treatment. The primary target parameter was the circumference of the leg measured just above the ankle. The second parameter was the summed score of subjective symptoms in the legs (sensation of heaviness or tension, pain, burning, itching, and paresthesias [pins and needles] affecting the legs). Plethysmography was also used to determine the venous refilling rate, caused by patients dangling legs after elevation at a 45 degree angle to empty them of blood.

Results
A statistically significant difference was observed in terms of the time course of the reduction in ankle edema ($p < 0.05$) that favored the test substance over the placebo. With respect to improvement in the subjective symptoms, only a small, statistically nonsignificant difference favoring the test substance was found. Photoplethysmographic measurement of the calf refilling favored the Aesculaforce tablets compared to placebo ($p = 0.0308$).

Side effects
Gastric complaints in one patient given test substance and two patients given placebo.

Authors' comments
The effectiveness of Aesculaforce was confirmed by the reduction or elimination of ankle edema and increase in venous capacity.

Reviewer's comments
The outcome measures were clear, and the sample size was appropriate. However, the data did not include standard deviations. The randomization was not adequately described. (3, 5)

Product Profile: Horse Chestnut (Generic)

Manufacturer	None
U.S. distributor	None
Botanical ingredient	**Horse chestnut seed extract**
Extract name	None given
Quantity	No information
Processing	Plant to extract ratio 5:1
Standardization	No information

Source(s) of information: Diehm et al., 1992.

Clinical Study: Horse Chestnut (Generic)

Extract name	Not given
Manufacturer	None
Indication	**Chronic venous insufficiency**
Level of evidence	**II**
Therapeutic benefit	**Yes**

Bibliographic reference
Diehm C, Vollbrecht D, Amendt K, Comberg HU (1992). Medical edema protection—clinical benefit in patients with chronic deep vein incompetence. *VASA* 21 (2): 188-192.

Trial design
Parallel. Pretrial period of one week with placebo.

Study duration	6 weeks
Dose	Approximately 780 mg dry extract containing 150 mg aescin daily

Route of administration	Oral
Randomized	Yes
Randomization adequate	Yes
Blinding	Double-blind
Blinding adequate	Yes
Placebo	Yes
Drug comparison	No
Site description	Single center
No. of subjects enrolled	40
No. of subjects completed	39
Sex	Male and female
Age	Mean: 51 ± 11 years

Inclusion criteria

Patients between ages 25 and 65 who were not liable to compression with chronic venous insufficiency of Stage 2 according to Hach, and venous flow impairment, obstructive edema, possible trophic skin changes, and venous capacity and/or venous return outside normal limits (venous capacity 3 to 6 ml per 100 ml tissue, venous return 27 ml/100 ml per minute).

Exclusion criteria

Patients younger than 25 or older than 65, primary venous insufficiency liable to compression, acute venous inflammation and/or acute thrombosis, venous ulcerations, edema due to cardiac insufficiency, renal functional disturbances or hepatic disorders, primary lymphatic edema, reflux in the region of the thigh, Hach Stage 3, diabetes for more than ten years, neuropathies, concurrent treatment with other venous agents/venous diuretics, cardiac glycosides, nonsteroidal antirheumatic agents, intolerance to horse chestnut seed extract, and pregnancy.

End points

Subjective symptoms such as feeling of heaviness/tenseness (both during day and night), leg fatigue, itching, and paresthesias, and the circumference of calves and ankles before and after edema provocation were measured at the end of the run-in phase and after each week during therapy. Leg volume (by hydroplethysmography before and after edema provocation) and venous occlusion (by plethysmography) were measured after two, four, and six weeks of therapy. Venous Doppler sonograms and phlebodynamometric measurements were taken at the beginning and end of treatment.

Results

After six weeks of therapy the mean leg volume in the horse chestnut group was statistically less than that of the placebo group ($p < 0.01$). The results were similar after edema provocation ($p < 0.01$). Additional measurements of leg circumference confirmed the results from hydroplethysmography (leg volume). Horse chestnut seed extract was also markedly more effective in alleviating subjective complaints than placebo.

Side effects
Both extract and placebo were well tolerated.

Authors' comments
Treatment with an edema protective agent of the horse chestnut type is a useful adjunct to compression therapy.

Reviewer's comments
This was a well-conducted trial, but the randomization and blinding could have been better explained. The sample size was appropriate, the inclusion/exclusion criteria were adequate, and the statistical methods were applied and described well. (5, 6)

Product Profile: Escin gel

Manufacturer	**Madaus AG, Germany**
U.S. distributor	None
Botanical ingredient	**Horse chestnut seed extract**
Extract name	None given
Quantity	No information
Processing	Extract incorporated into gel
Standardization	2% aescin
Formulation	Gel

Other ingredients: Lavender oil, orange flower oil, polyacrilic acid (Carbopol 940), polyethelyne glycol-6 caprylic/capric acid glycerides (Softigen 767), edetic acid disodium salt, trometamol, 2-propanol, water.

Source(s) of information: Calabrese and Preston, 1993; information provided by manufacturer.

Clinical Study: Escin gel

Extract name	Not given
Manufacturer	Madaus AG, Germany

Indication   **Hematoma** (induced)
Level of evidence **II**
Therapeutic benefit **Undetermined**

Bibliographic reference
Calabrese C, Preston P (1993). Report of the results of a double-blind, randomized, single-dose trial of a topical 2% escin gel versus placebo in the acute treatment of experimentally induced hematoma in volunteers. *Planta Medica* 59 (5): 394-397.

Trial design
Parallel. Experimental hematoma was induced by the subcutaneous injection of 2 ml of the subject's own blood.

Study duration	1 day
Dose	10 g gel (2% aescin)
Route of administration	Topical
Randomized	Yes
Randomization adequate	No
Blinding	Double-blind
Blinding adequate	Yes
Placebo	Yes
Drug comparison	No
Site description	Not described
No. of subjects enrolled	71
No. of subjects completed	70
Sex	Male and female
Age	21-47 years

Inclusion criteria
Healthy and normal weight patients between the ages of 18 and 50.

Exclusion criteria
Patients who were pregnant, with coagulation disorders, with allergy to aescin or allergic diathesis, or having significant current skin disorders. Use of nonsteroidal anti-inflammatory drugs, analgesics, or psychotropic agents in the week before the trial, and consumption of alcohol in the 24 hours before trial, were also excluded.

End points
Tonometric sensitivity measurements were taken at 1, 2.5, 4, 5.5, 7, and 9 hours after treatment.

Results
After hematoma induction and treatment, the aescin group responded with the first report of pain at higher mean adjusted tonometric pressure measurements (i.e., less tenderness) than did the placebo group at every time point ($p < 0.001$). The group treated with aescin had a significantly higher mean area under the curve (AUC) than placebo ($p < 0.001$), indicating less pain and a smaller difference from baseline.

Side effects
None mentioned.

Authors' comments
The results indicate efficacy of the 2 percent aescin gel in reducing tenderness in the injection hematoma model.

Reviewer's comments
This trial is technically well- and fairly rigorously done, but the underlying method is flawed: injected blood is not equal to a bruise or a hematoma acquired through trauma. It is not clear that this model is effective for the clinical parameter being tested. In addition, the randomization process was not described adequately. (3, 4)

Kava

Other Common Names: **Kava kava, kava peper, awa, yangona**
Latin Name: *Piper methysticum* **G. Forst.** [Piperaceae]
Plant Part: **Root**

PREPARATIONS USED IN REVIEWED CLINICAL STUDIES

A water extract of ground kava root (actually a rhizome or underground stem) has been used traditionally in the Pacific islands in religious ceremonies and at social events. Modern commercial preparations are usually made by extraction with ethanol or acetone. Pharmacological studies have profiled the constituent kavapyrones, also known as kavalactones, which are thought to be responsible for the anxiety-relieving effect of kava (Schulz, Hänsel, and Tyler, 2001).

Laitan®, produced by Dr. Willmar Schwabe GmbH & Co., Karlsruhe, Germany, contains an extract (WS 1490) prepared with acetone and standardized to 70 percent kavalactones.

Two studies used aqueous extracts prepared by soaking either 30 g root in 500 ml water or 200 g root in 1,000 ml water.

Kavatrol™, produced by Natrol, Inc., is sold in capsules containing 200 mg root extract including 60 mg kavalactones (30 percent) and 50 mg dried plant material each of hops (*Humulus lupulus* L.) flowers, passionflower (*Passiflora incarnata* L.) aerial parts (aboveground parts), schizandra [*Schisandra chinensis* (Turcz.) Baill.] fruits, and chamomile (*Matricaria recutita* L.) flowers.

SUMMARY OF REVIEWED CLINICAL STUDIES

Kava is used traditionally to make a ceremonial beverage. It has been tested clinically most often for its use to treat anxiety. Anxiety is

KAVA SUMMARY TABLE

Product Name	Manufacturer/ U.S. Distributor	Product Characteristics	Dose in Trials	Indication	No. of Trials	Benefit (Evidence Level-Trial No.)
Single Ingredient Products						
Laitan® (EU)	Dr. Willmar Schwabe GmbH & Co., Germany/ None	Acetone extract containing 70% kavalactones (WS 1490)	100 mg 3 times daily	Anxiety	5	Yes (I-3, II-1, III-1)
				Sleep quality	1	Undetermined (III-1)
				Cognitive functioning	1	Undetermined (II-1)
Generic	None/None	Aqueous extract	30-100 g root	Cognitive functioning	2	Undetermined (III-2)
Combination Product						
Kavatrol™	Natrol, Inc./ Natrol, Inc.	Extract containing 30% kavalactones; dried hops flowers, passionflower aerial parts, schizandra fruits, and chamomile flowers	2 (200 mg) 2 times daily	Anxiety	1	Trend (II-1)

a vague, unpleasant emotional state with qualities of apprehension, dread, stress, and uneasiness. The presence and severity of characteristic anxiety symptoms are often measured using the Hamilton Anxiety Rating Scale (HAM-A), a standard and well-established clinician rated scale with 14 items. The total item score is the "gold-standard" measure used to establish and compare the efficacy of new treatments for general anxiety disorder. Benzodiazepines are commonly used to treat anxiety, but are associated with adverse effects such as dependence, sedation, and memory impairment (Hardman et al., 1996).

Ten controlled trials on the use of kava were reviewed. Six studies were conducted on anxiety. Five of these studies, which used the product Laitan, were well-designed studies that reported significant effects. The sixth study, which used the product Kavatrol, showed a trend toward efficacy. The other four studies on cognitive functioning and sleep were poorly designed, and although kava had no obvious effect on cognitive performance, any definite conclusion would be premature.

Laitan (WS 1490)

Seven trials with Laitan are reviewed here, the majority (five) being for relief from anxiety. One study explored the effect on sleep, and another showed that kava, unlike oxazepam, did not slow reaction times. The usual dose was 100 mg extract (WS 1490) three times daily, or a total of 210 mg kavalactones per day.

Anxiety

A well-conducted, placebo-controlled trial included 52 adults with a HAM-A anxiety score greater than 18 who were given 100 mg extract three times daily or placebo for one month. A significant reduction in anxiety scores was observed in the treatment group compared to the placebo group after one week, and this difference increased over four weeks. The average HAM-A score in the kava group dropped from 25.6 at baseline to 12.6 at the end of the month. The score remained practically unchanged in the placebo group (24.5 to 21.0) (Lehmann, Kinzler, and Friedemann, 1996).

Another study with 73 adults with anxiety as defined by DSM-III-R and a HAM-A score of at least 19 compared the effects of 300 mg extract per day to placebo in a 25-week treatment period. A significant improvement was observed in the treatment group compared with the placebo group after eight weeks, with the improvement increasing over time. The baseline HAM-A total score in the kava group of 30.7 dropped to 9.7 by the end of the study. The placebo group scores also fell, but to a lesser extent, from 31.4 to 15.2 (Volz and Kieser, 1997). The quality of this study was reduced by the lack of detail in descriptions of both the randomization and blinding processes.

A good-quality, placebo-controlled study was conducted with 40 peri- and postmenopausal women with a HAM-A score of at least 18. Treatment was 300 mg extract per day for two months. There was a significant reduction in anxiety compared with placebo after one week that increased after four and eight weeks. In the kava group, the baseline HAM-A score of 31.1 was reduced to 5.5 after eight weeks. The placebo group score dropped from 30.2 to 22.5 after eight weeks (Warnecke, 1991).

A study investigated the efficacy of WS 1490 in patients treated previously with benzodiazepines for at least two weeks, with the purpose of assessing the potential of the extract to replace benzodiazepines in the treatment of anxiety. The placebo-controlled study included 37 subjects with anxiety according to DSM-III-R and a maximum HAM-A rating of 14 points. During the first two weeks of the trial, the benzodiazepines were tapered off and the dose of kava was increased. For the next three weeks patients received only kava, 300 mg extract per day, or placebo. At the end of five weeks, the kava group had a decrease in HAM-A scores of 7.5 points compared with a one point increase for placebo group. The kava group also had fewer benzodiazepine withdrawal symptoms (Malsch and Kieser, 2001).

A good-quality drug comparison trial with 164 participants with a HAM-A score of more than 18 compared the effects of Laitan (300 mg per day) with oxazepam (5 mg three times daily) and bromazepam (3 mg three times daily). The study reported that all three treatment groups showed a continuous reduction of anxiety from the first through the sixth week, with no significant difference between them (Woelk et al., 1993).

Sleep Quality

A small pilot study with 12 healthy subjects explored the effect of either 150 mg or 300 mg WS 1490, compared with placebo baselines, on sleep polysomnographic electroencephalograph (EEG) patterns. With both doses, the amount of sleep spindles (an EEG pattern) and the percentage of deep sleep increased, whereas REM sleep did not change. The time to fall asleep and the waking stage tended to decrease. There was a suggestion that the higher dose of kava produced more effects on sleep than the lower dose (Emser and Bartylla, 1991). The increase in sleep-spindle density is a typical effect of an anxiolytic. However kava did not cause a suppression of deep sleep and REM sleep, which is a typical effect of benzodiazepine and barbiturate sleep medications. However, poor study design and minimal details in the report led the reviewers to rate this study as having undetermined benefit.

Cognitive Functioning

A crossover-design pilot study with 12 healthy young men explored the effects of kava extract WS 1490 on memory performance as measured with a continuous word recognition task. The continuum of processes between stimulus and response was measured by recording event-related brain potentials (ERPs), scalp-recorded electrical potentials generated by neural activity associated with specific sensory, cognitive, and motor processes. A relatively high dose of kava, 200 mg three times daily for five days, was compared with placebo and oxazepam (15 mg the day before testing and 75 mg on the morning of testing). A significant slowing of reaction time and reduction in the number of correct responses were seen following administration of oxazepam. In contrast, a statistically insignificant trend toward improvement was observed following administration of kava compared to placebo. The results of the ERPs showed a similar pattern (Munte et al., 1993). Due to the use of relatively nonstandard techniques and lack of an a priori hypothesis, our reviewers, Drs. Lynn Shinto and Barry Oken, deemed the therapeutic benefit from kava as inconclusive.

Generic Extract

Cognitive Functioning

The effects of kava on cognitive function were tested in two poor-quality trials that used aqueous extracts of the root. The first study compared the effects of two different doses of kava to controls who consumed no kava in open-label experiments on 27 healthy college students. The lower dose was an aqueous extract prepared from 30 g root, and the second dose varied with the weight of the subject (1 g per kg body weight, or 70 g for a 150 lb person). After a single administration, neither kava dose altered the speed of activation of verbal information in long-term memory or alertness (Russell, Bakker, and Singh, 1987). The second study used a slightly higher dose of kava, equivalent to 100 g root. In this placebo-controlled study with 24 subjects, one dose of kava produced feelings of intoxication, body sway, and a trend toward reduced cognitive performance (Prescott et al., 1993).

Kavatrol

Anxiety

A kava product that also contains small amounts of four other botanicals, Kavatrol, was tested for its effect on anxiety in 60 subjects. A dose of two (200 mg) capsules were given twice daily, the equivalent of 800 mg extract per day, or 240 mg kavalactones. Subjects evaluated their own degree of stress in a Daily Stress Inventory and a State-Trait Anxiety Inventory. According to the authors, the study indicated that kava reduced the stress associated with the daily hassles of life (Singh et al., 1998). However, our reviewers deemed the study to be flawed due to a lack of description of the type of anxiety, coupled with the fact that no assessment of the anxiety state was made by a physician.

SYSTEMATIC REVIEWS

Pittler and Ernst (2000) conducted a systematic review of seven double-blind, randomized, placebo-controlled trials of oral kava extract for the treatment of anxiety. The superiority of kava extract (mostly WS 1490) over placebo was suggested by all seven trials. A meta-analysis of three of the trials suggests a significant difference in the reduction of the total score on the Hamilton Rating Scale for anxiety by approximately ten points in favor of kava. The studies lasted from 4 to 24 weeks, and the kava extract treatments ranged in kava-lactone content from 60 to 240 mg per day.

ADVERSE REACTIONS OR SIDE EFFECTS

Recently, kava products have been taken off the market in several countries due to concerns over possible liver toxicity. However, in the reviewed clinical studies, side effects reported for kava preparations were similar to those reported for placebos. Four of the reviewed studies (three with WS 1490 and one on a generic product) listed side effects that included gastric pressure, tiredness, and nausea (Volz and Kieser, 1997; Warnecke, 1991; Woelk et al., 1993; Prescott et al., 1993). Two postmarketing surveillance studies were undertaken, each involving more than 3,000 patients. The first study, in which patients were given a daily dose equivalent to 120 to 240 mg kavapyrones, reported adverse events in 2.3 percent of patients. The second study, in which patients were given a daily dose equivalent to 105 mg kavapyrones reported adverse events in 1.5 percent of patients. The adverse events reported most frequently were gastrointestinal complaints, allergic skin reactions, headache, and photosensitivity (Pittler and Ernst, 2000).

A systematic survey of the physical health of a case-controlled population study of Aborigines in Australia reported that heavy use of kava, more than 310 g root per week, caused (directly or indirectly) malnutrition, weight loss, liver and kidney dysfunction, a skin rash, red eyes, and shortness of breath. Very heavy use, more than 440 g root per week, was associated with increased plasma levels of gamma-glutamyl transferase, an indication of liver dysfunction (Mathews et al., 1988). Chronic heavy traditional use is reported to cause a particular scaly skin eruption (ichthyosiform eruption), which is reversible with discontinued use (Norton and Ruze, 1994). A study concluded that the dermopathy was not caused by niacin deficiency after heavy kava users were randomized to receive either 100 mg oral nicotinamide or placebo daily for three weeks (Ruze, 1990).

Kava may interact with alcohol, creating greater cognitive impairment than the alcohol alone, although the type of kava preparation may be important in this interaction. Forty men and women participated in a randomized, placebo-controlled, comparative study wherein participants received placebo, kava (1 g powdered root per kg body weight), alcohol (0.75 g per kg body weight), or kava plus alcohol. A battery of tests given 30, 60, and 90 minutes after consuming the beverage revealed that kava alone had no effect on subjective measures of sedation, cognition, coordination, intoxication, and willingness to drive. In contrast, subjects receiving alcohol, with blood levels beyond 0.05 percent, had marked changes in all measures. The combination of kava plus alcohol produced a significantly larger decrement in an attention performance test than alcohol alone (Foo and Lemon, 1997). In contrast, a similar study with 20 subjects that used kava extract WS 1490 (300 mg per day for eight days) and similar blood alcohol levels found no negative multiplicative effects in a battery of performance tests (Herberg, 1993).

Recently, a number of case reports of severe liver damage have been reported subsequent to taking kava preparations. In the majority of cases, various underlying diseases were present, or additional medication was being taken that is known to have hepatotoxic effects. It may be that this toxicity is idiosyncratic and not predictable. In any case, it needs to be further investigated (Loew, 2002). A study comparing the relative incidence of hepatoxicity of kava preparations with that of other anxiolytics (bromazepam, diazepam, oxazepam) found a comparable rate of toxicity (Schulze, Meng, and Siegers, 2001). However, several European governmental bodies have concluded that kava has a negative risk/benefit ratio based upon the available data on hepatotoxicity and the lack of data supporting efficacy. Following this conclusion, kava sales have been restricted in Germany, Switzerland, Canada, Australia, and France (Centers for Disease Control, 2003). The U.S. Food and Drug Administration Center for Food Safety and Applied Nutrition (FDA CFSAN) issued a warning in March 2002, citing that "although liver damage appears to be rare, FDA believes consumers should be informed of this potential risk" and that "persons who have liver disease or liver problems, or persons who are taking drug products that can affect the liver, should consult a physician before using kava-containing supplements" (FDA CFSAN, 2002).

INFORMATION FROM PHARMACOPOEIAL MONOGRAPHS

Source of Published Therapeutic Monographs

German Commission E

Indications

The dried rhizome (underground stem) is approved by the German Commission E for conditions of nervous anxiety, stress, and restlessness (Blumenthal et al., 1998).

Doses

Root and preparations equivalent to 60 to120 mg kavalactones per day (Blumenthal et al., 1998).

Treatment Period

The Commission E suggests that treatment not last more than three months without medical advice (Blumenthal et al., 1998).

Contraindications

The Commission E lists the following contraindications: pregnancy, nursing, and endogenous depression (Blumenthal et al., 1998).

Adverse Reactions

According to the Commission E, extended continuous intake can cause a temporary yellow discoloration of skin, hair, and nails. In this case, further application of this drug must be discontinued. In rare cases, allergic skin reactions can occur. Also, accommodative disturbances, such as enlargement of the pupils and problems with oculo-motor equilibrium, have been described (Blumenthal et al., 1998).

Precautions

The Commission E warns that even when administered within its prescribed dosages, this herb may adversely affect motor reflexes and judgment necessary for driving and/or operating heavy machinery (Blumenthal et al., 1998).

Drug Interactions

The Commission E states that potentiation of effectiveness is possible for substances acting on the central nervous system, such as alcohol, barbiturates, and psychopharmacological agents (Blumenthal et al., 1998).

REFERENCES

Blumenthal M, Busse W, Hall T, Goldberg A, Grünwald J, Riggins C, Rister S, eds. (1998). *The Complete German Commission E Monographs: Therapeutic Guide to Herbal Medicines.* Trans. S Klein. Austin: American Botanical Council.

Centers for Disease Control and Prevention (2003). Hepatic toxicity possibly associated with kava-containing products—United States, Germany, and Switzerland 1999-2002. *Journal of the American Medical Association* 289 (1): 36-37.

Emser W, Bartylla K (1991). Improvement in quality of sleep: Effect of kava extract WS 1490 on the sleep patterns in healthy people. *TW Neurologie Psychiatrie* 5: 636-642.

Foo H, Lemon J (1997). Acute effects of kava, alone or in combination with alcohol, in subjective measures of impairment and intoxication and on cognitive performance. *Drug and Alcohol Review* 16: 147-155.

Food and Drug Administration Center for Food Safety and Applied Nutrition (FDA CFSAN) (2002). *Consumer Advisory: Kava-Containing Dietary Supplements May Be Associated with Severe Liver Injury.* Rockville, MD: U.S. Department of Health and Human Services, Food and Drug Administration. Available at <http://www.cfsan.fda.gov/~dms/addskava.html>.

Hardman JG, Limbird LE, Molinoff PB, Ruddon RW, Goodman-Gillman A (1996). *Goodman and Gillman's The Pharmacological Basis of Therapeutics*, Ninth Edition. New York: McGraw-Hill.

Herberg KW (1993). The influence of kava special extract WS 1490 on safety-relevant performance alone and in combination with ethyl-alcohol. *Blutalkohol* 30 (2): 96-105.

Lehmann E, Kinzler E, Friedemann J (1996). Efficacy of a special kava extract *(Piper methysticum)* in patients with states of anxiety, tension and excitedness of non-mental origin—A double-blind placebo-controlled study of four weeks. *Phytomedicine* 3 (2): 113-119. (Also published in Kinzler E, Kromer J, Lehmann E [1991]. *Arzneimittel-Forschung/Drug Research* 41 [1]: 584-588.)

Loew D (2002). Kava kava extract: Risks, benefits, or a problem of society? *Deutsche Apotheker Zeitung* 9: 64-74.

Malsch U, Kieser M (2001). Efficacy of kava-kava in the treatment of non-psychotic anxiety, following pretreatment with benzodiazepines. *Psychopharmacology* 157 (3): 277-283.

Mathews JD, Riley MD, Fejo L, Munoz E, Milns NR, Gardner ID, Powers JR, Ganygulpa E, Gununuwawuy BJ (1988). Effects of the heavy usage of kava on physical health: Summary of a pilot survey in an aboriginal community. *The Medical Journal of Australia* 148 (11): 548-555.

Munte TF, Heinze HJ, Matzke M, Steitz J (1993). Effects of oxazepam and an extract of kava roots *(Piper methysticum)* on event-related potentials in a word recognition task. *Neuropsychobiology* 27 (1): 46-53. (Also published in Heinze HJ, Munthe TF, Steitz J, Matzke M [1994]. *Pharmacopsychiatry* 27 [6]: 224-230.)

Norton SA, Ruze P (1994). Kava dermopathy. *Journal of the American Academy of Dermatology* 31 (1): 89-97.

Pittler MH, Ernst E (2000). Efficacy of kava extract for treating anxiety: Systematic review and meta-analysis. *Journal of Clinical Psychopharmacology* 20 (1): 84-89.

Prescott J, Jamieson D, Emdur N, Duffield P (1993). Acute effects of kava on measures of cognitive performance, physiological function, and mood. *Drug and Alcohol Review* 12: 49-58.

Russell PN, Bakker D, Singh NN (1987). The effects of kava on alerting and speed of access of information from long-term memory. *Bulletin of the Psychonomic Society* 25 (4): 236-237.

Ruze P (1990). Kava-induced dermopathy: A niacin deficiency? *The Lancet* 335 (8703): 1442-1445.

Schulz V, Hänsel R, Tyler VE (2001). *Rational Phytotherapy: A Physicians' Guide to Herbal Medicine,* Fourth Edition. Trans. TC Telgar. Berlin: Springer-Verlag.

Schulze J, Meng G, Siegers CP (2001). Safety assessment of kavalactone-containing herbal drugs in comparison to other psychotropics. *Naunyn-Schmiedeberg's Archives of Pharmacology* 364 (3, Suppl.): R 22.

Singh NN, Ellis CR, Best AM, Eakin K (1998). Randomized, double-blind, placebo-controlled study on the effectiveness and safety of Kavatrol in a non-clinical sample of adults with daily stress and anxiety. Unpublished manuscript.

Volz HP, Kieser M (1997). Kava-kava extract WS 1490 versus placebo in anxiety disorders—A randomized placebo-controlled 25-week outpatient trial. *Pharmacopsychiatry* 30 (1): 1-5.

Warnecke G (1991). Psychosomatic disorders in the female climacterium, clinical efficacy and tolerance of Kava extract WS 1490. *Fortschritte der Medizin* 109 (4): 119-122. (Similar 12-week study published in Warnecke G, Pfaender H, Gerster G, Gracza E [1990]. Efficacy of an extract of kava root in patients with climacteric syndrome. *Zeitschrift für Phytotherapie* 11: 81-86.)

Woelk H, Kapoula O, Lehrl S, Schroter K, Weinholz P (1993). Treatment of patients suffering from anxiety. Double-blind study: Kava special extract versus benzodiazepines. *Zeitschrift für Allgemeinmedizin* 69: 271-277.

DETAILS ON KAVA PRODUCTS
AND CLINICAL STUDIES

Product and clinical study information is grouped in the same order as in the Summary Table. A profile on an individual product is followed by details of the clinical studies associated with that product. In some instances, a clinical study, or studies, supports several products that contain the same principal ingredient(s). In these instances, those products are grouped together.

Clinical studies that follow each product, or group of products, are grouped by therapeutic indication, in accordance with the order in the Summary Table.

Index to Kava Products

Product Profile: Laitan®

Manufacturer	**Dr. Willmar Schwabe GmbH & Co., Germany**
U.S. distributor	None
Botanical ingredient	**Kava root extract**
Extract name	**WS 1490**
Quantity	100 mg
Processing	No information
Standardization	70% kavalactones
Formulation	Capsule

Source(s) of information: Lehmann, Kinzler, and Friedemann, 1996.

Clinical Study: Laitan®

Extract name	WS 1490
Manufacturer	Dr. Willmar Schwabe GmbH & Co., Germany

Indication	**Anxiety**
Level of evidence	**I**
Therapeutic benefit	**Yes**

Bibliographic reference

Lehmann E, Kinzler E, Friedemann J (1996). Efficacy of a special kava extract *(Piper methysticum)* in patients with states of anxiety, tension and excitedness of non-mental origin—A double-blind placebo-controlled study of four weeks. *Phytomedicine* 3 (2): 113-119. (Also published in Kinzler E, Kromer J, Lehmann E [1991] *Arzneimittel-Forschung/Drug Research* 41 [1]: 584-588.)

Trial design

Parallel. A washout period of at least five half-lives of the medication was required before admittance to the study.

Study duration	1 month
Dose	1 (100 mg extract) capsule 3 times daily
Route of administration	Oral
Randomized	Yes
Randomization adequate	Yes
Blinding	Double-blind
Blinding adequate	Yes
Placebo	Yes
Drug comparison	No
Site description	Not described
No. of subjects enrolled	58
No. of subjects completed	52
Sex	Male and female
Age	31-55 years

Inclusion criteria

Total score of greater than 18 points on the Hamilton Anxiety Scale (HAM-A); age between 18 and 60 years.

Exclusion criteria
Suicidal tendencies; endogenous depression; organic psychoses; psychoses of the schizophrenic group; psychopathies; dementia syndrome; diseases of the kidneys, liver, lungs, heart, cardiovascular system, as well as neoplasia; pregnancy; and medications interfering with the effectiveness evaluation, and those not included as comedications (including medications such as psychotonics, neuroleptics, antidepressants, tranquilizers, and beta-blockers).

End points
Subjects were evaluated at the beginning of the study as well as after 7, 14, and 28 days using the HAM-A, the self-assessment Adjectives Check List (EWL), the Clinical Global Impression Scale (CGI), and Fischer's Somatic or Adverse Experiences Checklist (FSUCL).

Results
The HAM-A overall score of anxiety symptomatology was significantly reduced in the kava group compared to placebo after one week of treatment ($p < 0.02$). This difference between the two groups increased over four weeks. In the kava group, the average HAM-A score of 25.6 at baseline dropped to 12.6 at the end of the month. The score remained practically unchanged in the placebo group (24.5 to 21.0, respectively). The anxiety/depression subscale of the EWL dropped significantly compared to placebo ($p < 0.05$). The other subscales showed no changes. The CGI rating decreased compared to placebo. No undesirable events were documented by FSUCL.

Side effects
None documented.

Authors' comments
WS 1490 is suitable for general practitioners to use in treating states of anxiety, tension, and excitedness.

Reviewers' comments
Well-designed, randomized, double-blind, placebo-controlled trial on reducing anxiety. To improve the study even more, a comparison to a conventional treatment group (e.g., benzodiazepine) would help in the evaluation of recommending kava as an alternative treatment. A longer trial would also allow for the better characterization of adverse events. (5, 6)

Clinical Study: Laitan®

Extract name	WS 1490
Manufacturer	Dr. Willmar Schwabe GmbH & Co., Germany

Indication	**Anxiety**
Level of evidence	**III**
Therapeutic benefit	**Yes**

Bibliographic reference
Volz HP, Kieser M (1997). Kava-kava extract WS 1490 versus placebo in anxiety disorders—A randomized placebo-controlled 25-week outpatient trial. *Pharmacopsychiatry* 30 (1): 1-5.

Trial design
Parallel. Pretrial single-blind washout period with placebo of one week. After the 24-week randomized treatment period there was again a one-week washout period.

Study duration	24 weeks
Dose	1 (100 mg extract) capsule 3 times daily
Route of administration	Oral
Randomized	Yes
Randomization adequate	No
Blinding	Double-blind
Blinding adequate	No
Placebo	Yes
Drug comparison	No
Site description	10 general practices
No. of subjects enrolled	101
No. of subjects completed	73
Sex	Male and female
Age	Mean: 53.9 ± 16.3 years

Inclusion criteria
Patients suffering from anxiety and tension of nonpsychotic origin, with one of the following DSM-III-R diagnostic criteria: agoraphobia, specific phobia, social phobia, generalized anxiety disorder, or adjustment disorder with anxiety. In the Mehrfachwahl-Wortschatz test (multiple-choice vocabulary test) version B (MWT-B), a maximum of 13 mistakes were allowed. On the Hamilton Anxiety Scale (HAM-A) a score of at least 19 was required.

Exclusion criteria
Comedication with psychoactive compounds; hypotension (blood pressure lower than 90/60 mmHg); cerebellar ataxia; sleep apnea syndrome; a history or presence of substance abuse; clinically relevant cardiovascular, renal, hepatic, or respiratory diseases; and malignancies. Patients with an increase or decrease of more than six points on the HAMA at the end of the

one-week, single-blind, placebo washout period preceding the trial were also excluded.

End points
Evaluations were performed at the beginning of the placebo washout period, at weeks 0, 12, and 24, and after the final placebo washout period. The outcome criteria were the HAM-A, self-report symptom inventory (SCL-90-R), Clinical Global Impression (CGI), subjective well-being scale (Befindlichkeits-Scala, Bf-S) and registration of adverse events in a questionnaire. Additional HAMA ratings and adverse checks were carried out at weeks 4, 8, 16, and 20.

Results
A significant superiority of kava was observed in the HAM-A scores compared to placebo starting from week 8 ($p < 0.02$) that later increased (weeks 16, 20, 24; $p < 0.001$). HAMA values in the kava group fell from 30.7 at baseline to 9.7 after 24 weeks. The HAMA values for the placebo group fell from 31.4 to 15.2, respectively. WS 1490 was also found to be superior with respect to the secondary outcome variables: HAMA subscores somatic and psychic anxiety, CGI, SCL-90-R, and Bf-S.

Side effects
Nine patients in placebo group reported 15 adverse events; five patients in the kava group reported six events (stomach upset in two cases that may have been related to kava).

Authors' comments
The results support WS 1490 as a treatment alternative to tricyclic antidepressants and benzodiazepines in anxiety disorders, with proven long-term efficacy and none of the tolerance problems associated with those drugs.

Reviewers' comments
Overall, this is a well-designed study evaluating the effects of kava for patients suffering from anxiety (as determined by DSM-III-R diagnostic criteria). The study reports a significant reduction in anxiety (measured by HAM-A) starting from week 8 of treatment and continuing until week 24. HAM-A scores from week 25 (one-week posttreatment washout) were not included. Randomization and blinding procedures were not described adequately. (1, 6)

Clinical Study: Laitan®

Extract name	WS 1490
Manufacturer	Dr. Willmar Schwabe GmbH & Co., Germany

Indication	**Anxiety in menopausal women**
Level of evidence	I
Therapeutic benefit	**Yes**

Bibliographic reference

Warnecke G (1991). Psychosomatic disorders in the female climacterium, clinical efficacy and tolerance of Kava extract WS 1490. *Fortschritte der Medizin* 109 (4): 119-122. (Similar 12-week study published in Warnecke G, Pfaender H, Gerster G, Gracza E [1990]. Efficacy of an extract of kava root in patients with climacteric syndrome. *Zeitschrift für Phytotherapie* 11: 81-86.)

Trial design

Parallel. Pretrial washout period of one week (or at least five to six times the half-life of any prohibited medication) in which patients received placebo.

Study duration	2 months
Dose	1 (100 mg extract) capsule 3 times daily
Route of administration	Oral
Randomized	Yes
Randomization adequate	Yes
Blinding	Double-blind
Blinding adequate	Yes
Placebo	Yes
Drug comparison	No
Site description	Single center
No. of subjects enrolled	40
No. of subjects completed	40
Sex	Female
Age	Not given

Inclusion criteria

Women ages 45 to 60 years with menopausal symptoms, presence of psychoautonomic syndromes (anxiety, conditions of restlessness and sleep disturbances) and psychosomatic disturbances that manifested themselves as gynecological disorders, and Hamilton Anxiety Score (HAM-A) > 18.

Exclusion criteria

Constitutional hypotension with blood pressure < 90/79 mmHg; suicidal tendencies; endogenic depression; organic psychoses; schizophrenia; psychopathies; dementia or lacking sufficient intelligence to fill out forms; severe conditions of the kidneys, liver, lungs, heart/circulation, and neoplasma; pregnancy; and long-term treatment with medications such as psychotonics, neuroleptics, antidepressants, tranquilizers, and hormone preparations.

End points
Overall score of anxiety symptomatology according to the HAM-A score, Depressive Status Inventory (DSI), subjective well-being (patient diary), severity of the disease with the Clinical Global Impression, and climacteric symptomatology (Kuppermann Index and Schneider Scale). Examinations were carried out before the trial and after one, four, and eight weeks.

Results
The overall HAM-A score of anxiety symptomatology revealed a significant difference in the kava group compared to the placebo group after one week of treatment ($p < 0.001$). By the fourth and eighth week the significance increased ($p < 0.0005$). In the kava group, the baseline score of 31.1 was reduced to 5.5 after eight weeks. The placebo group score dropped from 30.2 to 22.5. The DSI decreased significantly compared to the placebo in the fourth and eighth week, $p < 0.01$. Other parameters, such as subjective well-being and CGI, demonstrated a high level of efficacy for the kava extract.

Side effects
Six adverse events were reported in the placebo group, and four in the kava group. Patients reported restlessness, tremor, gastric pressure, and tiredness (events reported were similar between the two groups).

Author's comments
This study demonstrates a high level of efficacy of kava extract WS 1490 in neurovegetative and psychosomatic dysfunctions in menopause, associated with very good tolerance.

Reviewers' comments
Well-designed and well-reported trial on the efficacy of kava (WS 1490) in reducing both anxiety (significant decreases in HAMA scores) and severity of menopausal symptoms (Kuppermann Index). (Translation reviewed) (5, 6)

Clinical Study: Laitan® 50

Extract name	WS 1490
Manufacturer	Dr. Willmar Schwabe GmbH & Co., Germany
Indication	**Anxiety**
Level of evidence	I
Therapeutic benefit	**Yes**

Bibliographic reference
Malsch U, Kieser M (2001). Efficacy of kava-kava in the treatment of non-psychotic anxiety, following pretreatment with benzodiazepines. *Psychopharmacology* 157 (3): 277-283.

Trial design
Parallel. Subjects had been taking benzodiazepines for at least two weeks prior to the trial start. During the first two weeks of the trial, the benzodiazepine treatment was tapered off at a steady rate. Simultaneously, during the first week of the study, the daily dose of the kava extract was increased from 50 mg to 300 mg. By weeks 3 through 5, subjects were only taking either 300 mg kava extract or placebo daily. A follow-up was conducted three weeks after the treatment phase.

Study duration	5 weeks
Dose	3 (50 mg) capsules twice daily
Route of administration	Oral
Randomized	Yes
Randomization adequate	Yes
Blinding	Double-blind
Blinding adequate	Yes
Placebo	Yes
Drug comparison	No
Site description	One hospital
No. of subjects enrolled	40
No. of subjects completed	37
Sex	Male and female
Age	21-75 years (mean: 40)

Inclusion criteria
Subjects suffering from nonpsychotic nervous anxiety, restlessness, and tension that results in impairment of work performance, relationships, and normal social activities (diagnoses according to the DSM-III-R of agoraphobia, simple or social phobia, generalized anxiety disorders, or adaptation disturbances). Prior to inclusion into the study, subjects had to have been taking 14 days of uninterrupted treatment with benzodiazepines. Subjects also needed a medical indication for the change to a different anxiolytic drug and therefore a discontinuation of the benzodiazepine treatment. Subjects had to score a total of at least 12 points on the verbal multiple-choice intelligence test (MWT-B) and a score of at most 14 on the Hamilton Anxiety Scale (HAM-A).

Exclusion criteria
Subjects were excluded if they had other anxiety disorders and psychiatric

diseases, drug abuse or addiction, suicidal tendencies, severe physical illness, constitutional hypotension, ocular disorders, need of medical treatment that could interfere with the trial evaluation, or known lactose intolerance or allergies to kava extract. Pregnant or nursing mothers were also excluded.

End points
The primary end points were overall changes from baseline to the trial end in the HAM-A and the Befindlichkeits-Skala (Bf-S, subjective well-being scale), and the incidence of withdrawal symptoms from the cessation of benzodiazepine treatment. Secondary end points included the Erlangen Anxiety and Aggression Scale (EAAS) and the Clinical Global Impression Scale (CGI).

Results
After five weeks of treatment, the group taking kava extract saw a decrease in the HAM-A total score (median improvement: 7.5 points; 60 percent were responders). This was significantly different from placebo (HAM-A scores: $p < 0.05$; percent responders: $p < 0.013$). The kava group also showed significantly greater improvement on the Bf-S total score compared to placebo (median improvement: 18.5 and 3 points, respectively; $p < 0.01$). More subjects in the placebo group (52.6 percent) experienced withdrawal symptoms than in the kava group (40 percent), but this difference was not significant. On the EAAS, the kava group showed a reduction in the total score by 3.5 points, whereas the placebo group's total score was reduced by 0.5 points ($p = 0.02$). The kava group also improved more according to Items 1 and 2 of the CGI: perceived severity decreased for the kava but remained unchanged for placebo ($p = 0.01$); and subjects' overall condition was much improved for the kava group versus unchanged for the placebo ($p = 0.02$).

Side effects
No serious adverse events occurred during the trial. Five subjects in the kava group and ten in the placebo group experienced adverse events, all of which were related to the withdrawal of benzodiazepine. No differences were observed in laboratory tests at the beginning and end of the trial.

Authors' comments
This trial demonstrates that kava special extract WS 1490 is significantly more effective than placebo in the treatment of moderately severe anxiety disorders of nonpsychotic origin. Beyond confirming the anxiolytic effect of kava-kava special extract WS 1490, the results of the study also show that a further alleviation of many patients' anxiety could be produced despite long previous treatment with benzodiazepines.

Reviewers' comments
Although the sample size is small (40 subjects), this is a very well-designed study evaluating the effects of a well-studied standardized extract of kava

(WS 1490) in the treatment of moderately severe anxiety. The study demonstrated that subjects on long-term benzodiazapine therapy could be safely switched to kava by tapering subjects off preexisting benzodiazapines while tapering up the kava dose. There were no serious adverse events reported after five weeks of treatment. However this intervention period was not long enough to assess long-term treatment efficacy or the potential addictive properties of kava. (5, 5)

Clinical Study: Laitan®

Extract name	WS 1490
Manufacturer	Dr. Willmar Schwabe GmbH & Co., Germany
Indication	**Anxiety**
Level of evidence	**II**
Therapeutic benefit	**Yes**

Bibliographic reference
Woelk H, Kapoula O, Lehrl S, Schroter K, Weinholz P (1993). Treatment of patients suffering from anxiety. Double-blind study: Kava special extract versus benzodiazepines. *Zeitschrift für Allgemeinmedizin* 69: 271-277.

Trial design
Parallel. After a one-week washout period, patients were divided into three groups and received either kava, oxazepam (3 × 5 mg daily), or bromazepam (3 × 3 mg daily) for six weeks. In a subsequent 14-week open-study phase, all patients were treated with Kava (results of this phase are reported in another paper and not included here).

Study duration	6 weeks
Dose	3 (100 mg extract) capsules daily
Route of administration	Oral
Randomized	Yes
Randomization adequate	Yes
Blinding	Double-blind
Blinding adequate	Yes
Placebo	No
Drug comparison	Yes
Drug names	Oxazepam and bromazepam
Site description	12 medical practices
No. of subjects enrolled	172

No. of subjects completed 164
Sex   Male and female
Age   Mean: 50 years

Inclusion criteria
Patients 18 to 65 years with conditions of anxiety, tension and agitation of nonpsychotic origin, a Hamilton Anxiety Scale (HAM-A) total score of more than 18, and Mehrfachwahl-Wortschatz-Intelligenztest (multiple-choice vocabulary intelligence test) IQ of at least 80.

Exclusion criteria
Patients lacking the mental or linguistic capacity to perform tests, or perform them with insufficient compliance; pregnant and nursing patients; patients with severe diseases of kidneys, liver, lung, heart and circulation, and neoplasia; myasthenia gravis; constitutional hypotension with RR values < 90/60 mmHg; cerebral ataxia; sleep apnea; lactose intolerance; psychoses and danger of suicide; acute intoxications with centrally sedating drugs or alcohol; known drug, alcohol, or medicament abuse; and treatment with therapeutics able to interfere with the assessment of efficacy, such as psychotonics, neuroleptics, antidepressants, or other plant-based anxiolytics.

End points
Anxiety was assessed using the HAM-A total score. Additional tests included: the physician's assessment of global therapeutic success (CGI); a self-assessment test; the KEPS (short test for evaluating personality); EAAS scale for anxiety, aggression and tension; and the EWL-60-S for recording patients' subjective feelings.

Results
In all three treatment groups, a continuous decrease of anxiety was found after the first week. No significant difference could be verified when comparing the HAM-A total score of kava to each of the other treatment groups during the six-week trial. A comparable action was measured by the EWL-60-S and EAAS.

Side effects
Adverse events related to medication were not collected. However, investigating physicians reported four cases of tiredness, one with mild reversible pruritis with Bromazepam; one patient with tiredness, pressure in head, vertigo, and unrest while taking oxazepam; and one case of gastric pressure and nocturnal nausea, as well as a lack of initiative and spasmodic state under stress.

Authors' comments
It can be concluded that the kava special extract WS 1490 is comparable to oxazepam or bromazepam with regard to anxiolytic effect. It should be in-

cluded as a possible therapy for anxiety, tension, and agitation of non-psychotic origin.

Reviewers' comments
Reasonably well-designed, randomized, double-blind trial showing kava comparable to oxazepam and bromazepam in reducing anxiety (measured by HAM-A). A comparison of all three therapies to a placebo group would increase the validity of the findings. (Translation reviewed) (5, 5)

Clinical Study: Laitan®

Extract name	WS 1490
Manufacturer	Dr. Willmar Schwabe GmbH & Co., Germany
Indication	**Sleep quality** in healthy volunteers
Level of evidence	**III**
Therapeutic benefit	**Undetermined**

Bibliographic reference
Emser W, Bartylla K (1991). Improvement in quality of sleep: Effect of kava extract WS 1490 on the sleep patterns in healthy people. *TW Neurologie Psychiatrie* 5: 636-642.

Trial design
Parallel. Dose comparison. Each group received placebo on days 1, 3, and 4, and kava (either 3 × 50 mg or 3 × 100 mg) on day 2.

Study duration	4 nights
Dose	3 (50 mg or 100 mg) capsules daily
Route of administration	Oral
Randomized	No
Randomization adequate	No
Blinding	Double-blind
Blinding adequate	Yes
Placebo	Yes
Drug comparison	No
Site description	Not described
No. of subjects enrolled	12
No. of subjects completed	12
Sex	Male and female
Age	20-31 years

Inclusion criteria
Healthy individuals.

Exclusion criteria
Patients with alcohol or medical abuse, pain, or suicidal tendencies.

End points
Primary objective: EEG sleeping patterns of the subjects. A long-time EEG system was used over the test period of four days and four nights. Enumeration of EEG sleep spindles during sleep Stage 2 was done visually. Subjects filled out a sleep questionnaire daily.

Results
EEG sleep spindle densities for 11 of the 12 subjects on the kava-extract night increased around 20 percent in comparison with the densities recorded for both placebo nights. The percentage of deep sleep (slow wave sleep) increased, and falling asleep latency was reduced compared to placebo. REM sleep did not change. The duration of sleep Stage 1 (falling asleep stage) as well as duration of the waking stage tended to decrease after higher doses of kava (3 x 100 mg). Sleep questionnaires were not always consistent with EEG measurements, but overall cited an improvement in deep sleep as well as an improvement in peace, calm, and well-being the morning after taking kava extract.

Side effects
None reported.

Authors' comments
The increase in sleep spindle density in sleep EEG measurements is a characteristic of conventional tranquilizers that is shared by the kava special extract WS 1490. Kava did not cause a suppression of deep sleep or REM sleep, which is typical of benzodiazepine-type and barbituate-type sleeping medications. The small number of subjects limits the statistical significance of the findings, but the study is useful in identifying trends.

Reviewers' comments
This is a small pilot trial using various polysomnographic EEG outcome measures, including spindles density, sleep latencies, sleep stages, and awakenings. Based on the polysomnographic data, the high-dose kava group showed a decrease in slow-wave sleep latency. Subjective sleep quality was assessed by questionnaire data, but not completely described in the study report. The subjective sleep latencies increased with drugs in contrast to the polysomnographic data; however, the subjects did report an improvement in deep sleep with drugs. Some of the study differences are hard to evaluate because the authors do not give variability measures. The data

suggest that the higher dose of kava produced more effects on sleep than the lower dose. (3, 4)

Clinical Study: WS 1490

Extract name	WS 1490
Manufacturer	Dr. Willmar Schwabe GmbH & Co., Germany
Indication	**Cognitive functioning** in healthy volunteers
Level of evidence	**II**
Therapeutic benefit	**Undetermined**

Bibliographic reference
Munte TF, Heinze HJ, Matzke M, Steitz J (1993). Effects of oxazepam and an extract of kava roots *(Piper methysticum)* on event-related potentials in a word recognition task. *Neuropsychobiology* 27 (1): 46-53. (Also published in Heinze HJ, Munthe TF, Steitz J, Matzke M [1994]. *Pharmacopsychiatry* 27 (6): 224-230.)

Trial design
Crossover study, Latin design. Experimental sessions were separated by 12 days. For five days prior to an experimental session, subjects took one capsule three times daily of one of three treatments: placebo; kava extract; or placebo on the first three days, then 15 mg oxazepam the day before testing, and 75 mg on the morning of testing.

Study duration	5 days
Dose	1 (200 mg) capsule 3 times daily
Route of administration	Oral
Randomized	No
Randomization adequate	No
Blinding	Double-blind
Blinding adequate	Yes
Placebo	Yes
Drug comparison	Yes
Drug name	Oxazepam
Site description	Single center
No. of subjects enrolled	12
No. of subjects completed	12
Sex	Male
Age	24-37 years

Inclusion criteria
Healthy subjects with normal vision or vision corrected to normal.

Exclusion criteria
Neurological conditions.

End points
Memory performance was evaluated with a continuous word-recognition task. Scalp-recorded electrical potentials or event-related brain potentials (ERPs), were also recorded.

Results
In the word-recognition test, a significant slowing of reaction time and a reduction in the number of correct responses was seen for oxazepam, whereas a nonsignificant increase in the number of correct responses was observed for kava. The results of the ERPs showed a similar pattern.

Side effects
None reported.

Authors' comments
The behavioral indices in the word-recognition test suggest enhanced memory performance under kava medication and a greatly impaired performance with oxazepam.

Reviewers' comments
Although oxazepam produced significant impairments on cognitive testing compared to placebo, no significant impairment was observed with kava. In addition to the cognitive testing, event-related potentials were recorded. Although the authors reported some differences, given their relatively nonstandard techniques and lack of a priori hypotheses, no definite effects of kava were observed. The strength of the study is reduced by the small sample size and the inadequate inclusion/exclusion criteria. Note: the dose in this study is twice that used in the anxiety study (Lehmann, Kinzler, and Friedemann, 1996). (3, 4)

Product Profile: Kava (Generic)

Manufacturer	None
U.S. distributor	None
Botanical ingredient	**Kava root extract**
Extract name	None given
Quantity	No information

Processing	30 g kava root powder from Fiji was soaked in water, twice filtered through a piece of fine muslin cloth, and the residue discarded. The remaining liquid was adjusted to 250 ml by the addition of water.
Standardization	No information
Formulation	Liquid

Source(s) of information: Russell, Bakker, and Singh, 1987.

Clinical Study: Kava (Generic)

Extract name	None given
Manufacturer	None
Indication	**Cognitive functioning** in healthy volunteers
Level of evidence	**III**
Therapeutic benefit	**Undetermined**

Bibliographic reference
Russell PN, Bakker D, Singh NN (1987). The effects of kava on alerting and speed of access of information from long-term memory. *Bulletin of the Psychonomic Society* 25 (4): 236-237.

Trial design
In two experiments, a control group and either a low-dose kava group or a high-dose kava group were tested twice, two to six days apart. The control group consumed no kava prior to either session. The low-dose kava group consumed a 250 ml preparation made from 30 g of root. The high-dose kava group consumed 500 ml preparation made up to a strength of 1 g kava/kg body weight.

Study duration	2 testing sessions
Dose	250 ml (30 g root); 500 ml at a strength of 1g/kg body weight.
Route of administration	Oral
Randomized	No
Randomization adequate	No
Blinding	Open
Blinding adequate	No

Placebo	No
Drug comparison	No
Site description	Single center
No. of subjects enrolled	27
No. of subjects completed	27
Sex	Male and female
Age	18-22 years

Inclusion criteria
Caucasian undergraduates.

Exclusion criteria
None mentioned.

End points
Stimuli were presented to subjects. Reaction time and accuracy were recorded on two testing occasions (one at baseline and a second after two to six days).

Results
Kava produced no effect on the speed of activation of verbal information in long-term memory or on the rise or magnitude of the alerting function of a warning signal. Neither dose, one associated with traditional social use and one much greater, had an effect on reaction times or errors.

Side effects
None mentioned.

Authors' comments
It would be unwise to conclude from this study alone that kava has no effect on cognitive function. More research is needed. At this stage, however, kava appears preferable to alcohol as a beverage to be consumed on social occasions, at least in terms of its effects on human performance.

Reviewers' comments
This open-label pilot trial is not well designed. Instead of using a placebo, the "no kava" group did not consume anything before the cognitive performance test. Flaws also included a small sample size, inclusion criteria not well defined, no exclusion criteria, inadequately described statistical methods, and no randomization or blinding. (0, 2)

Product Profile: Kava (Generic)

Manufacturer	None
U.S. distributor	None
Botanical ingredient	**Kava root extract**
Extract name	None given
Quantity	No information
Processing	200 g of commercially available Fijian powdered kava root, held inside a permeable nylon sack, was infused into 1,000 ml of water for 10 minutes while squeezing the sack repeatedly
Standardization	No information
Formulation	Liquid

Source(s) of information: Prescott et al., 1993.

Clinical Study: Kava (Generic)

Extract name	None given
Manufacturer	None
Indication	**Cognitive functioning** in healthy volunteers
Level of evidence	**III**
Therapeutic benefit	**Undetermined**

Bibliographic reference
Prescott J, Jamieson D, Emdur N, Duffield P (1993). Acute effects of kava on measures of cognitive performance, physiological function, and mood. *Drug and Alcohol Review* 12: 49-58.

Trial design
Subjects attended two sessions on consecutive days. The first session was without kava, and produced a baseline. On the second day, participants received either juice (1,000 ml) or kava (500 ml) plus juice (500 ml).

Study duration	2 sessions on successive days
Dose	500 ml water extract (100 g root)

Route of administration	Oral
Randomized	Yes
Randomization adequate	No
Blinding	Double-blind
Blinding adequate	No
Placebo	Yes
Drug comparison	No
Site description	University hospital
No. of subjects enrolled	24
No. of subjects completed	24
Sex	Male and female
Age	18-53 years (mean: 26.7)

Inclusion criteria
Subjects who were consumers of alcohol, but had never consumed kava.

Exclusion criteria
None mentioned.

End points
Subjects undertook tasks of acute cognitive functioning, including reaction time and tracking tasks, and a measure of body sway. Heart rate, respiration rate, and blood pressure were recorded. Subjects were also asked to rate their degree of intoxication and complete a stress/arousal checklist.

Results
Subjects taking kava reported low to moderate levels of intoxication that peaked one hour after consumption and declined thereafter. These levels were statistically significant compared to placebo ($p = 0.002$). Compared to placebo, the kava group had increased body sway ($p = 0.016$). Cognitive performance tasks showed slight impairment in complex tasks for the kava group, but no significant differences were found between the two groups.

Side effects
Three subjects reported nausea after consumption of kava.

Authors' comments
Overall, the effects of kava ingestion in naive volunteers were evident only in the sway test, and in subjective feelings of intoxication, with some trends in the complex cognitive tasks. The possibility that cognitive impairment may have been more evident with a larger sample size suggests that caution should be exercised in ingesting kava prior to tasks that are cognitively demanding.

Reviewers' comments
The methodology of this study has some serious flaws. The blinding of the kava drink was not well done. Kava taken as a drink can cause oral numbness—an effect that would have to be accounted for in the placebo drink; therefore, using only juice as placebo does not provide a proper placebo control. Randomization was done on an alternating basis, which presumably also limited blinding. The blinding of outcome assessments was never mentioned in this report. No exclusion criteria were mentioned. The trial did include some well-defined and appropriate objective outcome assessments, including: cognitive performance tasks; Sternberg memory scanning task; simple reaction time, choice reaction time, tracking, and divided attention; physiological recordings; respiratory and heart rate; blood pressure; and objective measures of body sway. Effects of kava were observed for self-rated intoxication and body sway. (1, 3)

Product Profile: Kavatrol™

Manufacturer	**Natrol, Inc.**
U.S. distributor	**Natrol, Inc.**
Botanical ingredient	**Kava root extract**
Extract name	None given
Quantity	200 mg
Processing	Plant/extract ratio 6:1, water-ethanol extraction
Standardization	30% kavalactones (including kawain, dihydrokawain, methysticin, dihydromethysticin
Botanical ingredient	**Schizandra fruit**
Extract name	N/A
Quantity	50 mg
Processing	No information
Standardization	No information
Botanical ingredient	**Hops flower**
Extract name	N/A
Quantity	50 mg
Processing	No information
Standardization	No information
Botanical ingredient	**Chamomile flower**
Extract name	N/A
Quantity	50 mg
Processing	No information

Standardization	No information
Botanical ingredient	**Passionflower aerial parts**
Extract name	N/A
Quantity	50 mg
Processing	No information
Standardization	No information
Formulation	Capsule

Recommended dose: Take two capsules 2 times per day, preferably before a meal or on an empty stomach.

DSHEA structure/function: Helps you relax naturally.

Cautions: Avoid using with alcohol or mixing with any prescription medication and/or OTC drugs. If pregnant or lactating, consult your physician prior to use. Do not use if diagnosed with liver disease. If any symptoms of jaundice (nausea, fever, dark urine, yellow eyes, etc.) occur, discontinue use and seek medical attention. Not recommended to exceed more than 4 capsules per day. Consult a physician if intending to use this product routinely.

Other ingredients: Magnesium stearate, silica, gelatin.

Comments: Also comes in tablet form.

Source(s) of information: Product label, product information (www.natrol.com/catalog); FAQ Kavatrol (www.natrol.com); information provided by distributor.

Clinical Study: Kavatrol™

Extract name	None given
Manufacturer	Natrol, Inc.
Indication	**Anxiety and stress**
Level of evidence	**II**
Therapeutic benefit	**Trend**

Bibliographic reference
Singh NN, Ellis CR, Best AM, Eakin K (1998). Randomized, double-blind, placebo-controlled study on the effectiveness and safety of Kavatrol in a non-clinical sample of adults with daily stress and anxiety. Unpublished manuscript.

Trial design
Parallel. Pretrial washout period of at least five half-life periods of participants' medications.

Study duration	1 month
Dose	2 (200 mg) capsules twice daily
Route of administration	Oral
Randomized	Yes
Randomization adequate	No
Blinding	Double-blind
Blinding adequate	Yes
Placebo	Yes
Drug comparison	No
Site description	Not described
No. of subjects enrolled	67
No. of subjects completed	60
Sex	Male and female
Age	Mean: 36.5 years

Inclusion criteria
State-Trait Anxiety Inventory (STAI) score of one standard deviation above the mean, ages between 18 and 60, and good physical health.

Exclusion criteria
Endogenous depression, mental conditions of organic origin, or psychoses; syndromes of the kidneys, liver, lungs, heart, cardiovascular system, as well as neoplasia, irrespective of its localization; pregnancy; on prescribed medications that may interact with the kavalactones or interfere with the assessment of efficacy and safety of Kavatrol (including neuroleptics, antidepressants, sedatives, anxiolytics, and beta-blockers).

End points
Efficacy measures included the Daily Stress Inventory (DSI) and STAI scores. Subjects completed the STAI and DSI once a week on the same day for four weeks. Safety and tolerance were also measured weekly using the Untoward Effects Checklist.

Results
The results showed that state anxiety of the subjects on Kavatrol decreased from baseline to week four, a statistically significant reduction compared to the placebo group, $p < 0.0001$. As expected, the levels of trait anxiety (trait anxiety is thought to be a relatively fixed attribute) for Kavatrol and placebo groups did not change.

Side effects
No serious or significant side effects.

Authors' comments
This is the first study to show that kava reduces the stress associated with the daily hassles of life. Findings confirm the belief that kava products may offer an alternative to benzodiazepines in the reduction of anxiety states in adults.

Reviewers' comments
It is not clear from the inclusion/exclusion criteria what type of anxiety is being evaluated—no physician assessment of anxiety state was made, and only a self-assessment based on STAI greater than 1 standard deviation above the mean was provided. Exclusions for prescription medications may affect study outcomes, but not other botanical use. No mention is made of alcohol or caffeine use in the study subjects. Data variability measures are not given, but type of analysis and data are described. (3, 5)

Lemon Balm

Other Common Names: **Balm, bee balm, Melissa balm**
Latin Name: *Melissa officinalis* **L.** [Lamiaceae]
Plant Part: **Leaf**

PREPARATIONS USED IN REVIEWED CLINICAL STUDIES

The genesis of the lemon balm product Herpilyn®, indicated for the topical treatment of herpes infections, was the discovery of antiviral properties of the herb in a cell culture assay. The traditional use for lemon balm is reflected in the German Commission E's approval of oral preparations for nervous sleeping disorders and gastrointestinal complaints (Schulz, Hänsel, and Tyler, 2001).

A standardized preparation of lemon balm leaves is manufactured by Lomapharm, Rudolf Lohmann GmbH KG, Emmerthal, Germany. Lomaherpan® cream contains 1 percent of a dried aqueous extract called Lo-701 (ratio of leaf to extract 70:1). The product in the United States, distributed by Enzymatic Therapy under the name of Herpilyn®, contains the same lemon balm extract, Lo-701. In addition, it contains 1 percent allantoin, which is a monographed ingredient for over-the-counter (OTC) fever blister medications. The product tested in the two clinical trials reviewed here did not contain allantoin.

SUMMARY OF REVIEWED CLINICAL STUDIES

We reviewed two controlled clinical studies that examined the ability of Lomaherpan to reduce the symptoms of herpes simplex, a viral lesion that can occur on the lips of the mouths (cold sores), on the genitals (genital herpes), or on the skin. Herpes infections are characterized by local outbreaks with itching followed by blisters and

LEMON BALM SUMMARY TABLE

Product Name	Manufacturer/ U.S. Distributor	Product Characteristics	Dose in Trials	Indication	No. of Trials	Benefit (Evidence Level-Trial No.)
Herpilyn® (US), Lomaherpan® (EU)	Lomapharm, Rudolf Lohmann GmbH KG/ Enzymatic Therapy	Cream containing 1% aqueous extract (Lo-701)	Apply 2-4 times daily	Herpes simplex	2	Trend (III-2)

inflammation, which usually heal in a few days, sometimes producing scabs in the process. Herpes is often treated with antiviral agents such as acyclovir, which, when given orally, can reduce virus shedding, symptoms, and time to healing. Such agents appear to have less benefit when given topically (Hardman et al., 1996).

Lomaherpan

Herpes simplex

A recent study included 66 adults with a history of recurrent herpes of the lips (orolabial herpes). The subjects were administered Lomaherpan or placebo cream (2 mm) four times daily at the first sign of an outbreak. Participants were monitored for five days following an outbreak, with symptoms on day 2 being the primary end point. The Lomaherpan cream produced a significant reduction in the symptom score compared with placebo on day 2. However, overall symptom scores for the five-day periods were not different for the two groups (Koytchev, Alken, and Dundarov, 1999). Our reviewer, Dr. Richard O'Connor, considered that the small improvement observed after two days might not be clinically relevant.

The second placebo-controlled, double-blind study examined a total of 116 outpatients, both children and adults, with herpes lesions on multiple sites, including the lips, skin, and genitals. Patients were instructed to apply cream two to four times daily to the affected site over a maximum of ten days (on average five) until the lesion was healed. A significant reduction in redness (rubor) and swelling was observed on day two, but no significant difference in symptoms of blisters, scabbing, erosion, pain, or course and extent of the lesions. However, a significant increase in healing time compared with placebo was seen in a subgroup of patients (67) with herpes on the lips of the mouth (Wolbling and Leonhardt, 1994). The evidence for benefit in this trial was weakened by poor methodological descriptions in the report.

ADVERSE REACTIONS OR SIDE EFFECTS

No adverse reactions due to treatment were reported in the reviewed studies, which included a total of 91 subjects in both treatment groups.

INFORMATION FROM PHARMACOPOEIAL MONOGRAPHS

Sources of Published Therapeutic Monographs

German Commission E
European Scientific Cooperative on Phytotherapy

Indications

The German Commission E approved preparations of the fresh or dried leaf for nervous sleeping disorders and functional gastrointestinal complaints (Blumenthal et al., 1998). According to the European Scientific Cooperative on Phytotherapy (ESCOP) monograph, the dried leaves can be taken internally to treat tenseness, restlessness, and irritability, as well as the symptomatic treatment of digestive disorders, such as minor spasms. The dried leaves can be used externally to treat herpes labialis (cold sores) (ESCOP, 1996).

Doses

Tea: 1.5 to 4.5 g of herb per cup, several times daily as needed (Blumenthal et al., 1998); 2 to 3 g of the drug as an infusion, two to three times daily (ESCOP, 1996)
Tincture: 1:5 in 45 percent alcohol, 2 to 6 ml three times daily (ESCOP, 1996)
Topical application: cream containing 1 percent of a lyophilized aqueous extract (70:1), two to four times daily (ESCOP, 1996)

Treatment Period

ESCOP lists no restriction for oral administration. In topical application for herpes labialis, ESCOP suggests use from prodromal signs to a few days after the healing of lesions, or a maximum of 14 days (ESCOP, 1996).

Contraindications

The Commission E and ESCOP list no known contraindications (Blumenthal et al., 1998; ESCOP, 1996).

Adverse Reactions

The Commission E and ESCOP list no known adverse reactions (Blumenthal et al., 1998; ESCOP, 1996).

Precautions

ESCOP states there are no precautions (ESCOP, 1996).

Drug Interactions

According to the Commission E and ESCOP, there are no known drug interactions (Blumenthal et al., 1998; ESCOP, 1996).

REFERENCES

Blumenthal M, Busse W, Hall T, Goldberg A, Grünwald J, Riggins C, Rister S, eds. (1998*). The Complete German Commission E Monographs: Therapeutic Guide to Herbal Medicines.* Trans. S Klein. Austin: American Botanical Council.

European Scientific Cooperative on Phytotherapy (ESCOP) (1996). *Melissae folium:* Melissa leaf. In *Monographs on the Medicinal Uses of Plant Drugs.* Exeter, UK: European Scientific Cooperative on Phytotherapy.

Hardman JG, Limbird LE, Molinoff PB, Ruddon RW, Gilman AG (1996). *Goodman and Gillman's The Pharmacological Basis of Therapeutics,* Ninth Edition. New York: McGraw-Hill.

Koytchev R, Alken RG, Dundarov S (1999). Balm mint extract (Lo-701) for topical treatment of recurring herpes labialis. *Phytomedicine* 6 (4): 225-230.

Schulz V, Hänsel R, Tyler VE (2001). *Rational Phytotherapy: A Physicians' Guide to Herbal Medicine,* Fourth Edition. Trans. TC Telgar. Berlin: Springer-Verlag.

Wolbling RH, Leonhardt K (1994). Local therapy of herpes simplex with dried extract from *Melissa officinalis. Phytomedicine* 1: 25-31. (Also published in Vogt HJ, Tausch I, Wolbling RH, Kaiser PM [1991]. *Der Allgemeinarzt* 13 [11]: 832-841.)

DETAILS ON LEMON BALM PRODUCTS AND CLINICAL STUDIES

Product and clinical study information is grouped in the same order as in the Summary Table. A profile on an individual product is followed by details of the clinical studies associated with that product. In some instances, a clinical study, or studies, supports several products that contain the same principal ingredient(s). In these instances, those products are grouped together.

Clinical studies that follow each product, or group of products, are grouped by therapeutic indication, in accordance with the order in the Summary Table.

Product Profile: Herpilyn®

Manufacturer	**Lomapharm, Rudolf Lohmann GmbH KG, Germany**
U.S. distributor	**Enzymatic Therapy**
Botanical ingredient	**Lemon balm leaf extract**
Extract name	**Lo-701**
Quantity	No information
Processing	Plant to extract ratio 70:1
Standardization	No information
Formulation	Cream
Botanical ingredient	**Comfrey extract**
Extract name	None given
Quantity	No information
Processing	No information
Standardization	1% allantoin

Recommended dose: Apply at first sign of burning, tingling, or itching. If a cold sore has already developed, apply two to four times daily, or as often as needed.

DSHEA structure/function: OTC label indication: natural cold sore and fever blister medication.

Cautions: Avoid contact with eyes. If condition worsens or does not improve in 7 days, consult a physician.

Other ingredients: White soft paraffin, benzyl alcohol.

Comments: Sold as Lomaherpam® in Europe.

Source(s) of information: Product package; information provided by distributor; Koytchev, Alken, and Dundarov, 1999; correspondence with Enzymatic Therapy.

Clinical Study: Lomaherpan®

Extract name	Lo-701
Manufacturer	Lomapharm, Rudolf Lohmann GmbH, Germany
Indication	**Herpes simplex** (labialis)
Level of evidence	**III**
Therapeutic benefit	**Trend**

Bibliographic reference
Koytchev R, Alken RG, Dundarov S (1999). Balm mint extract (Lo-701) for topical treatment of recurring herpes labialis. *Phytomedicine* 6 (4): 225-230.

Trial design
Parallel. Patients were instructed to start therapy no later than four hours after the onset of symptoms and to contact the physician within 24 hours for a visit.

Study duration	5 days
Dose	Cream (2 mm) applied 4 times daily
Route of administration	Topical
Randomized	Yes
Randomization adequate	No
Blinding	Double-blind
Blinding adequate	No
Placebo	Yes
Drug comparison	No
Site description	Single center
No. of subjects enrolled	66
No. of subjects completed	66
Sex	Male and female
Age	18-65 years (mean: 43)

Inclusion criteria
Caucasian; history of recurrent herpes (at least four episodes per year); ex-

perienced in observing symptoms of itching, tingling, burning, and tautness; outbreaks typically localized to the lip margin or perioral skin; and previously diagnosed with recurrent herpes labialis.

Exclusion criteria
Concomitant local or systemic treatment with antiherpetic or antiviral agents, as well as immunosuppressive agents, were generally not allowed.

End points
During each herpetic episode there were four visits: on the first, second, third and fifth day after onset of symptoms. The primary target parameter was a combined symptom score of the values for complaints, size of affected area, and blisters at day 2 of therapy. The secondary target parameter was total score of herpetic symptoms over five days of therapy.

Results
A significant difference was observed in the values of the primary target parameter between groups on day 2, with a mean value of 4.03 in the Lo-701 group and 4.94 in the placebo group ($p = 0.042$). In the secondary target parameter (symptoms over five days of therapy), the verum group had a mean value lower than the placebo group, but not significantly ($p = 0.16$).

Side effects
None mentioned.

Authors' comments
As a whole, the results of the present trial obtained both for the primary and secondary target parameters were coherent and demonstrated the efficacy of Lomaherpan cream for the treatment of herpes simplex labialis.

Reviewer's comments
The primary end point (symptom score on day 2) was significantly better in the treatment group compared to placebo. The small difference between treatment arms, although statistically significant, may not be clinically relevant. None of the other parameters (five-day symptom score, global evaluation by either patient or investigator, or number of blisters) were statistically different. The results suggest integral efficacy, at best. Neither the blinding nor randomization were described in any detail. (1, 6)

Clinical Study: Lomaherpan®

Extract name	Lo-701
Manufacturer	Lomapharm, Rudolf Lohmann GmbH, Germany
Indication	**Herpes simplex**

Level of evidence   **III**
Therapeutic benefit   **Trend**

Bibliographic reference
Wolbling RH, Leonhardt K (1994). Local therapy of herpes simplex with dried extract from *Melissa officinalis*. *Phytomedicine* 1: 25-31. (Also published in Vogt HJ, Tausch I, Wolbling RH, Kaiser PM [1991]. *Der Allgemeinarzt 13* [11]: 832-841.)

Trial design
This paper reported both a phase I open-label controlled study and a phase II double blind study. The second study is reported here. Parallel. Patients were instructed to apply cream for five to ten days subject to the healing time of the lesion. Placebo was the same cream base as the active drug, but without the active ingredient of lemon balm.

Study duration	5-10 days
Dose	Apply cream 2-4 times daily for 5-10 days
Route of administration	Oral
Randomized	Yes
Randomization adequate	No
Blinding	Double-blind
Blinding adequate	No
Placebo	Yes
Drug comparison	No
Site description	2 dermatological centers
No. of subjects enrolled	116
No. of subjects completed	113
Sex	Male and female
Age	Mean: 33.2 ± 14.8 (placebo); 40.3 ± 14.8 (Lomaherpan)

Inclusion criteria
Children and adults with herpes simplex infection of the skin or transitional mucosa, with clinical symptoms lasting for not more than 72 hours before admission to the study.

Exclusion criteria
Known hypersensitivity to the ingredients of the drug or control preparation; concomitant treatment (internal or external) with another antiviral preparation; other treatment of viral infection; limited legal capacity.

End points
Clinical symptoms were documented after two days and upon termination of treatment (usually five days). Global evaluation was carried out by the physician and the patient on the patient's last visit. Scores ranged from 1 (very good) to 5 (very bad). The dimensions of the lesions were also recorded.

Results
The sites of lesions were similar for the two groups, including a total of 67 cases of lesions on the lips and ten cases of genital herpes. Compared to placebo, symptoms in the Lomaherpan group declined significantly after two days ($p = 0.0055$). After five days, 24 of 58 patients in the Lomaherpan group had no symptoms compared to 15 of 58 patients in the placebo group. Physicians assessed healing as "very good" in 25 cases in the Lomaherpan group and ten cases in the placebo group ($p = 0.031$). Patients assessed healing as "very good" in 24 cases in the Lomaherpan group, and 11 in the placebo ($p = 0.022$).

Side effects
No difference between the two groups.

Authors' comments
The effect of Lomaherpan cream in the topical treatment of herpes simplex infections of the skin and transitional mucosa is statistically significant. To be effective, the treatment must be started in the very early stages of the infection. The achieved acceleration of healing, particularly in the first two days of the treatment, adds corroborative evidence to this phenomenon.

Reviewer's comments
The results showed slight improvement on day 2 only for redness and swelling, but not on day 5. None of the other parameters (vesicle formation, scabbing, erosion, or pain) were different from placebo. The phase II study is described as randomized, but no details are given, and the ages of the two groups were significantly different. The blinding was also described poorly, and the data were not summarized in sufficient detail to permit alternative analysis. (1, 4)

Milk Thistle

Other common names: **Mary's thistle**
Latin name: *Silybum marianum* **(L.) Gaertn.** [Asteraceae]
Plant part: **Seed**

PREPARATIONS USED
IN REVIEWED CLINICAL STUDIES

Milk thistle is native to southern Europe and northern Africa. The plant part that is used medicinally is the ripe fruit (seed) with the outer covering (pappus) removed. The seed contains about 2 to 3 percent of the active constituent silymarin, a mixture of four isomers: silybin (also spelled silybinin) (50 percent), isosilybinin, silydianin, and silychristin. Studies conducted on silymarin have shown that it promotes liver-tissue regeneration, and has antitoxic effects on the liver (Schulz, Hänsel, and Tyler, 2001).

Legalon® is manufactured in Germany by Madaus AG. Legalon contains a standardized extract of milk thistle seeds that is characterized as containing 80 percent silymarin (140 mg silymarin per 173 to 186.7 mg extract). Legalon was previously distributed in the United States by Nature's Way Products, Inc., under the name of Thisilyn®.

Silipide, produced by Inverni della Beffa in Italy, contains a milk thistle seed extract, IdB 1016, also known as Siliphos®, that is manufactured by Indena S.p.A. Siliphos is a complex of silybin combined with phosphatidylcholine containing 29.7 to 36.3 percent silybin. An initial pilot study was conducted on a product with a molar ratio of silybin to phosphatidylcholine of 1:1 (Buzzelli et. al., 1993). The current product is manufactured with a ratio of silybin to phosphatidylcholine of 1:2. Siliphos is sold in the United States under the

MILK THISTLE SUMMARY TABLE

Product Name	Manufacturer/ U.S. Distributor	Product Characteristics	Dose in Trials	Indication	No. of Trials	Benefit (Evidence Level-Trial No.)
Legalon® (EU)	Madaus AG, Germany/None	Extract containing 80% silymarin	210-800 mg daily, usually in 3 doses	Alcoholic liver disease	10	Yes (III-1) Trend (I-1, II-1, III-2) Undetermined (III-3) No (I-2)
				Liver damage caused by toxins other than alcohol	2	Undetermined (III-2)
Silipide (EU)	Inverni della Beffa, Italy (Indena S.p.A., Italy)/None	Extract IdB 1060 (Siliphos®) complexed with phosphatidylcholine containing 29.7-36.3% silybin	240 or 480 mg daily	Chronic hepatitis	1	Yes (II-1)
				Viral hepatitis	1	Trend (II-1)
Silimarina® (Romania)	Biofarm, Romania/ None	Extract containing 5% silybin (said to be a copy of Legalon)	4.2 g (210 mg silybin) daily	Hepatitis or cirrhosis	1	Undetermined (II-1)
Generic	None/None	Silymarin	800 mg daily	Drug-induced liver damage	1	Trend (III-1)

*Products that contain the Indena S.p.A. Siliphos® extract as a single ingredient. The extract has been tested clinically but the following final formulations have not.

Product Name	Manufacturer	Product characteristics
Maximum Milk Thistle™	Natural Wellness	240 mg each capsule
Ultra thistle™	Natural Wellness	360 mg each capsule

names UltraThistle™ and Maximum Milk Thistle™ by Natural Wellness.

Silimarina® is manufactured in Romania by Biofarm. Each 700 mg tablet contains the equivalent of 35 mg silybin. The clinical study report claims that Silimarina is a copy of Legalon.

One trial was conducted on a product simply described as silymarin, using a dose of 800 mg daily. No further description was available.

SUMMARY OF REVIEWED CLINICAL STUDIES

Milk thistle preparations have been tested for their ability to treat symptoms of liver disease caused by alcohol, other toxins, or viral infections. The major liver diseases are hepatitis, cirrhosis, and dysfunctions related to bile secretion. Hepatitis is characterized as an inflammation of the liver that can be present with or without cirrhosis. Forms of viral hepatitis include hepatitis A, B, and C. Cirrhosis is a state in which the tissue in the liver breaks down, becoming fatty and fibrous. Liver disease can be acute (short term) or chronic (long term) leading to cirrhosis and eventually to liver failure (Morazzoni and Bombardelli, 1995; Habib, Bond, and Heuman, 2001).

The clinical symptoms of liver disease are jaundice (yellowing of the skin), enlarged liver, ascites (pooling of fluid in the abdominal cavity), and encephalopathy (breakdown of brain tissue leading to impaired consciousness). Liver disease is characterized by a buildup of liver enzymes in the blood. These enzymes include aspartate aminotransferase (AST, also known as glutamic oxalacetic transaminase or GOT), alanine aminotransferase (ALT, also know as glutamic pyruvate transaminase or GPT), gamma-glutamyl transferase (GGT), and alkaline phosphatase. Three laboratory parameters are used routinely to assess liver function: serum bilirubin, serum albumin, and plasma prothrombin time. The yellow coloring characteristic of jaundice is caused by a buildup of bilirubin in the blood. Bilirubin is a yellow pigment formed by the breakdown of red blood cells that is normally secreted by the liver in bile. Plasma prothrombin time (international normalized ratio [INR], a blood clotting index) is a useful indicator of liver function, since it is dependent upon blood clotting factor VII, which is produced by the liver (Habib, Bond, and Heuman, 2001).

The presence and severity of cirrhosis has been graded using an index called the Child-Turcotte-Pugh (CTP) score. The CTP score is the sum of five parameter scores (prothrombin time, bilirubin, albumin, ascites, and encephalopathy). Lower CTP scores of relatively healthy subjects are classified as Child's Class A, moderate scores are classified as Child's Class B, and the high scores of subjects requiring liver transplants are classified as Child's Class C (Habib, Bond, and Heuman, 2001). Milk thistle has generally been used to treat those with cirrhosis categorized as Child's Class A.

Legalon

Twelve trials are reviewed that evaluate the potential benefit of Legalon on liver disease due to alcohol or other toxins. The usual dose was 420 mg silymarin, equivalent to 600 mg extract.

Alcoholic Liver Disease

The first trial included 36 adults with chronic alcoholic liver disease who were treated with 140 mg silymarin three times daily (420 mg per day) or placebo for six months. Significant improvement was reported for the silymarin group compared to baseline and to placebo. Serum bilirubin and liver enzymes AST and ALT were normalized, whereas GGT activity decreased (Feher et al., 1989).

In the second trial, 59 subjects with a history of alcoholism were treated with a lower dose of silymarin (140 mg twice daily, 280 mg per day) or placebo for 15 months. Those who ceased drinking had a significant fall in GGT, but more than half the subjects in both groups continued to drink. Overall there was no difference from placebo in mortality or laboratory tests (Bunout et al., 1992). Our reviewers, Drs. Karriem Ali and Richard Aranda, commented that there were some important differences existed in the two groups at the start of the study. GGT levels were different, indicating the silymarin group may have been heavier alcohol users. Differences in prothrombin time and total Child index indicated that the placebo group might have had more severe illness. They also commented that physicians conducting trials on alcoholic liver disease have a tendency to include the promotion of alcohol abstention in their protocol design. However, the deliberate alteration of alcohol consumption introduces a confounding variable that has the potential to affect agent pharmacokinetics, laboratory values, side effects, etc.

In a much shorter trial, 66 subjects with toxic liver damage, most often due to alcohol, were treated with 140 mg silymarin three times daily or placebo for one month. Elevated plasma transaminase levels (AST, ALT, and GGT) were significantly reduced in the silymarin group compared to the placebo group, and, in some cases, returning to normal values much sooner than in the placebo group (Fintelmann and Albert, 1980).

Another one-month study included 97 subjects with alcohol-induced slight acute and subacute liver disease with elevated serum transaminase levels (AST and ALT), despite the order to abstain from drinking alcohol. They were treated with 140 mg silymarin three times daily or placebo. As a result, a statistically significant reduction in ALT and AST levels was observed in the silymarin group in comparison to the placebo group. There was also a trend toward a reduction in bilirubin levels in the treatment group, although this change was not statistically significant (Salmi and Sarna, 1982).

A well-conducted trial with 81 subjects with alcoholic hepatitis, with or without cirrhosis, reported significant improvement after three months compared to baseline in liver biopsy histology scores and laboratory parameters in both the silymarin group (420 mg per day) and the placebo group. No significant difference was found between treatment groups. However, there were large statistical differences in both biopsy histology scores and serum transaminase levels between those who stopped drinking and those who continued to drink (Trinchet et al., 1989). Our reviewers commented that this finding illustrates the complication of promoting alcohol abstention as part of the study design.

A poor-quality trial, including 60 subjects with alcoholic cirrhosis, compared silymarin to a Hungarian hepatoprotective agent, Aica-P (4-amino-5-imidazol-carboxamid-phosphate) and placebo in a three-arm study lasting one month. Significant improvements were observed in both treatment groups (420 mg silymarin or 600 mg Aica-P per day) compared to placebo. Significant reductions in plasma transaminase levels (AST, ALT, and GGT) and bilirubin levels were observed in the silymarin group. Only AST and GGT were significantly reduced in the Aica-P group (Lang et al., 1990).

A well-conducted study included 125 alcoholics with cirrhosis of the liver who were asked to abstain from drinking alcohol. The subjects were given either 450 mg silymarin or placebo daily for two years. The study reported no difference in survival rate or disease state in alcoholics with cirrhosis given either treatment (Pares et al., 1998). Our reviewers pointed out that the majority of these patients were rated as having a disease severity of Child's Class B, but those rated as Child's Class A and C were also included. Disease severity may be an important variable to take into consideration in the efficacy of milk thistle.

The importance of disease severity was indicated in another good-quality trial that analyzed subgroups according to Child's Class. This study included 105 patients diagnosed as having alcoholic or non-alcoholic cirrhosis who were given either 420 mg silymarin per day or placebo and followed for two to six years (mean: 41 months). The four-year survival rate was significantly greater for the silymarin group compared to placebo, whereas the two-year survival rate showed only a trend toward benefit. When subgroups were analyzed, survival was significantly increased for those with alcoholic cirrhosis and those rated as Child's Class A. However, no statistical benefit was observed for those rated with more severe illness, Child's Classes B and C, or for those with nonalcoholic cirrhosis (Ferenci et al., 1989).

In another study, 138 patients with alcoholic or non-alcoholic cirrhosis were given either 420 silymarin mg per day or placebo for four years. The proportion of survivors was greater in the silymarin group compared to placebo, but not significantly. When patients were subdivided into cases of alcoholic and nonalcoholic cirrhosis, it was found that the survival rate was significantly improved for those with alcoholic cirrhosis. However, no significant increase in survival was seen for those with nonalcoholic cirrhosis taking silymarin (Benda et al., 1980).

Sixty non-insulin-dependent diabetics with alcoholic cirrhosis were given either silymarin (200 mg three times daily) or placebo for one year in addition to standard diabetic therapy. All subjects had given up alcohol for at least two years prior to the study. As a result of treatment with silymarin, there was a significant decrease in fasting blood glucose levels, mean daily blood glucose levels, glucosuria (glucose in urine), and glycosylated hemoglobin levels. In addition, levels of malondialdehyde were reduced, indicating improvement in liver function (Velussi et al., 1997). A fault of this trial was that the control group did not receive a placebo, and as a result the trial was not blinded.

Liver Disease Caused by Hepatoxins Other Than Alcohol

Two studies examined the effect of silymarin (Legalon) on liver damage induced by toxins other than alcohol. In the first study, 49 workers with liver disease attributable to toluene and/or xylene exposure were treated with 420 mg silymarin or placebo for one month. At the end of that time, signs of clinical improvement as well as significant decreases in serum AST and ALT and an increase in platelet counts in the silymarin group were observed. These parameters remained unchanged or worsened in the control group (Szilard, Szentgyorgyi, and Demeter, 1988).

In another study, 14 subjects exposed to an organophosphate pesticide (malathion) were matched with ten volunteers not exposed to the pesticide. Both groups were given 420 mg silymarin per day for one month. In the group exposed to pesticides, levels of GGT, cholinesterase, and leucine aminopeptidase increased significantly with silymarin treatment, whereas plasma levels of lipids and trigylcerides decreased significantly compared to baseline. Similar changes, also statistically significant, but to a lesser extent, were observed in the control group, with the exception that no change was seen in cholinesterase levels. Since the pesticide is known to have anticholinesterase activity, the authors speculated that silymarin may be reversing or blocking that action. By inhibiting the anticholinesterase activity, silymarin may reduce the toxic effect of organophosphates (Boari et al., 1981). However, the conclusion was weakened by the poor quality of the trial, which lacked a placebo group.

Silipide

Two double-blind, placebo-controlled studies were conducted with Silipide, a milk thistle extract (silybin) combined with phosphatidylcholine.

Chronic Hepatitis

A well-conducted study with 65 subjects with chronic persistent hepatitis proven with a biopsy were treated for three months with placebo or 240 mg silybin per day. As a result, a statistically significant reduction in serum aminotransferases (AST and ALT) was observed in the treatment group compared to placebo (Marcelli et al., 1992).

Viral Hepatitis

In a short pilot study, 20 patients with active viral hepatitis due to hepatitis B and/or C were treated with either 480 mg silybin or placebo for one week. A significant decrease in serum aminotransferases (AST, ALT, and GGT) and bilirubin levels was observed in the treated group compared to the placebo group (Buzzelli et al., 1993).

Silimarina

Hepatitis or Cirrhosis

A study with 177 subjects included those with chronic persistent hepatitis, chronic active hepatitis, or cirrhosis. Subjects with the three disease types were randomized to receive either placebo or Silimarina (210 mg silybin) daily for 40 days. Clinical improvement was reported for all groups in comparison to placebo. However, laboratory tests as a whole failed to show any improvement (Tanasescu et al., 1988). The published report of this study did not include any details of the 25 symptoms that were said to be included in the clinical assessment. Therefore, no details of the potential clinical benefit were available. The dose was also about half that used in most other studies.

Generic

Drug-Induced Liver Damage

The ability of silymarin to prevent liver damage due to psychotropic drugs was examined in a trial with 60 subjects who had been treated with phenothiazines and/or butyrophenones for at least five years. These subjects had AST and ALT activity more than twice the normal value. Half the participants suspended their intake of psychotropic drugs, and both groups were further divided into those who received silymarin, 800 mg per day, and those who received placebo. Serum levels of malondialdehyde (MDA) were used as indicators of oxidative liver damage, because MDA is an end product of the oxidation of polyunsaturated fatty acids. After three months, serum levels of MDA decreased significantly in subjects who suspended use of the psychotropic drugs. Little difference was observed between those subjects receiving silymarin and those receiving placebo. For those who continued to take the psychotropic drugs, a significant difference in MDA values was observed between those who also received silymarin and those who received placebo. The decrease in AST and ALT values was greatest for those who discontinued the use of psychotropic drugs, and there was little difference as to whether they received silymarin (Palasciano et al., 1994).

META-ANALYSES AND SYSTEMATIC REVIEWS

The Agency for Healthcare Research and Quality (AHRQ), U.S. Department of Health and Human Services, sponsored a systematic review of milk thistle through one of its evidence-based practice centers (EPC) (Lawrence et al., 2000). A synopsis of this report was published in the American Journal of Medicine (Jacobs, et al., 2002). The evidence report summarized the effects of milk thistle on liver disease and cirrhosis, as well as clinical adverse effects. Sixteen prospective trials were included—14 were randomized, blinded, and placebo-controlled. Four trials reported outcomes for mortality among 433 participants with an overall odds ratio for mortality of 0.8, showing a slight benefit for those taking milk thistle. Three trials involving 237 participants assessed the physical appearance of the liver using biopsy specimens. Variable results were reported, with the highest quality trial reporting no effect, and two others reporting positive benefits. The majority of trials reported a greater reduction in ALT and AST levels with milk thistle compared to placebo (11 trials with 840 participants and 12 trials with 838 participants, respectively). Five studies assessed serum albumin levels (476 participants) reporting a greater reduction with milk thistle compared to placebo (0.06

g/dl). Six trials involving 496 participants reported changes in prothrombin times, with a two-second greater reduction with milk thistle compared with placebo. In general, meta-analysis showed positive, but small and insignificant effect sizes. The AHRQ study concluded that the clinical efficacy of milk thistle is not clearly established. Interpretation of the evidence was hampered by poor study methods and/or poor quality of the published reports. Available evidence was not sufficient to suggest whether milk thistle may be more effective for some liver diseases than others, or if effectiveness might be related to duration of treatment or the length or severity of the liver disease (Lawrence et al., 2000). Jacobs and co-workers (2002) were more blunt in their analysis. They concluded that milk thistle has no effect on mortality or improvements in liver histology or biochemical markers of liver function among patients with chronic liver disease. They found insufficient evidence to recommend milk thistle to patients for the treatment of liver disease (Jacobs, et al., 2002).

ADVERSE REACTIONS OR SIDE EFFECTS

No significant side effects were reported in the trials conducted with Legalon that we reviewed. Eight trials reported no side effects or adverse reactions, and four trials reported minor complaints that were not different from that of the placebo group. These included arthralgias, pruritis, headache, urticaria, constipation, dryness of the mouth, nausea, abdominal discomfort, and a mild laxative effect (Bunout et al, 1992; Pares, et al., 1998; Ferenci et al, 1989; Boari et al, 1981). One of the trials on silipide did not report any side effects, and the other reported side effects similar to those reported previously and no different from placebo (Marcelli et al., 1992).

The AHRQ review found that milk thistle was associated with few, generally minor adverse effects, although little evidence was present to demonstrate that these effects were indeed caused by milk thistle. For randomized trials reporting adverse effects, the incidence of adverse effects was similar to that of placebo groups. The most common side effects were gastrointestinal problems, skin reactions, and headache. An extended review of the literature found three case reports of anaphylaxis, but in only one case was this reaction possibly attributed to milk thistle (Lawrence et al., 2000).

A drug monitoring study observed 2,637 patients treated for eight weeks with Legalon. The majority of patients took one tablet three times daily and almost a third of the subjects took two tablets three times daily (each tablet containing 70 mg silymarin each). Twenty-one patients (0.8 percent) reported adverse reactions that included mild diarrhea, nausea, gastric intolerance, pruritis, rash, and headache (Albrecht et al., 1992).

The possible interaction between milk thistle and indinavir was evaluated in an open study with ten healthy volunteers. Indinavir is a common therapy for patients with human immunodeficiency virus (HIV). This study was conducted because milk thistle is commonly taken by patients with HIV for the treatment or prevention of liver disease caused by hepatitis or hepatotoxic drugs. Blood levels of indinavir were established following four doses of indinavir (800 mg every eight hours). Subjects then took 175 mg milk thistle extract (Thisilyn) (containing 153 mg silymarin) three times a day for three weeks. Then administration of indinavir was added to the milk thistle treatment, and the blood sampling was repeated in the same pattern as before. Measurements of indinavir blood levels were again repeated after an 11-day washout period. As a result, milk thistle did not significantly alter the indinavir blood levels. The authors concluded that milk thistle, in commonly administered dosages, should not interfere with indinavir therapy (Piscitelli et al., 2002).

INFORMATION FROM PHARMACOPOEIAL MONOGRAPHS

Source of Published Therapeutic Monographs

German Commission E

Indications

The German Commission E approves of preparations of the ripe seed of milk thistle for dyspeptic complaints. An extract of the seed, standardized to at least 70 percent silymarin (a composite of silibinin, silydianin, and silychristin), is approved for treatment of toxic liver damage and for supportive treatment in chronic inflammatory liver disease and hepatic cirrhosis (Blumenthal et al., 1998).

Doses

> Seed: 12 to 15 g daily (Blumenthal et al., 1998)
> Extract: equivalent to 200 to 400 mg of silymarin, calculated as silibinin, daily (Blumenthal et al., 1998)

Contraindications

The Commission E lists no known contraindications (Blumenthal et al., 1998).

Adverse Reactions

The Commission E mentions that with the extract, a mild laxative effect has been observed in occasional instances (Blumenthal et al., 1998).

Drug Interactions

The Commission E lists no known drug interactions (Blumenthal et al., 1998).

REFERENCES

Albrecht M, Frerick H, Kuhn U, Strenge-Hesse A (1992). The treatment of toxic liver damage with Legalon. *Zeitschrift Klinische Medizin* 47 (2): 87-92.

Benda L, Dittrich H, Ferenzi P, Frank H, Wewalka F (1980). The efficacy of silymarin and the survival of patients with hepatic cirrhosis. *Wiener Klinische Wochenschrift* 92 (19): 678-983.

Blumenthal M, Busse W, Hall T, Goldberg A, Grünwald J, Riggins C, Rister S, eds. (1998). *The Complete German Commission E Monographs: Therapeutic Guide to Herbal Medicines.* Trans. S. Klein. Austin: American Botanical Council.

Boari C, Baldi E, Rizzoli O, Raffi GB, Caudarella R, Gennari P (1981). Silymarin in the protection against exogenous noxae. *Drugs Under Experimental and Clinical Research* 7 (2): 115-120.

Bunout D, Hirsch S, Petermann M, Pia de la Maza M, Silva G, Kelly M, Ugarte G, Iturriaga H (1992). Effects of silymarin on alcoholic liver disease (a controlled trial). *Revista Médica de Chile* 120 (12): 1370-1375.

Buzzelli G, Moscarella S, Giusti A, Duchini A, Marena C, Lampertico M (1993). A pilot study on the liver protective effect of silybinphosphatidylcholine complex (IdB1016) in chronic active hepatitis. *International Journal of Clinical Pharmacology, Therapy, and Toxicology* 31 (9): 456-460.

Feher J, Deak G, Muzes G, Lang I, Niederland V, Nekam K, Karteszl M (1989). The hepatoprotective effect of treatment with silymarin in patients with chronic alcoholic liver disease. *Orvosi Hetilap* 130 (51): 2723-2727.

Ferenci P, Dragosics B, Dittrich H, Frank H, Benda L, Lochs H, Mervn S, Base W, Schneider B (1989). Randomized controlled trial of silymarin treatment in patients with cirrhosis of the liver. *Journal of Hepatology* 9 (1): 105-113.

Fintelmann V, Albert A (1980). The therapeutic activity of Legalon in toxic hepatic disorders demonstrated in a double blind trial. *Therapiewoche* 30 (35): 5589-5594.

Habib A, Bond WM, Heuman DM (2001). Long-term management of cirrhosis: Appropriate supportive care is both critical and difficult. *Postgraduate Medicine* 109 (3): 101-113.

Jacobs BP, Dennehy C, Ramirez G, Sapp J, Lawrence VA (2002). Milk thistle for the treatment of liver disease: A systematic review and meta-analysis. *American Journal of Medicine* 113 (6): 506-515.

Lang I, Nekam K, Deak G, Muzes G, Gonzales-Cabello R, Gergely P, Csomos G, Feher J (1990). Immunomodulatory and hepatoprotective effects of in vivo treatment with free radical scavengers. *Italian Journal of Gastroenterology* 22 (5): 283-287.

Lawrence V, Jacobs B, Dennehy C, Sapp J, Ramirez G, Aguilar C, Montgomery K, Morbidoni L, Arterburn J, Chiquette E, et al. (2000). Milk thistle: Effects on liver disease and cirrhosis and clinical adverse effects. *Evidence Report/Technology Assessment* No. 21, AHRQ Publication No. 01-E025. Rockville, MD: Agency for Healthcare Research and Quality.

Marcelli R, Bizzoni P, Conte D, Lisena MO, Lampertico M, Marena C, De Marco MF, Del Ninno E (1992). Randomized controlled study of the efficacy and tolerability of a short course of IdB 1016 in the treatment of chronic persistent hepatitis. *European Bulletin of Drug Research* 1 (3): 131-135.

Morazzoni P, Bombardelli E (1995). *Silymarin marianum (Carduus marianus). Fitoterapia* 66 (1): 3-42.

Palasciano G, Portincasa P, Palmieri V, Ciani D, Vendemiale G, Altomare E (1994). The effect of silymarin on plasma levels of malon dialdehyde in patients receiving long-term treatment with psychotropic drugs. *Current Therapeutic Research* 55 (5): 537-545.

Pares A, Planas R, Torres M, Caballeria J, Viver JM, Acero D, Panes J, Rigau J, Santos J, Rodes J (1998). Effects of silymarin in alcoholic patients with cirrhosis of the liver: Results of a controlled, double-blind, randomized, and multicenter trial. *Journal of Hepatology* 28 (4): 615-621.

Piscitelli SC, Formentini E, Burstein AH, Alfaro R, Jagannatha S, Falloon J (2002). Effect of milk thistle on the pharmacokinetics of indinavir in healthy volunteers. *Pharmacotherapy* 22 (5): 551-556.

Salmi HA, Sarna S (1982). Effect of silymarin on chemical, functional, and morphological alterations of the liver. *Scandinavian Journal of Gastroenterology* 17 (4): 517-521.

Schulz V, Hänsel R, Tyler VE (2001). *Rational Phytotherapy: A Physicians' Guide to Herbal Medicine,* Fourth Edition. Trans. TC Telgar. Berlin: Springer-Verlag.

Szilard S, Szentgyorgyi D, Demeter I (1988). Protective effect of Legalon in workers exposed to organic solvents. *Acta Medica Hungarica* 45 (2): 249-256.

Tanasescu C, Petrea S, Baldescu R, Macarie E, Chiriloiu C, Purice S (1988). Use of the Romanian product Silimarina in the treatment of chronic liver diseases. *Revue Roumaine de Medecine-Medecine Interne* 26 (4): 311-322.

Trinchet JC, Coste T, Levy VG, Vivet F, Duchatelle V, Legendre C, Gotheil C, Beaugrand M (1989). Treatment of alcoholic hepatitis with silymarin: Comparative double-blind trial in 116 patients. *Gastroenterologie Clinique et Biologique* 13 (2): 120-124.

Velussi M, Cernigoi AM, De Monte A, Dapas F, Caffau C, Zilli M (1997). Long-term (12 month) treatment with an anti-oxidant drug (silymarin) is effective on hyperinsulinemia, exogenous insulin need and malondialdehyde levels in cirrhotic diabetic patients. *Journal of Hepatology* 26 (4): 871-879.

DETAILS ON MILK THISTLE PRODUCTS AND CLINICAL STUDIES

Product and clinical study information is grouped in the same order as in the Summary Table. A profile on an individual product is followed by details of the clinical studies associated with that product. In some instances, a clinical study, or studies, supports several products that contain the same principal ingredient(s). In these instances, those products are grouped together.

Clinical studies that follow each product, or group of products, are grouped by therapeutic indication, in accordance with the order in the Summary Table.

Index to Milk Thistle Products

Product Profile: Legalon®

Manufacturer	**Madaus AG, Germany**
U.S. distributor	None
Botanical ingredient	**Milk thistle seed extract**
Extract name	None given
Quantity	173-186.7 mg dry extract, equivalent to 140 mg silymarin
Processing	Plant to extract ratio 36-44:1, extracted with ethylacetate
Standardization	140 mg silymarin calculated as silibinin
Formulation	Capsule

Recommended dose: Take one capsule three times daily when starting treatment and also in serious cases. A maintenance dose of one capsule three times daily is recommended. The capsules should be swallowed whole with a small amount of liquid.

DSHEA structure/function: German drug indications include toxic liver damage and supportive treatment in cases of chronic inflammatory liver diseases and hepatic cirrhosis.

Cautions: Should jaundice become apparent (pale to dark yellow coloration of the skin, yellow coloration of the whites of the eyes) a doctor should be consulted. There have been no adequate investigations of the use of this medicine in children. It should therefore not be used in children under 12 years of age. No results are available regarding the use of Legalon 140 during pregnancy or lactation. It should therefore be used only after consultation with your doctor. If symptoms persist for any length of time you should consult your doctor.

Other ingredients: Mannitol, sodium carboxymethyl starch, polysorbate 80, polyvidone, magnesium stearate, gelatin, titanium dioxide E171, ferric oxide E172, dodecyl sodium sulphate.

Source(s) of information: Product information page (www.madaus. de); information provided by Nature's Way Products, Inc.

Clinical Study: Legalon®

Extract name	None given
Manufacturer	Madaus AG, Germany
Indication	**Alcoholic liver disease**
Level of evidence	**III**
Therapeutic benefit	**Yes**

Bibliographic reference
Feher J, Deak G, Muzes G, Lang I, Niederland V, Nekam K, Karteszl M (1989). The hepatoprotective effect of treatment with silymarin in patients with chronic alcoholic liver disease. *Orvosi Hetilap* 130 (51): 2723-2727.

Trial design
Parallel. Patients were encouraged to refrain from drinking alcohol.

Study duration	6 months
Dose	140 mg silymarin capsule 3 times daily
Route of administration	Oral
Randomized	Yes

Randomization adequate   No
Blinding   Double-blind
Blinding adequate   Yes

Placebo   Yes
Drug comparison   No

Site description   Single center

No. of subjects enrolled   36
No. of subjects completed 36
Sex   Male and female
Age   Mean: 46 ± 7 years

Inclusion criteria
Patients with chronic alcoholic liver disease in whom daily average alcohol consumption exceeded 60 g (men) and 30 g (women). The duration of the chronic alcohol consumption was 8 ± 4 years.

Exclusion criteria
Symptoms or signs of encephalopathy, malnutrition, or other alcohol-associated disease, positive tests for viral and immunological markers, or previous corticosteroid or other immunosuppressive treatment.

End points
Patients were assessed at entry into the trial and after three and six months of treatment. Laboratory parameters included: serum aspartate aminotransferase (AST); alanine aminotransferase (ALT); gamma-glutamyl transferase (GGT); alkaline phosphatase and bilirubin; as well as procollagen III peptide levels. Liver biopsies were also obtained.

Results
During silymarin treatment, serum bilirubin, AST, and ALT values were normalized, and GGT activity and procollagen III peptide level decreased. The changes from baseline levels, as well as the difference between posttreatment values of the two groups were significant. In the placebo group only GGT values decreased significantly but to a lesser extent than that in the silymarin group. The histological alterations showed an improvement in the silymarin group and were unchanged in the placebo group.

Side effects
None noted.

Authors' comments
These results indicate that silymarin exerts hepatoprotective activity and is able to improve liver function.

Reviewers' comments
Alcohol consumption was not measured quantitatively, and this may confound the results. The deliberate alteration of alcohol consumption introduces a confounding covariable that has the potential to affect agent pharmacokinetics, laboratory values, experienced side effects, etc. Biopsies were performed only on select patients in each group, creating a potential selection bias. The treatment length was adequate for a study of histology and serum biochemistry changes. (Translation reviewed) (2, 4)

Clinical Study: Legalon®

Extract name	None given
Manufacturer	Madaus AG, Germany
Indication	**Alcoholic liver disease**
Level of evidence	**III**
Therapeutic benefit	**Undetermined**

Bibliographic reference
Bunout D, Hirsch S, Petermann M, Pia de la Maza M, Silva G, Kelly M, Ugarte G, Iturriaga H (1992). Effects of silymarin on alcoholic liver disease (a controlled trial). *Revista Médica de Chile* 120 (12): 1370-1375.

Trial design
Parallel.

Study duration	15 months
Dose	2 (140 mg silymarin) capsules daily
Route of administration	Oral
Randomized	Yes
Randomization adequate	Yes
Blinding	Double-blind
Blinding adequate	No
Placebo	Yes
Drug comparison	No
Site description	Single center
No. of subjects enrolled	72
No. of subjects completed	59
Sex	Male and female
Age	Mean: 49.8 ± 2.4 years

Inclusion criteria
Patients having history of alcoholism (ingestion of at least 150 g/day alcohol or drinking attacks of more than three days at least once a month) and the presence of clinical signs (jaundice, ascites, edema, or encephalopathy) or lab values (total bilirubin more than 2 mg/dl, prothorombin time below 75 percent of control, or albumin below 3 mg/dl) indicating liver insufficiency.

Exclusion criteria
Patients with positive hepatitis B surface antigen, with renal or cardiac insufficiency, terminal liver damage.

End points
Patients were examined at least once a month for 15 months. Patients were asked about alcohol ingestion and possible adverse effects, and urine specimens were obtained. Hematocrit, albumin, creatinine, urea nitrogen, total bilirubin, aspartate aminotransferase, alkaline phosphatase, gamma-glutamyl transferase (GGT), prothrombin time (PT percent), and glycemia were measured every three months. Composite Clinical and Laboratory Index (CCLI) scoring was calculated from clinical and laboratory data as an indication of disease severity and prognosis.

Results
Ten patients died during the study, five taking placebo and five taking silymarin. Those patients who died had higher clinical CCLI and total baseline CCLI than those who survived. Final laboratory values and their changes revealed no difference between the placebo and silymarin groups. Twenty-two patients on placebo (65 percent) and 14 on silymarin (58 percent) continued to drink. Those who abstained had a significant fall in GGT during follow-up. No other significant differences were observed between these two groups.

Side effects
Adverse events included pruritus, cephalea, constipation, dryness of the mouth, and abdominal pain with no difference between the placebo and silymarin groups.

Authors' comments
This study did not show a beneficial effect of the treatment with silymarin on the evolution and mortality of patients affected by alcohol-induced liver damage.

Reviewers' comments
In contrast to what is stated in the paper, significant differences were observed in the baseline GGT and PT percent values between the placebo group and silymarin group. The GGT difference shows that silymarin group subjects may have been heavier alcohol users. The differences in PT per-

cent and CCLI show that placebo group subjects may have had more severe illness. Altogether, this implies that randomization did not yield well-matched groups. Deliberate reduction in alcohol consumption introduces a confounding covariable that has the potential to affect agent pharmacokinetics, laboratory values, experienced side effects, etc. Abstention from alcohol was not consistent for all subjects. The exclusion criteria should have also included other causes of cirrhosis by serology, etc., as well as drug exclusions (e.g., D-penicillamine, colchicine). The sample size may have been appropriate. However, no power calculation was presented. The dose of 280 mg is one-third smaller than most other studies. The adverse incidence of pruritis could have been related to alcohol abstention. The trial length is adequate. (Translation reviewed) (3, 4)

Clinical Study: Legalon®

Extract name	None given
Manufacturer	Madaus AG, Germany
Indication	**Alcoholic or nonalcoholic liver disease**
Level of evidence	**III**
Therapeutic benefit	**Undetermined**

Bibliographic reference
Fintelmann V, Albert A (1980). The therapeutic activity of Legalon in toxic hepatic disorders demonstrated in a double blind trial. *Therapiewoche* 30 (35): 5589-5594.

Trial design
Parallel. Patients received a "uniform reducing diet" high in protein and low in carbohydrates and fat (1,000 calories/day).

Study duration	1 month
Dose	1 (140 mg silymarin) capsule 3 times daily
Route of administration	Oral
Randomized	Yes
Randomization adequate	Yes
Blinding	Double-blind
Blinding adequate	No
Placebo	Yes
Drug comparison	No
Site description	Hospital

No. of subjects enrolled 70
No. of subjects completed 66
Sex Male and female
Age Not given

Inclusion criteria
Patients with clinical and serological diagnosis of toxic liver damage. The cause of toxic damage was not taken in account, but in most cases it was alcohol.

Exclusion criteria
None mentioned.

End points
Diagnosis of toxic liver damage was confirmed by liver biopsy. Laboratory parameters (aspartate aminotransferase [AST], alanine aminotransferase [ALT], and gamma glutamyl transferase [GGT]) were determined on days 1, 3, 7, 10, 14, 21, and 28. At the start of the trial, and on days 14 and 28, additional parameters were determined: glutamate dehydrogenase, alkaline phosphatase, leucine aminopeptidase (LAP), cholinesterase, bilirubin, total proteins, electrophoresis, as well as sonographic assessment of the liver size and internal structure.

Results
The parameters AST ($p < 0.1$), ALT ($p < 0.05$) and GGT ($p < 0.05$) were reduced significantly in the silymarin group compared to the placebo group, sometimes returning to normal in a much shorter time than in the placebo group. The differences for glutamate dehydrogenase, LAP, and alkaline phosphatase were not statistically significant. The sonographic findings were not exact enough to be relevant to the outcome of the trial.

Side effects
None attributed to Legalon.

Authors' comments
Previously reported investigations and the outcome of the present trial justify the conclusion that the therapeutic activity of Legalon in toxic disorders of the liver has definitively been established.

Reviewers' comments
No baseline data was presented, the diagnostic criteria was not thoroughly discussed, and the "uniform reducing diet" is a confounding covariable. The grouping of all toxic liver disorders together may have obscured the potential to demonstrate the efficacy of Legalon in the treatment of any particular liver disorder. The sample size may have been appropriate. However, no power calculation was presented. (Translation reviewed) (3, 3)

Clinical Study: Legalon®

Extract name	None given
Manufacturer	Madaus AG, Germany
Indication	**Alcoholic liver disease**
Level of evidence	**III**
Therapeutic benefit	**Trend**

Bibliographic reference

Salmi HA, Sarna S (1982). Effect of silymarin on chemical, functional, and morphological alterations of the liver. *Scandinavian Journal of Gastroenterology* 17 (4): 517-521.

Trial design

Parallel. Patients were treated for the first week in the hospital and thereafter as outpatients.

Study duration	1 month
Dose	420 mg daily
Route of administration	Oral
Randomized	Yes
Randomization adequate	No
Blinding	Double-blind
Blinding adequate	No
Placebo	Yes
Drug comparison	No
Site description	Military hospital
No. of subjects enrolled	106
No. of subjects completed	97
Sex	Male and female
Age	Mean: 37 ± 15.7 years

Inclusion criteria

Patients admitted to the hospital with an increase in the transaminase (serum aspartate aminotransferase [AST]; and serum alanine amino transferase [ALT]) levels of at least one month's duration, despite the order to abstain completely from alcohol. Patients had slight acute and subacute liver disease, mostly induced by alcohol abuse.

Exclusion criteria

None mentioned.

End points
Patients were examined before the trial, as well as after one, two, and three weeks. Laboratory tests included serum bilirubin, alkaline phosphatase, bromosulphalein (BSP), serum immunoglobulins, and blind liver biopsy.

Results
There was statistically a significantly greater decrease of ALT and AST in the treated group than in controls. Serum total and conjugated bilirubin decreased more in the treated group than in controls, but the differences were not statistically significant. BSP retention returned to normal significantly more often in the treated group. The mean percentage of decrease of BSP was also markedly higher in the treated group. Normalization of histological changes occurred significantly more often in the treated group than in controls.

Side effects
None reported.

Authors' comments
Silymarin appears to have a favorable effect on acute and subacute alcohol-induced liver disease of relatively slight degree. The results cannot be extrapolated to liver disease in general.

Reviewers' comments
The biopsy rate for the two groups was similar, but the reason for the low rate overall was not explained. The histological findings therefore may involve inadvertent selection bias. The trial may have been too short to allow resolution of a trend away from baseline. Transaminase levels remained very close, although the mean percentage decrease was reported to be significant. The deliberate promotion of abstention from alcohol consumption introduces a confounding covariable that has the potential to affect agent pharmacokinteics, laboratory values, experienced side effects, etc. At a minimum, a reevaluation should be conducted after a period of verifiable abstention to check baseline lab values. The sample size may have been adequate. However, no power calculation was presented. (1, 5)

Clinical Study: Legalon®

Extract name	None given
Manufacturer	Madaus AG, Germany
Indication	**Alcoholic hepatitis**
Level of evidence	**I**
Therapeutic benefit	**No**

Bibliographic reference
Trinchet JC, Coste T, Levy VG, Vivet F, Duchatelle V, Legendre C, Gotheil C, Beaugrand M (1989). Treatment of alcoholic hepatitis with silymarin: Comparative double-blind trial in 116 patients. *Gastroenterologie Clinique et Biologique* 13 (2): 120-124.

Trial design
Parallel.

Study duration	3 months
Dose	140 mg silymarin capsule 3 times daily
Route of administration	Oral
Randomized	Yes
Randomization adequate	Yes
Blinding	Double-blind
Blinding adequate	Yes
Placebo	Yes
Drug comparison	No
Site description	Multicenter
No. of subjects enrolled	116
No. of subjects completed	81
Sex	Male and female
Age	Mean 50.5 ± 10.5 years

Inclusion criteria
Patients with histologically proven alcoholic hepatitis confirmed by percutaneous liver biopsy, with or without cirrhosis.

Exclusion criteria
Patients with hepatic encephalopathy, diuretic-resistant ascites, or disorders of hemostasis contraindicating percutaneous liver biopsy, or hepatocellular carcinoma. The use of any other antihepatotoxic treatment or corticosteroid therapy was prohibited during the study.

End points
At the beginning and end of trial, the following lab parameters were measured: serum bilirubin, serum aspartateaminotransferase (AST) and gamma-glutamyl transpeptidase (GGT), PT, mean corpuscular volume (MCV) and serum albumin. A percutaneous liver biopsy was performed in all cases to determine the histological score at both times.

Results
Significant improvement in the score of alcoholic hepatitis and serum amino

transferase activity was noted in both groups during the trial, irrespective of treatment. At the end of the trial, 46 percent of patients had completely stopped drinking alcohol; these patients were equally distributed between the two groups. There were significant improvements in hepatitis scores, as well as in levels of serum AST ($p < 0.01$), GGT ($p < 0.0001$), and MCV ($p < 0.001$) in subjects who abstained compared to those who continued drinking.

Side effects
No side effects were noted.

Authors' comments
Silymarin treatment in patients with moderate alcoholic hepatitis, with or without cirrhosis, does not alter the biochemical or histological course of the disease.

Reviewers' comments
This is a well-conducted study. It illustrates the effect of promoting alcohol abstention as a confounding variable in protocol design. (Translation reviewed) (5, 6)

Clinical Study: Legalon®

Extract name	None given
Manufacturer	Madaus AG, Germany
Indication	**Alcoholic cirrhosis**
Level of evidence	**III**
Therapeutic benefit	**Trend**

Bibliographic reference
Lang I, Nekam K, Deak G, Muzes G, Gonzales-Cabello R, Gergely P, Csomos G, Feher J (1990). Immunomodulatory and hepatoprotective effects of in vivo treatment with free radical scavengers. *Italian Journal of Gastroenterology* 22 (5): 283-287.

Trial design
Parallel. Three treatment groups: Legalon; Aica-P (amino-imidazol-carbox-amid-phosphate) 200 mg three times daily; and placebo three times daily. All groups were discouraged from consuming alcohol.

Study duration	1 month
Dose	1 (140 mg silymarin) capsule 3 times daily
Route of administration	Oral
Randomized	Yes
Randomization adequate	No
Blinding	Double-blind
Blinding adequate	No
Placebo	Yes
Drug comparison	Yes
Drug name	Aica-P
Site description	Not described
No. of subjects enrolled	60
No. of subjects completed	Not given
Sex	Male and female
Age	Mean: 44.7 years

Inclusion criteria

Patients with alcoholic cirrhosis. The mean daily alcohol consumption exceeded 60 g in men and 30 g in women. The duration of alcohol consumption was between 6 and 11 years. Histological diagnosis was micronodular.

Exclusion criteria

Patients with symptoms of vascular and/or perenchymal decompensation and those positive to hepatitis B surface antigen (HbsAg).

End points

Patients were seen once a week, and alcohol consumption was recorded. Routine laboratory parameters, including aspartate aminotransferase, alanine aminotransferase, gamma-glutamyl transferase, alkaline phosphatase, and bilirubin, as well as cellular immunoreactivity, were determined before and after the treatment period. To evaluate cellular immunoreactivity, lectin-induced lymphoblast transformation, and antibody-dependent cell-mediated cytotoxicity (ADCC) and spontaneous natural killer (NK) lymphocytotoxicity tests were performed, and the percentages of peripheral T-, B-, CD4+, and CD8+ cells were determined.

Results

In the silymarin and Aica-P groups, hepatic functions showed marked improvement following one month of treatment compared to the placebo group. In the silymarin group, there were significant reductions in bilirubin ($p < 0.05$), AST ($p < 0.01$), ALT ($p < 0.02$), and GGT ($p < 0.05$). Only AST ($p < 0.01$) and GGT ($p < 0.0$) were reduced in the Aica-P group. The lectin-induced lymphoblast transformation was increased in both groups ($p <$ 0.01), and a decrease was observed in the percentage of suppressor cells (silymarin: $p < 0.05$; Aica-P: $p < 0.01$). Antibody-dependent cell mediated cytotoxicity was significantly decreased by silymarin, and both treatment groups had significantly reduced NK cell activity. None of these changes occurred in the placebo group.

Side effects
No side effects were seen.

Authors' comments
The hepatoprotective effects of silymarin and Aica-P are accompanied by changes in parameters of cellular immunoreactivity of treated patients.

Reviewers' comments
Only the AST and GGT differed significantly from placebo in the two treatment groups. The sample size may have been appropriate, but no power calculation was presented. The deliberate alteration of alcohol consumption introduces a confounding covariable that has the potential to affect agent pharmacokinetics, laboratory values, experienced side effects, etc. The trial length was adequate. The dose choice was standard in comparison to other trials. (0, 5)

Clinical Study: Legalon®

Extract name	None given
Manufacturer	Madaus Cerafarm, Spain (Madaus AG, Germany)
Indication	**Alcoholic cirrhosis**
Level of evidence	I
Therapeutic benefit	**No**

Bibliographic reference
Pares A, Planas R, Torres M, Caballeria J, Viver JM, Acero D, Panes J, Rigau J, Santos J, Rodes J (1998). Effects of silymarin in alcoholic patients with cirrhosis of the liver: Results of a controlled, double-blind, randomized and multicenter trial. *Journal of Hepatology* 28 (4): 615-621.

Trial design
Parallel. Patients were asked to abstain from alcohol.

Study duration	2 years
Dose	150 mg silymarin 3 times daily

Route of administration	Oral
Randomized	Yes
Randomization adequate	Yes
Blinding	Double-blind
Blinding adequate	Yes
Placebo	Yes
Drug comparison	No
Site description	6 hospitals
No. of subjects enrolled	200
No. of subjects completed	125
Sex	Male and female
Age	Mean: 50.5 ± 10.8 years

Inclusion criteria

Alcoholics with cirrhosis of the lever. Chronic alcoholism defined as a daily ethanol intake greater than 80 g in men and 60 g in women for a period longer than five years. Criteria for liver cirrhosis supported by histology after percutaneous liver biopsy, performed within the three months before inclusion in the trial, or by laparoscopic examination in those patients with very low prothrombin index or platelet count in whom percutaneous liver biopsy could not be performed.

Exclusion criteria

Patients with other known etiologies for liver cirrhosis, such as hepatitis B virus, primary biliary cirrhosis, autoimmunity or crytogenic cirrhosis; those treated with colchicine, malotilate, penicillamine, or corticosteroids; with a life expectancy of less than six months; drug addicted; or pregnant.

End points

The primary outcome was time to death, and the secondary outcome was progression of liver failure. At entry and every three months, a complete history, including alcohol consumption, was recorded. Serum levels of bilirubin, aspartate aminotransferase, alanine aminotransferase, gamma-glutamyl transferase, alkaline phophatase, albumin, gamma globulins, and the prothrombin index were measured.

Results

Twenty-nine patients (15 receiving silymarin and 14 receiving placebo) died during the trial. Survival was similar in patients receiving silymarin or placebo. The effect of silymarin on survival was not influenced by sex, the persistence of alcohol intake, the severity of liver dysfunction, the baseline Child's classification, or by the presence of alcoholic hepatitis. Silymarin did not have any significant effect on the course of the disease.

Side effects

Seven patients in the silymarin group and four in the placebo group reported side effects, but none were serious. These included: arthralgias, pruritis, headache, and urticaria.

Authors' comments

The results of this study indicate that silymarin has no effect on survival and the clinical course in alcoholics with liver cirrhosis.

Reviewers' comments

The majority of patients had a disease severity of Child's Class B. The effect of silymarin may vary distinctly between Classes A, B, and C. Including patients from all three classes may confound the data profile. The sample size may have been appropriate, however, no power calculation was presented. The deliberate alteration of alcohol consumption introduces a confounding covariable that has the potential to affect agent pharmacokinetics, laboratory values, experienced side effects, etc. The listed side effects could be caused, at least in part, by abstention from alcohol. The trial length was adequate. (5, 6)

Clinical Study: Legalon®

Extract name	None given
Manufacturer	Madaus AG, Germany
Indication	**Alcoholic or nonalcoholic cirrhosis**
Level of evidence	**I**
Therapeutic benefit	**Trend**

Bibliographic reference

Ferenci P, Dragosics B, Dittrich H, Frank H, Benda L, Lochs H, Mervn S, Base W, Schneider B (1989). Randomized controlled trial of silymarin treatment in patients with cirrhosis of the liver. *Journal of Hepatology* 9 (1): 105-113.

Trial design

Parallel. All patients were advised to abstain from alcohol.

Study duration	2-6 years (mean: 41 months)
Dose	140 mg silymarin 3 times daily
Route of administration	Oral
Randomized	Yes
Randomization adequate	Yes

Blinding	Double-blind
Blinding adequate	Yes
Placebo	Yes
Drug comparison	No
Site description	4 centers
No. of subjects enrolled	170
No. of subjects completed	105
Sex	Male and female
Age	Mean: 57.5 ± 12 years

Inclusion criteria
Patients with diagnosis of cirrhosis (alcoholic or nonalcoholic) made within two years of the study. All potential candidates were followed for three months before entry into study.

Exclusion criteria
Patients with end-stage liver failure, known malignancies, on immuno-suppressive treatment, and primary biliary cirrhosis. The use of D-peni-cillamine and steroids were not allowed.

End points
At subjects' entry into the study, the severity of the underlying liver disease was classified using the Child-Turcotte criteria, and the etiology was determined using clinical, biochemical, immunological, and histological criteria. At every three months each patient's bilirubin, serum aspartate amino-transferase (AST), alanine aminotransferase (ALT), alkaline phosphatase, gamma-glutamyl transferase (GGT), prothrombin time, albumin, pseudo-cholinesterase, and serum electrophoresis were determined.

Results
The four-year survival rate was 58 ± 9 percent in silymarin-treated patients and 39 ± 9 percent in the placebo group ($p = 0.036$). The two-year survival rate was 82 ± 4 percent for the treatment group and 68 ± 5 percent for the placebo group, an insignificant difference. For those with alcoholic cirrhosis, the number of deaths in the control group was twice that of the treatment group. In addition, treatment was associated with a better outcome ($p = 0.01$). Conversely, in nonalcoholic cirrhotics, the survival rates were not significantly influenced by treatment. In patients originally rated Child's Class A, survival was improved significantly by treatment with silymarin ($p = 0.03$). In those originally rated Classes B or C, survival rates did not differ in comparison to controls. Liver-function lab tests did not reveal a difference in the treatment and control groups.

Side effects
Four patients (two in each group) had side effects of epigastric discomfort and nausea.

Authors' comments
The results of this study suggest that mortality of patients with cirrhosis was reduced by treatment with silymarin. The effect was more pronounced in those with alcoholic cirrhosis.

Reviewers' comments
This is a good-quality study indicating the effectiveness of silymarin in reducing deaths for those with alcoholic cirrhosis and those initially diagnosed as Child's Class A. (5, 6)

Clinical Study: Legalon®

Extract name	None given
Manufacturer	Madaus AG, Germany
Indication	**Alcoholic or nonalcoholic cirrhosis**
Level of evidence	**II**
Therapeutic benefit	**Trend**

Bibliographic reference
Benda L, Dittrich H, Ferenzi P, Frank H, Wewalka F (1980). The efficacy of silymarin and the survival of patients with hepatic cirrhosis. *Wiener Klinische Wochenschrift* 92 (19): 678-983.

Trial design
Parallel. Patients received either silymarin plus a multivitamin mixture, or a multivitamin mixture alone (two capsules three times daily, as placebo).

Study duration	4 years
Dose	2 (70 mg silymarin + multivitamins) capsules 3 times daily
Route of administration	Oral
Randomized	Yes
Randomization adequate	Yes
Blinding	Double-blind
Blinding adequate	Yes
Placebo	Yes
Drug comparison	No

Site description   Not described

No. of subjects enrolled   172
No. of subjects completed 138
Sex   Not given
Age   Not given

Inclusion criteria
Patients with hepatic cirrhosis verified by biopsy, regardless of etiology.

Exclusion criteria
Patients who are moribund, on immunosuppressive therapy during the past year, prednisolone therapy during the past six months, D-penicillamine therapy during the past three months, or with primary biliary cirrhosis or Wilson's disease.

End points
Patients were followed-up every three months, observing the clinical course of cirrhosis and the value of various laboratory findings pertinent to chronic liver disease. The primary end point was survival rate.

Results
The mortality curve showed that the proportion of survivors in the treated group was consistently above the placebo group. Patients were subdivided into cases of alcoholic and nonalcoholic cirrhosis. The survival curves for silymarin and control groups are similar for patients with nonalcoholic forms of cirrhosis. For patients with alcoholic cirrhosis, the survival curve for the silymarin group is clearly above that of the control group ($p = 0.05$). For the control group, there was no difference in the survival curve for subjects with alcoholic or nonalcoholic cirrhosis. However, for subjects taking silymarin, the survival curve for those with alcoholic cirrhosis was clearly above that for those with nonalcoholic cirrhosis ($p < 0.05$). The results of the laboratory investigation were not published here.

Side effects
None observed in treatment group.

Authors' comments
A silymarin therapy for hepatic cirrhosis showed significant prolongation of survival in patients with alcoholic cirrhosis after four years of treatment.

Reviewers' comments
The study shows a trend toward increased survival for patients with alcoholic cirrhosis. Limitations of the study include a lack of baseline status of the patients, ensuring the treatment and control groups were matched as far as severity of illness, and no measurement of compliance to treatment or absti-

nence to alcohol. The dosage of silymarin was supported by reference to biochemical studies. (4, 5)

Clinical Study: Legalon®

Extract name	None given
Manufacturer	IBI Lorenzini, Italy (Madaus AG, Germany)
Indication	**Alcoholic cirrhosis in diabetics**
Level of evidence	**III**
Therapeutic benefit	**Undetermined**

Bibliographic reference
Velussi M, Cernigoi AM, De Monte A, Dapas F, Caffau C, Zilli M (1997). Long-term (12 month) treatment with an anti-oxidant drug (silymarin) is effective on hyperinsulinemia, exogenous insulin need, and malondialdehyde levels in cirrhotic diabetic patients. *Journal of Hepatology* 26 (4): 871-879.

Trial design
Parallel. Treatment group received silymarin plus standard therapy. Control group received standard therapy alone.

Study duration	1 year
Dose	200 mg silymarin 3 times daily 2 hours after meals
Route of administration	Oral
Randomized	Yes
Randomization adequate	No
Blinding	Open
Blinding adequate	No
Placebo	No
Drug comparison	No
Site description	Diabetes clinic
No. of subjects enrolled	60
No. of subjects completed	60
Sex	Male and female
Age	Mean: 62.5 ± 4 years

Inclusion criteria
Ages 45 to 70 years; non-insulin-dependent diabetics with alcoholic liver cirrhosis; body mass index < 29 kg/m²; diabetes diagnosed for a period of at

least five years and treated with insulin only; stable insulin therapy for a period of at least two years; raised endogenous insulin secretion; fasting insulin levels and basal and stimulated C-peptide levels above normal range (above 15 mU/ml for insulin, above 1 ng/ml for basal C-peptide levels, and 3 ng/ml stimulated C-peptide levels); negative for markers of hepatitis A, B, and C; not addicted to alcohol for a period of at least two years prior to the start of the study; no bleeding from variceal esophagus; liver biopsy, performed no more than four years prior to enrollment, demonstrating liver cirrhosis.

Exclusion criteria
Not mentioned.

End points
Every 30 days, fasting and mean daily blood glucose levels, glucosuria (glucose in urine), and mean daily insulin requirements were recorded. Every 60 days, glycosylated hemoglobin (HbA1c) levels were recorded. Every 90 days, fasting insulin, basal and stimulated C-peptide, malondialdehyde, serum aspartate aminotransferase (AST), alanine aminotransferase (ALT), alkaline phosphatase, gamma-glutamyl transferase (GGT), bilirubin, triglycerides, and total and high-density-lipoprotein (HDL) cholesterol were recorded. Every 180 days, creatinine, microalbuminuria, and hemochrome were recorded.

Results
A significant decrease ($p < 0.01$) was observed in fasting blood glucose levels, mean daily blood glucose levels, daily glucosuria, and HbA1c levels after four months of treatment in the silymarin group. In addition, a significant decrease ($p < 0.01$) was observed in fasting insulin levels and mean exogenous insulin requirements in the treated group, whereas the untreated group showed a significant increase ($p < 0.05$) in fasting insulin levels and a stabilized insulin need. These findings are consistent with the significant decrease ($p < 0.01$) in basal and glucagon-stimulated C-peptide levels in the treated group and the significant increase in both parameters in the control group. A significant decrease ($p < 0.01$) in malondialdehyde levels was observed in the treated group.

Side effects
None reported.

Authors' comments
These results show that treatment with silymarin may reduce the lipoperoxidation of cell membranes and insulin resistance, significantly decreasing endogenous insulin overproduction and the need for exogenous insulin administration.

Reviewers' comments
The control group did not receive a placebo, and therefore the trial was not blinded. The sample size may have been appropriate, however, no power calculation was presented. The trial length was adequate. (1, 4)

Clinical Study: Legalon®

Extract name	None given
Manufacturer	Madaus AG, Germany
Indication	**Toxin-induced liver disease**
Level of evidence	**III**
Therapeutic benefit	**Undetermined**

Bibliographic reference
Szilard S, Szentgyorgyi D, Demeter I (1988). Protective effect of Legalon in workers exposed to organic solvents. *Acta Medica Hungarica* 45 (2): 249-256.

Trial design
Parallel. Control group received no treatment. Both groups continued to work in conditions that exposed them to toluene and/or xylene.

Study duration	1 month
Dose	1 (140 mg silymarin) capsule 3 times daily
Route of administration	Oral
Randomized	No
Randomization adequate	No
Blinding	Open
Blinding adequate	No
Placebo	No
Drug comparison	No
Site description	Single center
No. of subjects enrolled	49
No. of subjects completed	49
Sex	Male
Age	30-45 years

Inclusion criteria
Workers who had symptoms of liver disease attributable to toluene and/or

xylene exposure, including hepatomegaly, increased AST and ALT (aspartate and alanine aminotransferase) levels, relative lymphocytosis, and decreased platelet counts.

Exclusion criteria
Alcoholics.

End points
Before and after the observation period, the workers were submitted to medical physicals and laboratory tests, including blood cell count, serum AST and ALT, gamma-glutamyl transferase (GGT), cholesterol, and urine urobilinogen.

Results
Workers treated with silymarin reported that appetite improved significantly, headaches were reduced, three of ten cases of moderate hepatomegaly regressed, and tympanites ceased in 13 cases. One case of hemorrhagic predisposition and two cases of gingivitis disappeared or improved by the end of treatment. Laboratory results showed a significant decrease in serum AST and ALT, and a trend toward decrease in GGT. The same parameters increased slightly in the control group. Relative lymphocytosis decreased, and platelet counts increased in the silymarin group. These parameters remained unchanged or showed slight worsening in the control group.

Side effects
None reported.

Authors' comments
Under the influence of Legalon, elevated levels of plasma enzymes associated with liver function and low platelet counts significantly improved. Leukocytosis and relative lymphocytosis showed a trend toward improvement.

Reviewers' comments
Serum levels of liver enzymes and platelet counts improved in patients exposed to toluene and/or xylene for more than five years. However, the trial had a poor experimental design—it was not blinded or randomized. The sample size may have been appropriate, however, no power calculation was presented. (1, 4)

Clinical Study: Legalon IBI

Extract name	None given
Manufacturer	Madaus AG, Germany

Indication **Toxin-induced liver damage**
Level of evidence **III**
Therapeutic benefit **Undetermined**

Bibliographic reference
Boari C, Baldi E, Rizzoli O, Raffi GB, Caudarella R, Gennari P (1981). Silymarin in the protection against exogenous noxae. *Drugs Under Experimental and Clinical Research* 7 (2): 115-120.

Trial design
Parallel. Fourteen subjects were chronically exposed to phosphor esters and ten subjects were healthy volunteers. The study medication was given to all subjects.

Study duration	1 month
Dose	1 (140 mg silymarin) capsule 3 times daily
Route of administration	Oral
Randomized	No
Randomization adequate	No
Blinding	Open
Blinding adequate	No
Placebo	No
Drug comparison	No
Site description	Not described
No. of subjects enrolled	24
No. of subjects completed	24
Sex	Not given
Age	Not given

Inclusion criteria
Subjects chronically exposed to organophosphate pesticide (malathion) (14 in number) and healthy volunteers not exposed to pesticides (ten in number).

Exclusion criteria
None mentioned.

End points
Laboratory measures were tested before the study period and after 30 days. Measures included alkaline phosphatase, gamma-glutamyl transferase (GGT), leucine aminopeptidase (LAP), pseudocholinesterase, total lipemia, and triglyceridemia.

Results

In the group exposed to pesticides, silymarin treatment caused a significant increase in GGT, cholinesterase, and LAP ($p < 0.01$). No change was observed in alkaline phosphatase levels. In nonexposed subjects, there was an increase in GGT and LAP only ($p < 0.05$). Thus, the increase in cholinesterase activity was seen in the exposed group only. The response of lipidemic indices were identical in the two groups, with a marked decrease in serum levels of total lipids and triglycerides after treatment.

Side effects

Mild laxative effect reported in both study groups (by 4 out of 24 subjects).

Authors' comments

Silymarin has a therapeutic efficacy in cases of chronic exposure to phosphor esters, since a clear-cut increase in cholinesterase activity of the serum was found in the subjects studied.

Reviewers' comments

This study had a poor experimental design—it had no placebo, no blinding, and it was not randomized. It is essential to have an exposed, placebo-treated or standard-therapy group to provide a clear and unbiased comparison of treatment efficacy. (1, 3)

Product Profile: Silipide

Manufacturer	**Inverni della Beffa, Italy (Indena S.p.A., Italy)**
U.S. distributor	None
Botanical ingredient	**Milk thistle seed extract**
Extract name	**IdB 1016 (Siliphos®)**
Quantity	120 mg
Processing	Lipophilic complex of silybin combined with phosphatidylcholine from soy in a molar ratio of 1:2
Standardization	29.7-36.3% silybin
Formulation	Capsule

Other ingredients: Phosphatidylcholine from soy bean.

Source(s) of information: Buzzelli et al., 1993; information provided by Indena USA, Inc.

Product Profile: Maximum Milk Thistle™

Manufacturer	**Natural Wellness (Indena S.p.A., Italy)**
U.S. distributor	**Natural Wellness**
Botanical ingredient	**Milk thistle seed extract**
Extract name	**Siliphos®**
Quantity	240 mg
Processing	1 part silybin to 2 parts phosphatidylcholine
Standardization	29.7-36.3% silybin
Formulation	Capsule

Recommended dose: 3 capsules per day, either all at once or at separate times, with or without food (or as recommended by your health care professional).

DSHEA structure/function: Clinically shown to support and promote normal liver function.

Other ingredients: Rice powder, magnesium stearate, silicon dioxide, gelatin capsule.

Source(s) of information: Product label; information provided by Indena USA, Inc.

Product Profile: UltraThistle™

Manufacturer	**Natural Wellness (Indena S.p.A., Italy)**
U.S. distributor	**Natural Wellness**
Botanical ingredient	**Milk thistle seed extract**
Extract name	**Siliphos®**
Quantity	360 mg
Processing	1 part silybin to 2 parts phosphatidylcholine
Standardization	29.7-36.3% silybin
Formulation	Capsule

Recommended dose: One capsule three times per day as a dietary supplement (or as recommended by your health care professional).

DSHEA structure/function: Clinically shown to support and promote normal liver function.

Other ingredients: Rice powder, magnesium stearate, silicon dioxide.

Source(s) of information: Product label; information provided by Indena USA, Inc.

Clinical Study: Silipide

Extract name	IdB 1016
Manufacturer	Inverni della Beffa, Italy (Indena S.p.A., Italy)

Indication	**Chronic hepatits**
Level of evidence	**II**
Therapeutic benefit	**Yes**

Bibliographic reference
Marcelli R, Bizzoni P, Conte D, Lisena MO, Lampertico M, Marena C, De Marco MF, Del Ninno E (1992). Randomized controlled study of the efficacy and tolerability of a short course of IdB 1016 in the treatment of chronic persistent hepatitis. *European Bulletin of Drug Research* 1 (3): 131-135.

Trial design
Parallel.

Study duration	3 months
Dose	1 (120 mg silybin) capsule twice daily
Route of administration	Oral
Randomized	Yes
Randomization adequate	No
Blinding	Double-blind
Blinding adequate	Yes
Placebo	Yes
Drug comparison	No
Site description	2 gastroenterology units
No. of subjects enrolled	65
No. of subjects completed	65
Sex	Male and female
Age	24-66 years (mean: 47.7)

Inclusion criteria
Outpatients with biopsy-proven chronic persistent hepatitis, not previously under established treatment, with serum alanine aminotransferase and/or

serum aspartate aminotransferase values at least 1.5 times greater than the upper limit of the normal range on two occasions during the year before treatment.

Exclusion criteria
Patients with decompensated liver diseases, or under therapy with interferon, antivirals, immunosuppressants, or immunomodulators within six months before enrollment.

End points
Patients were examined before and after three months of treatment. Serum aminotransferase activity, white blood cell count, direct and total bilirubin, total protein, and albumin, as well as prothrombin activity, were determined.

Results
A statistically significant decrease of mean serum activity of both aspartate ($p < 0.05$) and alanine ($p = 0.01$) aminotransferases was observed in the treatment group compared to the placebo group. Serum bilirubin, albumin, total protein, and prothrombin time were normal at baseline in the majority of patients and did not change in any clinically relevant way.

Side effects
No serious side effects were noted. Three patients in the treated group complained of nausea, heartburn, and transient headache. Five in the control group reported nausea, heartburn, dyspepsia, and skin rash.

Authors' comments
The results of the present study show that IdB 1016, over a period of three months, can induce positive changes in serum aspartate and alanine aminotransferases in patients with chronic persistent hepatitis.

Reviewers' comments
Based on the ALT, AST, and PT percent, the study group appears to have had more severe illness than the control group. There was no intent-to-treat analysis and no measure of compliance to protocol regimen. The sample size may have been appropriate given the significant finds, however, no power calculation was presented. The treatment length was adequate. (3, 6)

Clinical Study: Silipide

Extract name	IdB 1016
Manufacturer	Inverni della Beffa, Italy (Indena S.p.A., Italy)

Indication   **Viral hepatitis (B or C)**
Level of evidence   **II**
Therapeutic benefit   **Trend**

Bibliographic reference

Buzzelli G, Moscarella S, Giusti A, Duchini A, Marena C, Lampertico M (1993). A pilot study on the liver protective effect of silybinphosphatidylcholine complex (IdB1016) in chronic active hepatitis. *International Journal of Clinical Pharmacology, Therapy, and Toxicology* 31 (9): 456-460.

Trial design

Parallel.

Study duration   1 week
Dose   2 (120 mg silybin) capsules twice daily
Route of administration   Oral

Randomized   Yes
Randomization adequate   No
Blinding   Double-blind
Blinding adequate   No

Placebo   Yes
Drug comparison   No

Site description   Hospital

No. of subjects enrolled   20
No. of subjects completed   20
Sex   Male and female
Age   31-70 years (mean: 53)

Inclusion criteria

Patients with chronic active hepatitis (histologically proven), increased aspartate aminotransferase (AST) and/or alanine aminotransferase (ALT) serum activities (two to six times the upper limit of range) for more than 12 months.

Exclusion criteria

Patients who have the following: portal hypertension; hepatic encephalopathy; ascites; hepatocellular carcinoma; cholestasis; drug addiction; positive antinuclear, antimitochondrial, and antismooth muscle antibodies; ethanol intake > 30 g per day; malabsorption syndromes; cardiovascular, renal or endocrine disorders; pregnancy; and any pharmacological treatment three months before the beginning of the trial.

End points
Blood samples were collected before and after seven days of treatment, and several liver function tests were performed, as well as measurements of malonaldehyde as an index of liver peroxidation, and copper and zinc, two trace elements involved in protecting cells against free radical-mediated lipid peroxidation.

Results
A statistically significant reduction of mean serum concentrations of AST ($p < 0.01$), ALT ($p < 0.01$), gamma-glutamyl transpeptidase (GGT) ($p < 0.02$), and total bilirubin ($p < 0.05$) was observed in the treated group. The changes in AST, ALT, and GGT were also significant in comparison to the placebo group, in which these levels did not change significantly compared to baseline. There were no significant changes in malonaldehyde, copper, or zinc serum concentrations.

Side effects
None mentioned.

Authors' comments
These results show that Silipide may improve the biochemical signs of hepatocellular necrosis and/or increased cellular permeability in patients affected by chronic active hepatitis. However, it should be considered that this is a pilot study carried out on a small number of patients treated for only one week.

Reviewers' comments
This was an inpatient study, and fasting and controlled diet introduces a potential confounding covariable. The sample size may have been appropriate given the significant findings, however, no power calculation was presented. The dosage of 480 mg/day is twice that used in the study by Marcelli et al. (1992). The treatment length was adequate for a pilot study. (3, 6)

Product Profile: Silimarina®

Manufacturer	**Biofarm S.A., Romania**
U.S. distributor	None
Botanical ingredient	**Milk thistle seed extract**
Extract name	None given
Quantity	700 mg, equivalent to 35 mg silybin
Standardization	No information
Formulation	Tablet

Comments: According to the trial report, Silimarina is a reproduction of Legalon® (Madaus AG).

Source(s) of information: Tanasescu et al., 1988.

Clinical Study: Silimarina®

Extract name	None given
Manufacturer	Biofarm S.A., Romania
Indication	**Liver disease**
Level of evidence	**II**
Therapeutic benefit	**Undetermined**

Bibliographic reference
Tanasescu C, Petrea S, Baldescu R, Macarie E, Chiriloiu C, Purice S (1988). Use of the Romanian product Silimarina in the treatment of chronic liver diseases. *Revue Roumaine de Medecine-Medecine Interne* 26 (4): 311-322.

Trial design
Subjects were split into three groups according to their therapeutic indications (Group A: chronic persistent hepatitis; Group B: chronic active hepatitis; and Group C: hepatic cirrhosis). Patients in each group were randomized to receive either Silimarina or placebo.

Study duration	40 days
Dose	2 tablets (700 mg, containing 35 mg silybin) 3 times daily 1 hour after meals
Route of administration	Oral
Randomized	Yes
Randomization adequate	No
Blinding	Double-blind
Blinding adequate	Yes
Placebo	Yes
Drug comparison	No
Site description	Not described
No. of subjects enrolled	180
No. of subjects completed	177
Sex	Male and female
Age	Mean: 45.2 ± 11.5 years

Inclusion criteria
Patients between the ages of 20 and 60 years with chronic persistent hepatitis, chronic active hepatitis, or hepatic cirrhosis. Diagnosis was based on biopsy (with the exception of some with hepatic cirrhosis—Group C) correlated with clinical and laboratory data. The disease is in its medium state (monotherapy will not be detrimental to subjects), and the length of basic disease is from one to ten years.

Exclusion criteria
None mentioned.

End points
At the beginning and end of the study, clinical examination included 25 symptoms, objective signs characteristic for the disease, and the lab analyses of alanine aminotransferase, gamma-glutanmyl transpeptidase (GTP), zinc sulfate, bilirubin, alkaline phosphatase, serum proteins, IgG, and prothrombin concentration.

Results
The clinical aspect of liver disease was improved in all three groups compared with placebo. The improvement was proportionally similar in those with chronic persistent hepatitis (65 percent compared with 50 percent for controls), chronic active hepatitis (70 percent compared with 60 percent for controls), and in those with hepatic cirrhosis (55 percent compared with 45 percent for controls). Laboratory tests of groups as a whole failed to give conclusive evidence of treatment. However, activity was demonstrated within subgroups.

Side effects
No adverse events were observed.

Authors' comments
The results demonstrate the partial favorable effect of treatment with Silimarina on some clinical and laboratory parameters, as compared with placebo in patients with various forms of chronic liver disease.

Reviewers' comments
The "clinical parameters" were not well described or presented, and the secondary analysis of data was somewhat spurious. The sample size may have been appropriate, however, no power calculation was presented. Only part of Group C was biopsied—this was not explained. The dose of 210 mg/day was much lower than most other studies. Given the lack of side effects, a larger dose could have been used and perhaps yielded a clearer picture of efficacy. A longer duration may have allowed for clear resolution of the data profile. (2, 5)

Product Profile: Milk Thistle (Generic)

Manufacturer	None
U.S. distributor	None
Botanical ingredient	**Milk thistle seed extract**
Extract name	None given
Quantity	No information
Processing	No information
Standardization	No information
Formulation	No information

Clinical Study: Milk Thistle (Generic)

Extract name	None given
Manufacturer	None
Indication	**Drug-induced liver damage**
Level of evidence	**III**
Therapeutic benefit	**Trend**

Bibliographic reference

Palasciano G, Portincasa P, Palmieri V, Ciani D, Vendemiale G, Altomare E (1994). The effect of silymarin on plasma levels of malon dialdehyde in patients receiving long-term treatment with psychotropic drugs. *Current Therapeutic Research* 55 (5): 537-545.

Trial design

Parallel. Four treatment groups included Group IA: psychotropic drugs and silymarin (800 mg/d); Group IB: psychotropic drugs and placebo; Group IIA: suspension of psychotropic drugs and silymarin (800 mg/d); Group IIB: suspension of psychotropic drugs and placebo.

Study duration	3 months
Dose	400 mg silymarin twice daily
Route of administration	Oral
Randomized	Yes
Randomization adequate	No
Blinding	Double-blind
Blinding adequate	No
Placebo	Yes

Drug comparison   No

Site description   Hospital psychiatric department

No. of subjects enrolled   60
No. of subjects completed 60
Sex   Female
Age   40-60 years (mean: 51.9)

Inclusion criteria
Patients ages 40 to 60 years receiving chronic psychotropic drug therapy such as phenothiazines and/or butyrophenones for at least five years, and with aspartate aminotransferase (AST) or alanine aminotransferase (ALT) activity more than twice the normal value.

Exclusion criteria
Patients treated with other drugs that could influence the progress of hepatopathy (e.g., interferons or cortisone); other types of hepatopathies (e.g., viral, autoimmune hepatopathy, alcoholic, hemochromatosis, porphyria cutanea tarda, Wilson's disease, or primary or secondary hepatic neoplasia); altered renal function (blood urea nitrogen > 60 mg/dl and/or serum creatinine > 2.5 mg/dl); cardiac and circulatory insufficiency; diabetes; other extrahepatic diseases; pregnancy; or alcohol (> 30 g/d) or opiate abuse.

End points
Serum levels of malondialdehyde (MDA) (an end product of oxidation of polyunsaturated fatty acids) and indices of hepatocellular function were assessed at baseline and 15, 30, 60, and 90 days after beginning treatment, as well as one month after completion of treatment.

Results
The suspension of therapy with psychotropic drugs led to a reduction in serum MDA levels in both placebo- and silymarin-treated patients, with little difference between the two groups (IIA and IIB). There was an increase in serum MDA levels with placebo (group IB). Group IIB's serum MDA levels decreased until rebound occurred when psychotropic drug therapy was reinstated. The decrease over time in ALT and AST was greater in Group II compared with Group I. For those who continued to take the psychoactive drugs (Groups IA and IB), there was a significant improvement with silymarin at the end of three months.

Side effects
No adverse reactions were reported.

Authors' comments
Silymarin, used at submaximal dose, reduced the lipoperoxdative hepatic

damage that occurs during treatment with butyrophenones and pheno-thiazines. This protective effect is greater in suspended psychotropic drugs.

Reviewers' comments
The study groups were not well-matched at baseline with respect to labora-tory test results or age. Based upon the data, the most powerful effect was found with the withdrawal of neuroleptics. Some protection from lipoperoxi-dation may have been induced by certain phenothiazines and butyro-phenones conferred by co-treatment with silymarin, as indicated by the data that showed a significant decrease in MDA levels. The sample size may have been appropriate, however, no power calculation was presented. The dosage of 800 mg/day was significantly beyond the standard range (per Blumenthal et al., 1998). This choice was not discussed in the paper nor substantiated by reference(s). The treatment length was adequate. (1, 5)

Pygeum

Other common names: **African plum**
Latin name: *Prunus africana* (**Hook. f.**) **Kalkman** [Rosaceae]
Latin synonyms: *Pygeum africanum* **Hook. f.**
Plant part: **Bark**

PREPARATIONS USED
IN REVIEWED CLINICAL STUDIES

Pygeum bark has been traditionally used in central and southern Africa to assist bladder and urinary function. In this traditional use, the bark is ground into powder and mixed with milk. Modern formulation of this botanical is a lipophilic extract of the bark. At least three types of active compounds may be responsible for the therapeutic action of the extract: pentacyclic terpenes, phytosterols, and ferulic acid esters (Schulz, Hänsel, and Tyler, 2001).

Tadenan® is manufactured in France by Laboratoires Fournier. The capsules contain 50 mg of a lipophilic extract of pygeum bark. Tadenan is not sold in the United States.

Pigenil contains a pygeum bark extract (PrunuSelect™) manufactured by Indena S.p.A., Italy. This extract has a plant to extract ratio of 180:1, and is standardized to contain 11.7 to 14.3 percent sterols as beta-sitosterol. Pigenil, in 50 mg capsules, was originally manufactured by Inverni della Beffa in Italy. This product is not available in the United States.

Prostatonin® contains extracts of both pygeum bark and nettle (*Urtica dioica* L. spp. *dioica*) roots. This product is manufactured by Pharmaton S.A. in Switzerland, and is sold in the United States by Pharmaton Natural Health Products. It is available in softgel capsules containing 25 mg pygeum extract, PY102 (200:1), and 300 mg nettle extract, UR102 (5:1).

PYGEUM SUMMARY TABLE

Product Name	Manufacturer/ U.S. Distributor	Product Characteristics	Dose in Trials	Indication	No. of Trials	Benefit (Evidence Level-Trial No.)
Single Ingredient Products						
Tadenan® (EU)	Laboratoires Fournier, France/ None	Lipidic sterol extract	100 to 200 mg/day	Benign prostatic hyperplasia	8*	Yes (II-2) Trend (III-3) No (II-1) Undetermined (III-2)
Pigenil (EU)	Inverni della Beffa, Italy (Indena S.p.A., Italy)/None	Soft extract (PrunuSelect™)	100 mg/day	Benign prostatic hyperplasia	2	Yes (II-1) Undetermined (III-1)
Combination Product						
Prostatonin®	Pharmaton S.A., Switzerland/ Pharmaton Natural Health Products	Pygeum bark extract (PY102), Nettle root extract (UR102)	2 capsules twice daily	Benign prostatic hyperplasia	2	Undetermined (II-2)

*The trial information for one of these studies (Dutkiewicz, 1996) is included after the grass pollen summary, since it is reviewed primarily in that section.

SUMMARY OF REVIEWED CLINICAL STUDIES

Pygeum preparations have been assessed in clinical studies for the treatment of symptomatic benign prostatic hyperplasia (BPH), also known as benign prostatic hypertrophy and prostatic adenoma. BPH is a nonmalignant enlargement of the prostate common in men over 40 years of age. The symptoms of BPH include increased urinary urgency and frequency, urinary hesitancy, intermittency, sensation of incomplete voiding, and decreased force of the stream of urine. BPH is linked with a normal change in hormone levels that occurs with aging. Testosterone levels decrease while estrogen levels remain constant. This change is implicated in BPH, since estrogens induce hyperplasia (cell growth) in laboratory experiments. Further, BPH is associated with an increase in the activity of 5-alpha-reductase, the enzyme that converts testosterone to dihydrotesterone (DHT). The levels of DHT are not increased, but the number of androgen receptors seems to be. DHT has a greater affinity for androgen receptors than testosterone, and is thought to modulate prostatic growth. However, the pathology of BPH is not completely understood, and although BPH is associated with prostate enlargement, the size of the gland is not necessarily indicative of the degree of obstruction of the urethra and the extent of symptoms (Barrett, 1999).

Predominant pharmaceutical treatments for BPH include alpha-receptor blockers and 5-alpha-reductase inhibitors. Alpha-receptor blockers (e.g., prozosin, terazosin) are thought to relax smooth muscle in the bladder neck and within the prostate, and thus reduce symptoms. Five-alpha reductase inhibitors (e.g., finasteride) prevent the transformation of testosterone into DHT. The rationale for this treatment is that prostate enlargement may be linked to activation of androgen receptors by DHT and a reduction in testosterone levels (Barrett, 1999).

The clinical mode of action of pygeum has not been established, but biochemical studies indicate that it has anti-inflammatory activity and may inhibit 5-alpha-reductase. Nettle root extract, which is combined with pygeum extract in the product Prostatonin®, may have similar activity. Preparations of grass pollen and saw palmetto have also been assessed clinically for treatment of BPH, and more information about these botanicals is given in their sections in this book. The mechanism of action of these botanicals is also not established, but grass pollen has demonstrated anti-inflammatory activity, and may reduce the growth of epithelial cells and fibroblasts. Suggested pharmacological actions for saw palmetto include antiandrogenic, anti-inflammatory, antiproliferative, and smooth muscle relaxation (Marandola, et al., 1997; Awang, 1997; Barrett, 1999).

Tadenan

Benign Prostatic Hyperplasia

Tadenan was examined for the treatment of BPH in eight controlled clinical studies, including a total of 812 men. The studies suggest a moderate benefit with a reduction in symptoms after a month of treatment. Three of the studies were good-sized, including more than 100 men each, and four were smaller studies of 20 to 40 men each. Five of the studies were placebo controlled, two studies compared Tadenan to other agents, and one study was a dose comparison. One study that compared Tadenan to grass pollen extract (Cernilton®) is primarily included in that file.

The largest placebo-controlled study included 255 men and was rated by our reviewers, Drs. Elliot Fagelman and Franklin Lowe, as well conducted. Treatment with Tadenan, 100 mg per day for two months, led to a statistically significant increase in urinary volume and maximum urinary flow with a decrease in residual urine volume, compared with placebo. Urinary frequency during the day and night was also reduced (Barlet et al., 1990). A smaller, good-quality study with 39 men also reported a significant increase in urinary flow following treatment with 200 mg daily for two months compared to baseline and to placebo. A decrease in urinary frequency and a decrease in painful urination was observed in the treatment group compared to baseline. In addition, the diameter of the prostate was reduced by 11 percent, compared with a 5 percent reduction in the placebo group (Ranno et al., 1986). Two low-quality studies, according to the Jadad criteria, included 20 and 40 participants, respectively, treated with 200 mg pygeum per day or placebo for two months. Both studies reported a significant reduction in symptoms compared to baseline, not shared by the placebo group (Rizzo et al., 1985; Frasseto et al., 1986). A large (120 men) but short (six weeks) study of good quality reported reductions in symptoms for both the treatment group given 200 mg per day and the placebo group. Despite the very large placebo effect, there was an indication of benefit due to Tadenan (DuFour et al., 1984).

A large study including 209 men compared two dosage regimens, 50 mg twice daily to 100 mg once daily. Both dose regimens reduced symptom scores and increased quality of life scores. Although both forms were equally effective, the lack of a placebo group meant that efficacy could not be determined (Chatelain, Autet, and Brackman, 1999).

A comparison study with 40 participants compared 200 mg Tadenan to standard therapy with nonsteroidal anti-inflammatory drugs (NSAIDs) alone or with antibiotics. After one month of treatment, Tadenan was more effective than NSAIDs in improving symptoms of polyuria (excess urine), urinary frequency at night, urinary retention, and painful urination. The NSAID therapy was only comparable in improving strangury, the constricted passage of urine (Gagliardi et al., 1983).

A trial reviewed in the grass pollen section compared Tadenan with grass pollen extract (Cernilton). The Tadenan group received two tablets twice daily, and the Cernilton group received one to two tablets of Cernilton three times daily. In this trial, which included a total of 89 men, positive therapeutic response was reported for both treatments, with improved peak flow rate, decreased residual urine volume, decreased prostate volume, and improved obstructive and irritative symptom scores. Scores indicated more improvement for the Cernilton group than the Tadenan group (Dutkiewicz, 1996).

Pigenil

Benign Prostatic Hyperplasia

Two trials examined the efficacy of Pigenil on men with symptomatic BPH. Both studies reported a decrease in symptoms following two months of treatment with 50 mg twice daily. The first, a well-conducted, placebo-controlled study with 40 men, reported a decrease in urinary frequency, urgency, and painful urination, as well as an increase in urinary flow, with no change in prostate size compared with placebo (Bassi et al., 1987).

The second study compared Pigenil with mepartricin, an agent that lowers levels of circulating estrogen levels without causing changes in the levels of other hormones, including testosterone. The authors of a recent review concluded that mepartricin was as effective as alpha-adrenoceptor agonists and 5-alpha-reductase inhibitors in reducing symptoms of BPH (Boehm, Nirnberger, and Ferrari, 1998). The comparison study conducted with Pigenil and mepartricin included 40 men and demonstrated a reduction in urinary frequency, painful urination, and residual urine compared to baseline for both treatments. Pigenil was slightly more effective in reducing painful urination. In addition, after two months treatment, Pigenil reduced the size of the prostate by 11 percent, whereas mepartricin had no effect on prostate size (Scarpa et al., 1989).

A third trial described in this section compared Pigenil with Prostatonin and an extract of *Epilobium parviflorum* (Montanari et al., 1991).

Prostatonin

Benign Prostatic Hyperplasia

Two trials explored the efficacy of Prostatonin, a product containing extracts of both pygeum and nettle. The first study was a dose comparison study, and the second was a treatment comparison study. Unfortunately, neither study included a placebo group, an omission that caused the trials' efficacy to be rated undetermined by our reviewers. The first, a fairly large study of 124 men, compared the usual dose of two capsules twice daily to half that dose and found both to be equally effective in increasing urinary flow and decreasing residual urine and nighttime frequency following two months of treatment (Krzeski et al., 1993). The second, smaller study, including 59 men, compared the combination product Prostatonin (two capsules twice daily) with Pigenil (pygeum alone, 50 mg twice daily) and an extract of *Epilobium parviflorum* (250 mg extract twice daily). Strength of urinary flow was increased with all three treatments, with the combination product being more effective than pygeum alone, and both more effective than *Epilobium*. Both Prostatonin and Pigenil were more effective than *Epilobium* in reducing nighttime urination frequency. No change in prostate size was observed in any of the groups (Montanari et al., 1991).

SYSTEMATIC REVIEWS

A systematic review evaluated 18 randomized, controlled trials including 1,562 men with symptomatic BPH. The mean treatment duration was two months, with a range from one to four months. The doses of pygeum extract ranged from 75 to 200 mg per day. Of the 13 placebo-controlled studies, 12 reported a beneficial effect on at least one measure of effectiveness (overall symptoms, nighttime urination frequency, peak urine flow, or residual volume). Only one small trial with 20 men lasting 12 weeks found no benefit compared to placebo. Six studies involving a total of 474 participants could be pooled in a statistical evaluation of effectiveness. Five of these six studies used Tadenan as the test preparation. The statistical evaluation of the overall effect indicated a significant improvement in symptoms compared with placebo (standard deviation [SD] –0.8; 95 percent confidence interval [CI]: –1.4 to –0.3). The authors concluded that the evidence suggests that pygeum improves urologic symptoms and flow measures modestly, but significantly (Ishani et al., 2000).

ADVERSE REACTIONS OR SIDE EFFECTS

Pygeum extracts were well tolerated with only an occasional report of gastrointestinal discomfort in the trials discussed previously. A systematic review of 18 trials including 1,562 men reported that adverse reactions were mild and similar to those with the placebo. The most frequently reported side effects were gastrointestinal complaints (Ishani et al., 2000).

REFERENCES

Awang DVC (1997). Saw palmetto, African prune and stinging nettle for benign prostatic hyperplasia. *Canadian Pharmaceutical Journal, Revue Pharmaceutique Canadienne (CPJ RPC)* 130 (9): 37-62.

Barlet A, Albrecht J, Aubert A, Fischer M, Grof F, Grothuesmann HG, Masson JC, Mazeman E, Mermon R, Reichelt H, Schonmetzler F, Suhler A (1990). Efficacy of *Pygeum africanum* extract in the treatment of micturitional disorders due to benign prostatic hyperplasia: Evaluation of objective and subjective parameters. *Wiener Klinische Wochenschrift* 102 (22): 667-672.

Barrett, M (1999). The pharmacology of saw palmetto in treatment of BPH. *Journal of the American Nutraceutical Association* 2 (3): 21-24.

Bassi P, Artibani W, De Luca V, Zattoni F, Lembo A (1987). Estratto standardizzato di *Pygeum africanum* nel trattamento dell'ipertrofia prostatica benigna [Standardized *Pygeum africanum* extract in the treatment of benign prostatic hypertrophy]. *Minerva Urologica e Nefrologica* 39 (1): 45-50.

Boehm S, Nirnberger G, Ferrari P (1998). Estrogen suppression as a pharmacotherapeutic strategy in the medical treatment of benign prostatic hyperplasia: Evidence for its efficacy from studies with mepartricin. *Wiener Klinische Wochenschrift* 110 (23): 817-823.

Chatelain C, Autet W, and Brackman F (1999). Comparison of once and twice daily dosage forms of *Pygeum africanum* extract in patients with benign prostatic hyperplasia: A randomized, double-blind study, with long-term open label extension. *Urology* 54 (3): 473-478.

DuFour B, Choquenet C, Revol M, Faure G, Jorest R (1984). Controlled study of the effects of *Pygeum africanum* extracts on the symptoms of benign prostatic hypertrophy. *Annales d'Urologie* 18 (3): 193-195.

Dutkiewicz S (1996). Usefulness of Cernilton in the treatment of benign prostatic hyperplasia. *International Urology and Nephrology* 28 (1): 49-53.

Frasseto G, Bertoglio S, Mancuso S, Ervo R, Mereta F (1986). Study of the efficacy and tolerance of *Pygeum africanum* in patients with prostatic hypertrophy. *Il Progresso Medico* 42: 49-53.

Gagliardi V, Apicella F, Pino P, Falchi M (1983). Medical treatment of prostatic hypertrophy: A controlled clinical investigation. *Archivio Italiano di Urologia e Nefrologia* 55: 51-69.

Ishani A, MacDonald R, Nelson D, Rutks I, Wilt TJ (2000). *Pygeum africanum* for the treatment of patients with benign prostatic hyperplasia: A systematic review and quantitative meta-analysis. *The American Journal of Medicine* 109 (8): 654-664.

Krzeski T, Kazon M, Borkowski A, Witeska A, Kuczera J (1993). Combined extracts of *Urtica dioica* and *Pygeum africanum* in the treatment of benign prostatic hyperplasia: Double-blind comparison of two doses. *Clinical Therapeutics* 15 (6): 1011-1020.

Marandola P, Jallous H, Bombardelli E, Morazzoni P (1997). Main phytoderivatives in the management of benign prostatic hyperplasia. *Fitoterapia* 68 (3): 195-204.

Montanari E, Mandressi A, Magri V, Dormia G, Pisani E (1991). Benign prostatic hyperplasia: Differential therapy with phytopharmacological agents—A randomized study of 63 patients. *Separatum Der Informierte Arzt/Gazette Medicale* 6a: 593-598.

Ranno S, Minaldi G, Viscusi G, Di Marco G, Consoli C (1986). Efficacy and tolerability of treatment of prostatic adenoma with Tandenan 50. *Il Progresso Medico* 42: 165-169.

Rizzo M, Tosto A, Paoletti MC, Raugei A, Favini P, Nicolucci A, Paolini R (1985). Medical therapy of prostate adenoma: Comparative clinical evaluation between high dose *Pygeum africanum* extract and placebo. *Farmaci & Terapia* 2 (2): 105-110.

Scarpa RM, Migliari R, Campus G, De Lisa A, Sorgia M, Usai M, Usai E (1989). Medical treatment of benign prostatic hypertrophy with extract of *Pygeum africanum. Stampa Medica* (Suppl. 465): 25-39.

Schulz V, Hänsel R, Tyler VE (2001). *Rational Phytotherapy: A Physicians' Guide to Herbal Medicine,* Fourth Edition. Trans. TC Telgar. Berlin: Springer-Verlag.

DETAILS ON PYGEUM PRODUCTS
AND CLINICAL STUDIES

Product and clinical study information is grouped in the same order as in the Summary Table. A profile on an individual product is followed by details of the clinical studies associated with that product. In some instances, a clinical study, or studies, supports several products that contain the same principal ingredient(s). In these instances, those products are grouped together.

Clinical studies that follow each product, or group of products, are grouped by therapeutic indication, in accordance with the order in the Summary Table.

Index to Pygeum Products

Product Profile: Tadenan®

Manufacturer	**Laboratoires Fournier, France**
U.S. distributor	None
Botanical ingredient	**Pygeum bark extract**
Extract name	None given
Quantity	50 mg
Processing	Lipidic sterol extract
Standardization	No information
Formulation	Capsule

Recommended dose: One capsule taken in the morning and evening, preferably before meals.

DSHEA structure/function: French drug indication: treatment of mild micturition disorders caused by benign prostatic hyperplasia.

Cautions: Treatment duration is generally 6 weeks; it can be prolonged up to 8 weeks and can be repeated if necessary. The effect of Tadenan on functional disorders does not dispense from routine medical checkups since Tadenan cannot replace necessary surgery. Diagnosis and surveillance of benign prostatic hyperplasia must include periodic digital rectal examination for the early detection of a possible prostate cancer.

Other ingredients: Peanut oil, gelatin, glycerol, titanium dioxide (E 171), hydrosoluble copper complexes of chlorophyll (E 141).

Source(s) of information: Barlet et al., 1990; Banque de Données Automatisée sur les Médicaments (BIAM) (2000) Tadenan 50 mg capsules molles, <http://www3.biam2.org/www/lspe.html>.

Clinical Study: Tadenan®

Extract name	None given
Manufacturer	Laboratories Fournier, France
Indication	**Benign prostatic hyperplasia**
Level of evidence	**II**
Therapeutic benefit	**Yes**

Bibliographic reference
Barlet A, Albrecht J, Aubert A, Fischer M, Grof F, Grothuesmann HG, Masson JC, Mazeman E, Mermon R, Reichelt H, Schonmetzler F, Suhler A (1990). Efficacy of *Pygeum africanum* extract in the treatment of micturitional disorders due to benign prostatic hyperplasia: Evaluation of objective and subjective parameters. *Wiener Klinische Wochenschrift* 102 (22): 667-672.

Trial design
Parallel.

Study duration	2 months
Dose	50 mg capsule twice daily
Route of administration	Oral
Randomized	Yes
Randomization adequate	No
Blinding	Double-blind
Blinding adequate	Yes
Placebo	Yes
Drug comparison	No
Site description	8 centers
No. of subjects enrolled	263
No. of subjects completed	255

Sex   Male
Age   50-85 years

Inclusion criteria
Outpatients older than 50 years old with urinary disorders attributable to Stage I benign prostatic hyperplasia that had been present for at least six months, but not over four years. Nocturia had to be marked enough to allow quantitative recording (number of nightly urinations).

Exclusion criteria
Prostatic carcinoma or suspected carcinoma; residual urine over 100 ml, recurrent pollakiuria; urea in blood over 0.8 g/l; acute infections of the urinary tract, or patients' clinical or bacteriologic clearance within the prior four weeks; kidney failure or other recurrent diseases that might affect urinary flow; treatment in the last six months, or concomitant medication, with drugs that might improve the symptoms of bladder-emptying, such as anti-inflammatories, diuretics, and hormones.

End points
Primary end points were objective measurements of residual urine, micturition volume, maximum urine flow rate, and the number of daily and nightly urinations over 24 hours. Secondary subjective symptoms evaluated by patients were delayed urination, weak urine flow, stasis after urination, intermittent flow, and sense of residual urine.

Results
Treatment with pygeum extract led to a significant decrease in the volume of residual urine ($p = 0.001$), and an increase in micturition volume and maximum urine flow rate (both $p = 0.001$). The average number of nightly urination decreased significantly, both quantitatively and subjectively. Daytime urination decreased with treatment. Overall assessment at the end of therapy showed that micturition improved in 66 percent of the patients treated with pygeum extract compared with an improvement of 31 percent in the placebo group. The difference was significant at the statistical level of $p < 0.001$.

Side effects
During therapy with pygeum extract, gastrointestinal side effects occurred in five patients. Treatment was discontinued in three of those cases.

Authors' comments
The use of *Pygeum africanum* appears justified, especially because of its favorable risk-benefit ratio.

Reviewers' comments
Overall, this is a good study demonstrating a benefit in taking *Pygeum africanum* for BPH. (Translation reviewed) (3, 6)

Clinical Study: Tadenan® 50

Extract name	None given
Manufacturer	Roussel Maestretti S.p.A., Italy
	(Laboratoires Fournier, France)

Indication	**Benign prostatic hyperplasia**
Level of evidence	**II**
Therapeutic benefit	**Yes**

Bibliographic reference
Ranno S, Minaldi G, Viscusi G, Di Marco G, Consoli C (1986). Efficacy and tolerability of treatment of prostatic adenoma with Tandenan 50. *Il Progresso Medico* 42: 165-169.

Trial design
Parallel.

Study duration	2 months
Dose	2 (50 mg) capsules twice daily
Route of administration	Oral
Randomized	Yes
Randomization adequate	No
Blinding	Double-blind
Blinding adequate	Yes
Placebo	Yes
Drug comparison	No
Site description	Single practice
No. of subjects enrolled	39
No. of subjects completed	39
Sex	Male
Age	Mean: 70 years

Inclusion criteria
Patients suffering from adenoma of the prostate in the first and second stages, not requiring surgery, and with disorders of micturition of moderate severity.

Exclusion criteria
Hormone-based drugs, antiprostatics, anti-inflammatory drugs, diuretics, or antibiotics were not allowed during treatment.

End points
Symptoms such as dysuria, diurnal and nocturnal pollakiuria, and urinary flow

were evaluated at the beginning and end of the study. Echographs of the prostate were performed before the trial, after 30 days, and after 60 days.

Results
Treatment with pygeum led to a statistically significant reduction in symptoms (dysuria, diurnal pollakiuria, and nocturnal pollakiuria) ($p < 0.01$, compared to baseline). In contrast, the placebo did not cause any significant change. Pygeum also caused improvement in mean and maximal urinary flow as well as duration of micturition ($p < 0.01$, compared to baseline and placebo). It also caused a slight reduction (11 percent) in the diameter of the prostate in comparison with placebo (5 percent).

Side effects
None observed.

Authors' comments
In comparison with placebo, the extract of pygeum caused appreciable and significant improvement in symptoms.

Reviewers' comments
The study is limited because of the small number of patients and short treatment length. However, symptoms and peak urinary flow were improved with treatment. (Translation reviewed) (3, 4)

Clinical Study: Tadenan® 50

Extract name	None given
Manufacturer	Laboratoires Fournier, France
Indication	**Benign prostatic hyperplasia**
Level of evidence	**III**
Therapeutic benefit	**Trend**

Bibliographic reference
Rizzo M, Tosto A, Paoletti MC, Raugei A, Favini P, Nicolucci A, Paolini R (1985). Medical therapy of prostate adenoma: Comparative clinical evaluation between high dose *Pygeum africanum* extract and placebo. *Farmaci & Terapia* 2 (2): 105-110.

Trial design
Parallel.

Study duration	2 months
Dose	2 (50 mg) capsules twice daily

Route of administration	Oral
Randomized	Yes
Randomization adequate	No
Blinding	Double-blind
Blinding adequate	No
Placebo	Yes
Drug comparison	No
Site description	Single practice
No. of subjects enrolled	40
No. of subjects completed	40
Sex	Male
Age	42-72 years (mean: 62)

Inclusion criteria
Patients with a diagnosis of an adenoma of prostate for no more than five years, and with urination problems.

Exclusion criteria
None mentioned.

End points
Clinical symptomatology were evaluated subjectively (dysuria, daytime frequency, nocturia, decreased urinary flow) and objectively (rectal exam, uroflow meter, echography). Examination were completed at inclusion into the study, after 30 days, and after 60 days.

Results
A significant improvement for dysuria was observed in the treatment group after 60 days ($p < 0.01$). There was an improvement in nocturia after 30 and 60 days ($p < 0.05$ and $p < 0.01$, respectively). No statistically significant improvement in daytime frequency was observed. According to the uroflow measurements, there was a statistically significant increase in average and maximal flow after 60 days ($p < 0.01$). No change in prostate size was observed. No significant changes in these parameters were seen in the placebo group.

Side effects
None. Treatment was very well tolerated.

Authors' comments
Pygeum africanum is a valid and current therapy for prostate adenoma.

Reviewers' comments
The data show some benefit for *Pygeum africanum,* but a poor study design limits their usefulness. The authors state that patients had symptoms due to prostatic enlargement, but the average maximum uroflow prior to treatment was 715 ml/sec. With such a high maximum flow, and without performing pressure flow studies, the diagnosis of BPH is in doubt. Sixty days is a short duration of therapy. (Translation reviewed) (1, 3)

Clinical Study: Tadenan® 50

Extract name	None given
Manufacturer	Roussel Maestretti S.p.A., Italy
	(Laboratoires Fournier, France)
Indication	**Benign prostatic hyperplasia**
Level of evidence	**III**
Therapeutic benefit	**Trend**

Bibliographic reference
Frasseto G, Bertoglio S, Mancuso S, Ervo R, Mereta F (1986). Study of the efficacy and tolerance of *Pygeum africanum* in patients with prostatic hyper-trophy. *Il Progresso Medico* 42: 49-53.

Trial design
Parallel.

Study duration	2 months
Dose	2 (50 mg) capsules twice daily
Route of administration	Oral
Randomized	No
Randomization adequate	No
Blinding	Single-Blind
Blinding adequate	No
Placebo	Yes
Drug comparison	No
Site description	Single practice
No. of subjects enrolled	20
No. of subjects completed	20
Sex	Male
Age	51-89 years

Inclusion criteria
Men with an enlarged prostate and subjective symptoms of nocturia, pollackiuria, and decreased flow of urine.

Exclusion criteria
Patients affected by neoplasia of the urinary tract, lithiasis of the urinary tract, urinary infection, sphincter malfunction, urinary tract malfunction, and prostatic hypertrophy needing surgery.

End points
A transrectal echographic test was performed at the beginning and end of treatment. The subjective symptom of dysuria was evaluated before the trial, after 30 days, and at the end of treatment (60 days).

Results
A statistically significant reduction in symptoms of nocturia, pollackiuria, and decreased urinary flow was observed after 60 days of treatment ($p < 0.001$, $p < 0.05$, $p < 0.05$ respectively). There was no significant change in these parameters in the placebo group. Changes in the size of the prostate in the treatment group were insignificant.

Side effects
None observed.

Authors' comments
It is inferred from this study that pygeum acts on the periurethral inflammatory component of prostate hypertrophy and has no noticeable effect on the fibrosclerotic component.

Reviewers' comments
This was a limited study, since it was not randomized and the blinding was not described. A statistical benefit was noted with *Pygeum africanum,* but the differences are small and may not be clinically significant. The study also had a small sample. (Translation reviewed) (1, 4)

Clinical Study: Tadenan®

Extract name	None given
Manufacturer	Laboratoire Dabat., France (Laboratoires Fournier, France)
Indication	**Benign prostatic hyperplasia**
Level of evidence	**II**
Therapeutic benefit	**No**

Bibliographic reference
DuFour B, Choquenet C, Revol M, Faure G, Jorest R (1984). Controlled study of the effects of *Pygeum africanum* extracts on the symptoms of benign prostatic hypertrophy. *Annales d'Urologie* 18 (3): 193-195.

Trial design
Parallel.

Study duration	6 weeks
Dose	4 (50 mg) capsules daily
Route of administration	Oral
Randomized	Yes
Randomization adequate	No
Blinding	Double-blind
Blinding adequate	Yes
Placebo	Yes
Drug comparison	No
Site description	Multicenter
No. of subjects enrolled	120
No. of subjects completed	120
Sex	Male
Age	Not given

Inclusion criteria
Prostatic hypertrophy subjects with related urination difficulties that do not require surgery.

Exclusion criteria
None mentioned.

End points
Symptoms of benign prostatic hyperplasia, including nocturnal frequency, urine flow, daily frequency, difficulty in initiating urination, sensation of incomplete emptying of the bladder, terminal drip, sense of residual urine, and interrupted flow.

Results
Statistically greater improvement was observed in the pygeum group in nocturnal frequency, difficulty in starting micturition, and incomplete emptying of the bladder. A large placebo effect was present, with 34 to 55 percent improvement of symptoms.

Side effects
None mentioned.

Authors' comments
The placebo effect is so pronounced that a statistical analysis of each symptom is necessary. The study showed a statistically significant improvement in three functional symptoms with the use of pygeum.

Reviewers' comments
This study did not show a difference in symptoms after treatment of pygeum africanum compared with placebo. The study was short, however, and in a longer study the placebo effect would remain constant, and it is possible a therapeutic benefit would be seen. (Translation reviewed) (3, 5)

Clinical Study: Tadenan®

Extract name	None given
Manufacturer	Laboratoires Fournier, France
Indication	**Benign prostatic hyperplasia**
Level of evidence	**III**
Therapeutic benefit	**Undetermined**

Bibliographic reference
Chatelain C, Autet W, and Brackman F (1999). Comparison of once and twice daily dosage forms of *Pygeum africanum* extract in patients with benign prostatic hyperplasia: A randomized, double-blind study, with long-term open label extension. *Urology* 54 (3): 473-478.

Trial design
Parallel, with three phases. One-month run-in phase without treatment preceding a two-month dose comparison trial, followed by a ten-month open phase period (100 mg once daily).

Study duration	2 months
Dose	50 mg twice daily or 100 mg once daily
Route of administration	Oral
Randomized	Yes
Randomization adequate	No
Blinding	Double-blind
Blinding adequate	No
Placebo	No

Drug comparison	No
Site description	Single center
No. of subjects enrolled	235
No. of subjects completed	209
Sex	Male
Age	58-74 years

Inclusion criteria
Age 50 years or older; clinical symptoms of benign prostatic hyperplasia (urinary symptoms, International Prostate Symptom Score [IPSS] 10 or greater, and quality of life [QOL] 3 or greater) confirmed by digital rectal examination and transrectal ultrasound (prostate volume 30 cm^3 or greater); maximum urinary flow rate (Qmax) 15 ml/s or less (voided volume 140 ml or greater); residual volume 150 ml or less; serum prostate-specific antigen (PSA) less than 10 ng/ml; and serum creatinine less than 160 µmol/l.

Exclusion criteria
Indication for or previous prostate or bladder surgery; prostate and/or bladder cancer; urinary symptoms due to other causes; and treatment during the three months preceding inclusion with finasteride, *Pygeum africanum,* or *Serenoa repens,* or with any alpha-blocker during one month before inclusion.

End points
Patients were evaluated at inclusion, after the run-in phase, after one and two months of treatment, and after 5, 8, and 12 months as part of the open phase extension. The IPSS, quality of life, vital signs, and side effects were assessed at all visits. Digital rectal examinations, Qmax, voided volume, postvoid residual volume, and sexual function were assessed at entry and after 2 and 12 months. Prostate volume and serum PSA levels were assessed at entry and after 12 months.

Results
Both treatments had similar efficacy. IPSS (baseline 17 in both groups) improved by 38 percent in Group A (50 mg twice daily) and 35 percent in Group B (100 mg once daily). QOL improved by 28 percent in both. Qmax increased by 1.63 ml/s (16 percent) in Group A and 2.02 ml/s (19 percent) in Group B. After 12 months, the IPSS fell from 16 to 9. Half of the patients had an IPSS less than 8. Mean Qmax increased by 1.65 ml/s (15 percent).

Side effects
The safety profile was similar between groups and study phases. Treatment-emergent side effects were mostly gastrointestinal. Most effects were not treatment related.

Authors' comments
Pygeum africanum extract at 50 mg twice daily and 100 mg once daily proved equally effective and safe at two months. Further improvements in efficacy with a satisfactory safety profile were documented after 12 months.

Reviewers' comments
This study compared two different dosing regimens of *Pygeum africanum* and found their efficacy and safety similar. The therapeutic benefit of this extract cannot be determined from this study. Neither the randomization nor the blinding were adequately described. The treatment length was adequate. (1, 6)

Clinical Study: Tadenan®

Extract name	None given
Manufacturer	Laboratoires Fournier, France
Indication	**Benign prostatic hyperplasia**
Level of evidence	**III**
Therapeutic benefit	**Trend**

Bibliographic reference
Gagliardi V, Apicella F, Pino P, Falchi M (1983). Medical treatment of prostatic hypertrophy: A controlled clinical investigation. *Archivio Italiano di Urologia e Nefrologia* 55: 51-69.

Trial design
Parallel. Comparison trial of pygeum versus standard treatment with nonsteroidal anti-inflammatory drugs (NSAIDs). (NSAIDs were given alone or with antibiotics.)

Study duration	30-35 days
Dose	2 (50 mg) capsules twice daily
Route of administration	Oral
Randomized	Yes
Randomization adequate	No
Blinding	Open
Blinding adequate	No
Placebo	No
Drug comparison	Yes
Drug name	NSAIDs

Site description   Single practice

No. of subjects enrolled   40
No. of subjects completed   40
Sex   Male
Age   50-84 years

Inclusion criteria

Patients with prostatic hypertrophy and symptoms associated with micturition and a variable amount of residual urine in the bladder.

Exclusion criteria

None mentioned.

End points

Symptoms of polyuria (excess urine), strangury (constricted passing of urine), dysuria, nocturia, retention of urine, and prostatic volume were assessed at the start and end of treatment.

Results

Tadenan was more effective than anti-inflammatory agents in improving symptoms. Tadenan administration improved symptoms of polyuria, strangury, dysuria, and nocturia ($p < 0.01$). The only symptom improved by anti-inflammatory agents was strangury ($p < 0.05$). Tadenan also decreased residual urine ($p < 0.01$). No statistical improvement was observed in the control group.

Side effects

None observed.

Authors' comments

Since it has been shown to be effective and safe, Tadenan is regarded as a drug of choice for medical treatment of prostatic adenoma prior to surgery.

Reviewers' comments

The inclusion/exclusion criteria were not explained in detail, and the lack of double-blinding limits the utility of the study. In addition, 30 to 35 days is a short treatment length. No adverse effects were noted with either treatment, which is surprising given the known side effects of non-steroidal anti-inflammatory drugs. (Translation reviewed) (1, 4)

Product Profile: Pigenil

Manufacturer	**Inverni della Beffa, Italy (Indena S.p.A., Italy)**
U.S. distributor	None
Botanical ingredient	**Pygeum bark soft extract**
Extract name	**PrunuSelect™**
Quantity	50 mg
Processing	Plant to extract ratio 180:1
Standardization	11:7-14.3% sterols as beta-sitosterol

Source(s) of information: Scarpa et al., 1989; information provided by Indena USA, Inc.

Clinical Study: Pigenil

Extract name	PrunuSelect™
Manufacturer	Inverni della Beffa, Italy (Indena S.p.A., Italy)
Indication	**Benign prostatic hyperplasia**
Level of evidence	**II**
Therapeutic benefit	**Yes**

Bibliographic reference
Bassi P, Artibani W, De Luca V, Zattoni F, Lembo A (1987). Estratto standardizzato di *Pygeum africanum* nel trattamento dell'ipertrofia prostatica benigna [Standardized *Pygeum africanum* extract in the treatment of benign prostatic hypetrophy]. *Minerva Urologica e Nefrologica* 39 (1): 45-50.

Trial design
Parallel.

Study duration	2 months
Dose	50 mg twice daily
Route of administration	Oral
Randomized	Yes
Randomization adequate	No
Blinding	Double-blind
Blinding adequate	Yes

Placebo	Yes
Drug comparison	No
Site description	Single center
No. of subjects enrolled	40
No. of subjects completed	40
Sex	Male
Age	Mean: 66.8 years

Inclusion criteria
Patients with prostatic hypertrophy and symptoms of obstruction and irritation with minimal residual urine who had not received any treatment for the ailment.

Exclusion criteria
Severe illnesses, especially of renal and/or hepatic origin, hypertrophy of the median lobe, urinary infection, bladder stones, or dilution of the superrenal excretory pathways due to kidney insufficiency.

End points
Patients were assessed before and after treatment for urological symptoms (daytime and nighttime frequency, urgency, posturination drip, dysuria, as well as force and caliber of flow) and objective measurements (physical exam, uroflow measurements).

Results
The preliminary results demonstrate a significant improvement of the frequency ($p < 0.001$), urgency ($p < 0.02$), dysuria ($p < 0.02$), and urinary flow ($p < 0.05$) in patients treated with pygeum compared to placebo. No significant change was observed in the quality of urination, posturination drip, nor the size or consistency of the prostate gland.

Side effects
One patient in 20 had gastric symptoms that resolved on their own.

Authors' comments
This study shows the therapeutic efficacy of the *Pygeum africanum* extract in the treatment of prostatic hypertrophy of mild to moderate degree.

Reviewers' comments
This is a good study demonstrating a benefit of Pigenil. The study was limited, however, by a small sample size, lack of details on randomization, and a short treatment length. (Translation reviewed) (3, 5)

Clinical Study: Pigenil 50

Extract name	PrunuSelect™
Manufacturer	Inverni della Beffa, Italy (Indena S.p.A., Italy)
Indication	**Benign prostatic hyperplasia**
Level of evidence	**III**
Therapeutic benefit	**Undetermined**

Bibliographic reference
Scarpa RM, Migliari R, Campus G, De Lisa A, Sorgia M, Usai M, Usai E (1989). Medical treatment of benign prostatic hypertrophy with extract of *Pygeum africanum. Stampa Medica* (Suppl. 465): 25-39.

Trial design
Parallel. Drug comparison with mepartricin (one tablet containing 50,000 U three times daily).

Study duration	2 months
Dose	1 (50 mg) capsule twice daily
Route of administration	Oral
Randomized	Yes
Randomization adequate	No
Blinding	Double-blind
Blinding adequate	No
Placebo	No
Drug comparison	Yes
Drug name	Mepartricin
Site description	Single center
No. of subjects enrolled	40
No. of subjects completed	40
Sex	Male
Age	42-80 years

Inclusion criteria
Both inpatients and outpatients with specific and mild to medium symptoms of benign prostatic hypertrophy, which impedes the normal voiding of the bladder, but does not require surgical intervention in the short term.

Exclusion criteria
Patients with concomitant diseases of the genitourinary tract (including urinary tract infections), except for morphofunctional sequels directly due to bladder output obstruction.

End points

Before and after treatment, patients were assessed using ultrasound for bladder volume, residual urine, and prostate size. Clinical symptoms (the number of daytime voidings, nighttime voidings, dysuria, sensation of incomplete bladder emptying, perineal or retropubic tenderness or pressure) were assessed at baseline and after 30 and 60 days.

Results

Both treatments reduced urinary frequency, painful urination, and residual urine compared to baseline. After 60 days, the effect on dysuria (painful urination) was significantly greater with Pigenil ($p < 0.01$). In addition, a statistically significant reduction of prostate size (11 percent) was found only in patients treated with *Pygeum africanum* (comparison between groups $p < 0.05$). No statistically significant changes were observed in a panel of laboratory tests.

Side effects

Tolerance was rated as good or very good in all cases.

Authors' comments

Although the medical treatment of benign prostatic hyperplasia with *Pygeum africanum* extract cannot be considered definitive and does not completely remove the cause of the disorder, the maintenance of an acceptable quality of life for long periods is no small achievement.

Reviewers' comments

This study was limited by design, small numbers of patients, and a lack of placebo control. Neither the blinding nor the randomization was adequately described. No difference was observed after treatment with pygeum or mepartricin. However, the treatment length was short. (1, 5)

Product Profile: Prostatonin®

Manufacturer	**Pharmaton S.A., Switzerland**
U.S. distributor	**Pharmaton Natural Health Products**
Botanical ingredient	**Pygeum bark extract**
Extract name	**PY102**
Quantity	25 mg
Processing	Plant to extract ratio 200:1
Standardization	No information
Formulation	Softgel capsule
Botanical ingredient	**Nettle root extract**

Extract name   **UR102**
Quantity   300 mg
Processing   Plant to extract ratio 5:1
Standardization   No information

Recommended dose: Adult males: Take one softgel capsule twice a day with water (in the morning and evening with meals). Optimal effectiveness has been shown after six weeks with continuous uninterrupted use.

DSHEA structure/function: Promotes normal urinary patterns, helps manage frequent urination at night, supports prostate health.

Cautions: In case of accidental overdose, seek the advice of a professional immediately. Consult a physician if receiving medical treatment and taking medication for a prostate problem, or experiencing symptoms of a prostate problem, such as painful, frequent, or difficult urination.

Other ingredients: Rape oil, gelatin, triglycerides, glycerol, sorbitol, soya lecithin, synthetic iron oxides, titanium dioxide.

Source(s) of information: Product package (© Boehringer Ingelheim Pharmaceuticals, Inc., 1999); Krzeski et al., 1993.

Clinical Study: Prostatonin®

Extract name   PY102, UR102
Manufacturer   Pharmaton S.A., Switzerland

Indication   **Benign prostatic hyperplasia**
Level of evidence   **II**
Therapeutic benefit **Undetermined**

Bibliographic reference
Krzeski T, Kazon M, Borkowski A, Witeska A, Kuczera J (1993). Combined extracts of *Urtica dioica* and *Pygeum africanum* in the treatment of benign prostatic hyperplasia: Double-blind comparison of two doses. *Clinical Therapeutics* 15 (6): 1011-1020.

Trial design
Parallel. Dose comparison: Either the standard dose of two capsules containing 300 mg of Urtica dioica extract and 25 mg pygeum extract twice daily, or two capsules containing half that amount twice daily.

Study duration	2 months
Dose	2 (either 162 or 325 mg) capsules twice daily
Route of administration	Oral
Randomized	Yes
Randomization adequate	No
Blinding	Double-blind
Blinding adequate	Yes
Placebo	No
Drug comparison	No
Site description	2 medical centers
No. of subjects enrolled	134
No. of subjects completed	124
Sex	Male
Age	53-84 years

Inclusion criteria

Patients showed at least one symptom of benign prostatic hyperplasia: residual urine, decreased urine flow, or nocturia.

Exclusion criteria

Patients with serious diseases, such as diabetes mellitus or recent myocardial infarction.

End points

Data on three target criteria (urine flow, residual urine, and nocturia) were obtained on three pretreatment control days and after four and eight weeks of treatment.

Results

After 28 days of treatment, a significant increase in urinary flow and residual urine was observed. Nocturia was significantly reduced in both treatment groups. After 56 days of treatment, further significant decreases were found in residual urine (half-dose group) and nocturia (both groups). No between-group differences were observed in these measures of efficacy.

Side effects

One case of gastrointestinal discomfort was attributed to the treatment.

Authors' comments

It was concluded that half doses of the Prostatonin extract are as safe and effective as the recommended full doses.

Reviewers' comments
This study demonstrated equivalent effectiveness of therapy of the two different doses. However, since there was no placebo group, it cannot be determined whether the drug has a therapeutic benefit. Eight weeks is also a relatively short duration of treatment. (3, 6)

Clinical Study: Prostatonin®

Extract name	PY102, UR102
Manufacturer	Pharmaton S.A., Switzerland
Indication	**Benign prostatic hyperplasia**
Level of evidence	**II**
Therapeutic benefit	**Undetermined**

Bibliographic reference
Montanari E, Mandressi A, Magri V, Dormia G, Pisani E (1991). Benign prostatic hyperplasia: Differential therapy with phytopharmacological agents— A randomized study of 63 patients. *Separatum Der Informierte Arzt/Gazette Medicale* 6a: 593-598.

Trial design
Parallel. Three treatment groups. Group 1 received two capsules (25 mg pygeum extract and 300 mg nettle root extract, trade name: Prostatonin) twice daily. Group 2 received two capsules (125 mg of *Epilobium parviflorum* Schreb. extract) daily. Group 3 received two capsules (25 mg of *Pygeum africanum* extract, trade name: Pigenil) twice daily.

Study duration	2 months
Dose	2 (25 mg pygeum extract + 300 mg nettle root extract) capsules twice daily
Route of administration	Oral
Randomized	Yes
Randomization adequate	No
Blinding	Double-blind
Blinding adequate	Yes
Placebo	No
Drug comparison	Yes
Drug name	*Epilobium parviflorum* extract; Pigenil
Site description	Single center
No. of subjects enrolled	63

No. of subjects completed 59
Sex   Male
Age   57-77 years

Inclusion criteria
Patients with micturition disorders attributed solely to benign prostatic hyperplasia.

Exclusion criteria
Patients with other urological diseases.

End points
Patients were interviewed at baseline and after 60 days. Alcohol and coffee consumption, as well as sexual activity, frequency of nocturia, intervals between individual micturitions, strength of urinary flow, and urinary urgency, were noted. Measurements of blood pressure, heart rate, general physical exam, and size and consistency of the prostate were made.

Results
All three treatment groups showed significant extension of micturition interval with no significant difference between them. No significant difference was observed between pygeum and the pygeum/nettle combination therapy in regard to the success of treatment for nocturia. However, treatment with *Epilobium* was notably less successful. Strength of urinary flow was improved in more than half the patients given the combination treatment, followed by 30 percent improvement with pygeum extract and 20 percent improvement with *Epilobium*. There was no significant change in prostate size with any of the treatments. Urinary volumes and maximum and average flow were increased in all three groups, with the greatest improvement being with the combination therapy.

Side effects
Nonspecific epigastric complaints in one patient in the combination group.

Authors' comments
Two months of treatment with a combination of the extracts of nettle root and pygeum bark proved to be superior both to the extract of *Epilobium* and to that of pyguem alone in respect to elimination of improvement of the different symptoms of benign prostatic hyperplasia.

Reviewers' comments
Although the combination of nettle root and pygeum was superior to pygeum alone or the *Epilobium* extract, a lack of a placebo group limits the usefulness of the study. Two months is a short treatment length. (4, 4)

Red Clover

Latin name: ***Trifolium pratense* L.** [Fabaceae]
Plant part: **Leaf**

PREPARATIONS USED IN REVIEWED CLINICAL STUDIES

Red clover is a member of the pea family, and is an extensive agricultural crop. The leaves and flowers contain a class of compounds called isoflavones that includes formononetin, daidzein, and genistein. Red clover products are characterized and standardized according to the quantity and composition of these isoflavones (Kelly, Husband, and Waring, 1998).

Clinical studies have been conducted with a standardized extract of red clover leaves. This extract is incorporated into tablets called Promensil™, manufactured by Novogen Laboratories Pty Ltd., NSW, Australia, and distributed in the United States by Novogen Inc., Stamford, Connecticut. The tablets are characterized as containing 40 mg isoflavones, including biochanin (24.5 mg), formononetin (8.0 mg), genistein (4 mg), and daidzein (3.5 mg). One of the studies (Samman, 1999) used an unnamed Novogen product with a very similar composition. The tablets contained 43 mg isoflavones, consisting of biochanin A (25.7 mg), formononectin (9.3 mg), genistein (4.3 mg), and daidzein (3.7 mg).

SUMMARY OF REVIEWED CLINICAL STUDIES

Some plants in the pea family, including red clover and soy, contain isoflavones that have weak estrogenic activity. With the waning of estrogen levels in menopause, these phytoestrogens are thought to help compensate and thus reduce the symptoms that may include hot flashes, sweating, cardiovascular complaints, fatigue, vertigo, mus-

RED CLOVER SUMMARY TABLE

Product Name	Manufacturer/ U.S. Distributor	Product Characteristics	Dose in Trials	Indication	No. of Trials	Benefit (Evidence Level-Trial No.)
Promensil™	Novogen Laboratories, Pty Ltd., Australia/Novogen Inc.	Tablets contain 40 mg isoflavones	1-4 tablets daily	Menopausal symptoms	2	No (II-2)
			1-2 tablets daily	Cardiovascular risk factors	2	Undetermined (II-1, III-1)

cle and joint pain, urinary incontinence, vaginal dryness, and atrophy of the vaginal epithelium. Other symptoms of a psychological nature may include irritability, forgetfulness, anxiety, depression, sleep disturbances, and reduced libido. Menopausal symptoms occur when a woman's ovaries no longer contain eggs. The resulting decline in ovarian function causes a reduced production of estrogen and progesterone, and a corresponding increase in follicle stimulating hormone (FSH) and luteinizing hormone (LH) (Murray and Pizzorno, 1999).

An Asian diet is estimated to deliver 25 to 45 mg total isoflavones per day, whereas the Western diet is estimated to contain less than 5 mg. Epidemiological data imply that the lower incidence of menopausal symptoms in Japanese women compared with Western women may be related to an enhanced dietary intake of soy isoflavones. A soy-based diet is also thought to explain the relatively low incidence of cardiovascular disease in Southeast Asia, since the diet is correlated with low levels of plasma cholesterol (Glazier and Bowman, 2001; Barnes, 1998).

Promensil™

The effects of Promensil on menopausal symptoms and risk factors for cardiovascular disease in women have been tested in four clinical trials. Two clinical studies on menopausal symptoms failed to show any significant improvement over placebo. No changes in vaginal cytology or serum hormone levels were noted. Two studies that addressed the use of red clover extracts to reduce the risk of cardiovascular incidents (heart attack and stroke) through improvement of plasma lipid profiles in pre- and postmenopausal women were inconclusive. Further studies are necessary to evaluate any potential beneficial effects on lipid profiles.

Menopausal Symptoms

The first menopausal study was a well-designed, three-month trial including 35 women (40 to 65 years of age) with at least three hot flashes a day, who were distributed into three groups: placebo; 40 mg red clover extract (one tablet Promensil); and 160 mg red clover extract (four tablets Promensil). No significant difference was observed in the incidence of flashes between the three groups after three months. There was also no difference in vaginal pH or serum levels of FSH or sex hormone binding globulin (SHBG), a hormone-binding protein (Knight, Howes, and Eden, 1999). Our reviewer, Dr. Tieraona Low Dog, noted that the control group had increased urinary iso-flavone levels, indicating an inadvertent intake of dietary isoflavones that would be a major flaw for the study.

The second study was a relatively good, randomized, double-blind crossover study that enrolled 51 women with more than three hot flashes a day. Subjects were given either one tablet Promensil daily or placebo for three months, with the two treatment phases separated by a month's washout period. No significant difference was observed between groups in reduction of hot flashes, levels of SHBG, vaginal swab, or ultrasound examinations (Baber et al., 1999). Again the study lacked control of dietary sources of isoflavones.

Cardiovascular Risk Factors

Plasma lipid profiles and elasticity of the main arteries were mea-sured in a study that addressed a heightened cardiovascular risk asso-ciated with menopause. A small, double-blind, placebo-controlled pilot study included 13 women who had been clearly postmenopausal for at least one year and free of cardiovascular disease. In this study, a three-week run-in period included a controlled diet. The treatment group received placebo for five weeks, one tablet Promensil for five weeks, and then two tablets Promensil for another five weeks, whereas the control group received placebo only for the 15 weeks. The study concluded that arterial compliance (elasticity of the main arteries as measured using blood flow and blood pressure) was in-creased by treatment compared to placebo, but that there was no sig-nificant difference between dosage of one or two Promensil tablets. Plasma lipid levels were not significantly affected (Nestel et al., 1999). Assessment of the results was complicated by the placement of the participants on a low-fat diet, encouragement to engage in exercise, and the small sample size.

In another small, crossover, single-blind trial, 14 healthy pre-menopausal women were given either placebo or two tablets red clo-ver (similar to Premensil) per day for two menstrual cycles before switching to the other treatment. The study failed to show any change in low-density lipoprotein (LDL) oxidation, total cholesterol, or triglycerides. However, an increase of high-density lipoprotein (HDL)-3 was noted (Samman et al., 1999).

ADVERSE REACTIONS OR SIDE EFFECTS

No significant side effects or adverse reactions were noted in the four reviewed trials.

INFORMATION FROM PHARMACOPOEIAL MONOGRAPHS

Source of Published Therapeutic Monographs

British Herbal Compendium, Volume 1

Indications

The *British Herbal Compendium (BHC)* states that red clover flowers (dried flowerheads) are used externally to treat skin conditions, such as psoriasis, eczema, and rashes, as well as taken internally for coughs and bronchitis (Bradley, 1992).

Doses

Infusion: dried flowerheads, 2 to 4 g three times daily (Bradley, 1992)
Liquid extract: (1:1, 25 percent ethanol), 2 to 4 ml three times daily (Bradley, 1992)
Externally: ointment prepared from infusion or liquid extract containing 10 to 15 percent of flowerheads or equivalent (Bradley, 1992)

Contraindications

The *BHC* lists no known contraindications (Bradley, 1992).

REFERENCES

Baber RJ, Templeman C, Morton T, Kelly GE, West L (1999). Randomized placebo-controlled trial of an isoflavone supplement and menopausal symptoms in women. *Climateric* 2 (2): 85-92.

Barnes S (1998). Evolution of the health benefits of soy isoflavones. *Proceedings of the Society for Experimental Biology and Medicine* 217 (3): 386-392.

Bradley PR, ed. (1992). *British Herbal Compendium: A Handbook of Scientific Information on Widely Used Plant Drugs,* Volume 1. Dorset: British Herbal Medicine Association.

Glazier MG, Bowman MA (2001). A review of the evidence for the use of phytoestrogens as a replacement for traditional estrogen replacement therapy. *Archives of Internal Medicine* 161 (9): 1161-1172.

Kelly G, Husband A, Waring M (1998). *Standardized Red Clover Extract.* Seattle, WA: Natural Product Research Consultants.

Knight DC, Howes JB, Eden JA (1999). The effect of Promensil, an isoflavone extract, on menopausal symptoms. *Climateric* 2 (2): 79-84.

Murray MT, Pizzorno JE (1999). Menopause. In *Textbook of Natural Medicine,* Second Edition, Volume 2. Eds. HE Pizzorno, MT Murray. Edinburgh: Churchill Livingstone.

Nestel PJ, Pomeroy S, Kay S, Komesaroff P, Behrsing J, Cameron JD, West L (1999). Isoflavones from red clover improve systemic arterial compliance but not plasma lipids in menopausal women. *The Journal of Clinical Endocrinology and Metabolism* 84 (3): 895-898.

Samman S, Lyons Wall PM, Chan GSM, Smith SJ, Petocz P (1999). The effect of supplementation with isoflavones on plasma lipids and oxidisability of low density lipoprotein in premenopausal women. *Atherosclerosis* 147 (2): 277-283.

DETAILS ON RED CLOVER PRODUCTS
AND CLINICAL STUDIES

Product and clinical study information is grouped in the same order as in the Summary Table. A profile on an individual product is followed by details of the clinical studies associated with that product. In some instances, a clinical study, or studies, supports several products that contain the same principal ingredient(s). In these instances, those products are grouped together.

Clinical studies that follow each product, or group of products, are grouped by therapeutic indication, in accordance with the order in the Summary Table.

Product Profile: Promensil™

Manufacturer	**Novogen Laboratories Pty Ltd., Australia**
U.S. distributor	**Novogen Inc.**
Botanical ingredient	**Red clover leaf extract**
Extract name	None given
Quantity	40 mg (isoflavone phytoestrogens)
Processing	Plant to extract ratio 5:1, ethanol extraction
Standardization	40 mg isoflavones, including genistein (4 mg), biochanin A (24.5 mg), daidzein (3.5 mg), formononetin (8 mg)
Formulation	Tablet

Recommended dose: Take one tablet daily with a meal. It may take four to five weeks of daily use to achieve the desired and full effect. Continue to use to maintain benefits.

DSHEA structure/function: Natural plant estrogens for women experiencing normal midlife changes.

Cautions: Not recommended for pregnant women or for children under the age of 15 years.

Other ingredients: Dicalcium phosphate, microcrystalline cellulose, hydroxypropyl methylcellulose, magnesium stearate, mixed tocopherols, silica, soy polysaccharide, titanium dioxide, polyethylene glycol, organic coloring containing: red 40, yellow 6, yellow 5, blue 1.

Source(s) of information: Product package; information provided by distributor; Nestel et al., 1999.

Clinical Study: Promensil™

Extract name	None given
Manufacturer	Novogen Laboratories Pty Ltd., Australia
Indication	**Menopausal symptoms**
Level of evidence	**II**
Therapeutic benefit	**No**

Bibliographic reference
Knight DC, Howes JB, Eden JA (1999). The effect of Promensil, an iso-flavone extract, on menopausal symptoms. *Climateric* 2 (2): 79-84.

Trial design
Parallel. Pretrial observation period of one week. Three treatment groups: one tablet (40 mg) Promensil; four tablets (160 mg) Promensil; and placebo. All subjects consumed a total of four tablets daily.

Study duration	3 months
Dose	1 or 4 (40 mg isoflavone) tablets daily
Route of administration	Oral
Randomized	Yes
Randomization adequate	Yes
Blinding	Double-blind
Blinding adequate	Yes
Placebo	Yes
Drug comparison	No
Site description	University hospital
No. of subjects enrolled	37
No. of subjects completed	35
Sex	Female
Age	40-65 years

Inclusion criteria
Postmenopausal women ages 40 to 65 years who were symptomatic, having at least three hot flashes per day. Menopause was defined by bilateral oophorectomy or amenorrhea for at least six months with typical symptoms

of menopause, and a serum follicle stimulating hormone (FSH) level greater than 40 IU/l.

Exclusion criteria
Hormone replacement therapy (HRT) use within the previous six weeks; allergy to foodstuffs known to contain isoflavones; current history of active bowel, liver, or gallbladder disease; diabetes requiring drug therapy; and malignancy (excluding skin cancers). Women with contraindications to HRT use, vegetarians and/or regular soy product users, and those receiving medications that result in liver enzyme induction.

End points
Pretrial flushing was assessed using a daily diary of hot flashes for the week prior to trial entry. The severity of menopausal symptoms was assessed during this period using the Greene Menopause Scale. A 24-hour urine collection for isoflavone measurement was also performed during this week. After screening and assignment to treatment groups, physical and vaginal examinations were performed. Blood was examined for hematological profile, liver function, and serum levels of FSH and sex hormone binding globulin (SHBG). Subjects were seen every four weeks for clinical assessment. In the final week, physical and vaginal examinations, and urine and blood tests were repeated.

Results
No significant difference was observed in the incidence of hot flashes between the three groups at trial conclusion. There was no difference in the incidence between the groups in Greene Menopause Symptom Scores, vaginal pH, levels of FSH, SHBG, total cholesterol, liver function, or blood parameters. A statistically significant increase in high-density lipoprotein (HDL) cholesterol of 18.1 percent ($p = 0.038$) occurred in the 40 mg group.

Side effects
None mentioned.

Authors' comments
A large placebo response and inadvertent use of dietary isoflavones in the placebo group may have obscured a significant change in hot flash frequency. Previous uncontrolled studies claiming a beneficial effect of foods with a high isoflavone content on menopausal symptoms may have been confounded by a large placebo response.

Reviewer's comments
This was a well-designed and well-conducted study. The red clover preparation had no effect. However, there were some important flaws. The sample size was small (no power calculation), and the control group had increased urinary isoflavone levels, indicating a likely dietary breach in the trial. (5, 5)

Clinical Study: Promensil™

Extract name	None given
Manufacturer	Novogen Laboratories Pty Ltd., Australia
Indication	**Menopausal symptoms**
Level of evidence	**II**
Therapeutic benefit	**No**

Bibliographic reference
Baber RJ, Templeman C, Morton T, Kelly GE, West L (1999). Randomized placebo-controlled trial of an isoflavone supplement and menopausal symptoms in women. *Climateric* 2 (2): 85-92.

Trial design
Crossover. Subjects were assessed for one week before the start of trial to ensure entry qualifications. Treatment periods were separated by a one-month washout period.

Study duration	3 months
Dose	1 (40 mg isoflavone) tablet daily
Route of administration	Oral
Randomized	Yes
Randomization adequate	No
Blinding	Single-Blind
Blinding adequate	Yes
Placebo	Yes
Drug comparison	No
Site description	Hospital clinic
No. of subjects enrolled	51
No. of subjects completed	43
Sex	Female
Age	Mean: 54 years

Inclusion criteria
Women with more than three hot flashes per day.

Exclusion criteria
Intercurrent medical problems; hormone replacement therapy or antibiotics in previous three months; FSH < 30 mIU/ml; menstruation in previous six months; hysterectomy; or vegetarian (>10 g legumes per day).

End points
Tests were completed at the start and completion of the first treatment period and at the end of the second treatment period. They included a routine medical examination, blood collection, 24-hour urine sample for isoflavone analysis, endometrial thickness determined by transvaginal ultrasound, and vaginal smear to assess vaginal maturation index. In addition, a nurse examined subjects on a monthly basis, and subjects kept a daily symptom diary.

Results
No significant difference was observed between active and placebo groups in the reduction in hot flashes between start and finish time-points. Analysis performed on interim data time-points revealed a substantially greater reduction in hot flashes in the active group than placebo at four and eight weeks after commencement of treatment, but this was not statistically significant. No significant differences were observed between groups for Greene Menopause Symptom Scores, sex hormone binding globulin levels, hematological or biochemical parameters, and vaginal swab or ultrasound findings. The combined values for all subjects, regardless of treatment group, revealed a strong negative correlation between the level of urinary isoflavone excretion and the incidence of hot flashes.

Side effects
No adverse events.

Authors' comments
These data do not indicate a therapeutic benefit from dietary supplementation with isoflavones in women experiencing menopausal symptoms, but do indicate that the apparent placebo effect in many studies of menopausal symptoms may be attributable to dietary sources of isoflavones. The study also demonstrates that three months of isoflavone supplementation did not cause adverse events or endometrial changes.

Reviewer's comments
Although this was a relatively well-run study, the randomization was not adequately described, and no power calculation was provided for sample size. The Promensil treatment failed to show benefit. (3, 5)

Clinical Study: Promensil™

Extract name	None given
Manufacturer	Novogen Laboratories Pty Ltd., Australia

Indication   **Cardiovascular risk factors** in
                              postmenopausal women
Level of evidence   **II**
Therapeutic benefit   **Undetermined**

Bibliographic reference
Nestel PJ, Pomeroy S, Kay S, Komesaroff P, Behrsing J, Cameron JD, West
L (1999). Isoflavones from red clover improve systemic arterial compliance
but not plasma lipids in menopausal women. *The Journal of Clinical Endocrinology and Metabolism* 84 (3): 895-898.

Trial design
Parallel. A three-week run-in phase with placebo and controlled diet preceded randomization into two groups. The active group received placebo for
five weeks, one Promensil tablet daily for another five weeks, then two
Promensil tablets for the remaining five weeks. The other group, one-fifth the
size, received placebo throughout.

Study duration   15 weeks
Dose   1 or 2 (40 mg isoflavone) tablets daily
Route of administration   Oral

Randomized   Yes
Randomization adequate   No
Blinding   Double-blind
Blinding adequate   Yes

Placebo   Yes
Drug comparison   No

Site description   Not described

No. of subjects enrolled   26
No. of subjects completed   13
Sex   emale
Age   41-71 years

Inclusion criteria
Women who had been clearly postmenopausal for at least one year, FSH
level greater than 40, plasma cholesterol level between 5 to 7 mmol/l, and
free of cardiovascular disease.

Exclusion criteria
Over 70 years of age; hormone replacement therapy in preceding six weeks;
supplements such as evening primrose oil or vitamin E in preceding four to
six weeks; medication that might affect plasma lipids or cardiovascular func-

tion; smoking, and drinking more than 14 standard alcoholic drinks weekly; and body mass index greater than 32.

End points

Measurements were made at the end of each treatment phase (i.e., after run-in, placebo, and two active periods). Plasma lipid profiles were determined on two consecutive days. Isoflavone excretion in urine was measured to monitor absorption. Systemic arterial compliance, measurement of elasticity of the main conduit arteries, was determined near the end of each period.

Results

Arterial compliance rose by 23 percent with the 80 mg dose relative to the placebo period, and only slightly less with the 40 mg dose. The mean arterial compliance values for the active substance group were: run-in, 18.5; placebo, 19.7; 40 mg isoflavones, 23.7; and 80 mg isoflavones, 24.4 (mmHg/ml/min). The corresponding mean arterial compliance values for the four placebo individuals were: 17, 16, 16, and 16, respectively. For the active treatment group, differences were significant between placebo phase and 40 and 80 mg isoflavone doses (by paired t-tests: placebo versus 40 mg, $p = 0.039$; placebo versus 80 mg, $p = 0.018$). No significant difference was observed between the two treatment phases or between the placebo and run-in periods for the active treatment group. Plasma lipids were not significantly affected. The high dropout rate, higher during placebo phases than intervention phases, was due in part to intolerable menopausal symptoms.

Side effects

None mentioned.

Authors' comments

An important cardiovascular risk factor, arterial compliance, which diminishes with menopause, was significantly improved with red clover isoflavones. Since diminished compliance leads to systolic hypertension and may increase left ventricular work, the findings indicate a potential new therapeutic approach for improved cardiovascular function after menopause.

Reviewer's comments

This is an interesting study. However, participants were placed on a low-fat diet and "encouraged" to exercise, in addition to taking isoflavones. The placebo group had only three participants; the study was too small to draw any significant conclusions. (3, 4)

Clinical Study: Red Clover

Extract name	None given
Manufacturer	Novogen Laboratories Pty Ltd., Australia
Indication	**Cardiovascular risk factors** in premenopausal women
Level of evidence	**III**
Therapeutic benefit	**Undetermined**

Bibliographic reference
Samman S, Lyons Wall PM, Chan GSM, Smith SJ, Petocz P (1999). The effect of supplementation with isoflavones on plasma lipids and oxidisability of low density lipoprotein in premenopausal women. *Atherosclerosis* 147 (2): 277-283.

Trial design
Crossover. Subjects took either placebo or red clover for two menstrual cycles, then switched to the other treatment for the following two cycles. Each subject served as her own control. Subjects were requested to maintain their normal eating patterns and alcohol consumption throughout the trial. The tablets used in this study are not Promensil, although the isoflavonoid profile is similar to two Promensil tablets.

Study duration	2 menstrual cycles
Dose	2 (43 mg isoflavone) tablets daily
Route of administration	Oral
Randomized	Yes
Randomization adequate	No
Blinding	Single-Blind
Blinding adequate	Yes
Placebo	Yes
Drug comparison	No
Site description	Not described
No. of subjects enrolled	21
No. of subjects completed	14
Sex	Female
Age	Mean: 27.5 ± 8.2 years

Inclusion criteria
Premenopausal, healthy women, regular menstrual cycle (23 to 35 days), ages 18 to 45.

Exclusion criteria
History of chronic illness; taking medications or oral contraceptives; suffering from liver, bowel, or gall bladder disorders; unstable body weight and exercise patterns; and regular intake of soy products (more than one serving per week).

End points
Normal ovulatory cycles were confirmed by measurement of luteinizing hormone in urine. Blood and urine samples were taken at baseline and during Cycles 2 and 4 to determine lipoprotein profiles and isoflavone concentrations.

Results
Supplementation resulted in a fivefold increase in urinary isoflavone excretion. No significant changes in oxidizability of low-density lipoprotein (LDL), or plasma concentrations of total cholesterol or triglyceride, were observed, with the exception of high-density lipoprotein (HDL) 3, which showed a significant period effect ($p = 0.024$) and a trend toward a carryover effect ($p = 0.086$).

Side effects
None mentioned.

Authors' comments
Supplementation of normocholesterolemic premenopausal women with isoflavones does not affect plasma cholesterol or LDL cholesterol concentrations, but may increase the concentration of HDL3 cholesterol. This observation, together with favorable effects on other cardiovascular risk factors reported previously, namely arterial compliance, supports the notion that isoflavones are cardioprotective.

Reviewer's comments
The therapeutic benefit was not determined. The report did not include a discussion of randomization, and the study was single-blinded. A further flaw was the small sample size. (1, 5)

Red Yeast Rice

Other common names: *Hong qu*
Latin name: *Monascus* purpureus **Went.** [Monascaceae]

PREPARATIONS USED
IN REVIEWED CLINICAL STUDIES

Red yeast rice is a traditional Chinese fermented product made from a red yeast, *Monascus purpureus* Went., that is grown on rice. Documentation of the use of red yeast rice extends back to the Tang dynasty in 800 A.D. Red yeast rice products contain a group of compounds called the monacolins, which are a family of polyketides. The monacolins have been identified as inhibitors of an enzyme involved in the endogenous biosynthesis of cholesterol, 3-hydroxy-3-methylglutaryl coenzyme A (HMG-CoA) reductase. One of the monacolins, monacolin K, is identical to lovastatin. Lovastatin is a common cholesterol-lowering statin drug that is manufactured by Merck and Co., Inc., West Point, Pennsylvania (Heber et al., 1999; Schulz, Hänsel, and Tyler, 2001).

Cholestin™ capsules are manufactured by Pharmanex, a subsidiary of Nu Skin Enterprises, Provo, Utah. The capsules contained 600 mg red yeast rice product, including 0.4 percent monacolins by weight (RY-2), approximately half of which (0.2 percent) were monacolin K. Recent court action by Merck, due to the similarity of monacolin K in Cholestin to lovastatin (mevinolin) in Mevacor®, blocked the sale of Cholestin as originally formulated in the United States. The original Cholestin, containing red yeast rice, is still available in other countries. The new U.S. formulation includes, as a substitute, a beeswax extract called policosanol. According to Pharmanex, policosanol is a safe and effective ingredient that successfully maintains existing normal cholesterol levels, although the new formulation has not been tested clinically. Each capsule of Cholestin

RED YEAST SUMMARY TABLE

Product Name	Manufacturer/ U.S. Distributor	Product Characteristics	Dose in Trials	Indication	No. of Trials	Benefit (Evidence Level-Trial No.)
Cholestin™/No longer available in the United States in its original form	Pharmanex LLC/Pharmanex Natural Healthcare	Capsules containing 600 mg extract: 2.4 mg monacolins (RY-2)	1.2-2.4 g daily	Hyperlipidemia (elevated blood lipid levels)	2	Yes (I-1, II-1)
Xue-zhi-kang	Wei-Xin Company, China/None	1.2 g contains 13.5 mg total monacolins (RY-1)	1.2 g daily	Hyperlipidemia (elevated blood lipid levels	1	Trend (III-1)
Zhitai	WBL Peking Univ Biotech Co. Ltd., China/None	5 g contains 10-13 mg total monacolins	5 g daily	Hyperlipidemia (elevated blood lipid levels)	1	Yes (II-1)

sold in the United States now contains 15 mg policosanol (beeswax extract 5:1).

Monascus purpureus Went. yeast is called Xue-zhi-kang in Chinese. The Xue-zhi-kang product (RY-1) produced by Wei-Xin Company (China) delivered a daily dose of 1.2 g red yeast rice containing 13.5 mg total monacolins.

The red yeast rice product called Zhitai, produced by WBL Peking University Biotech Co. Ltd. (China) delivered 10-13 mg total monacolins in a 5 g daily dose. According to a spokesperson from Pharmanex, the former two products were prototypes studied in the development of the original Cholestin.

SUMMARY OF REVIEWED CLINICAL STUDIES

Red yeast rice products have been tested in clinical studies for their effect in reducing elevated serum cholesterol levels. High cholesterol levels, total serum cholesterol more than 200 mg/dl and low-density lipoprotein (LDL) cholesterol more than 130 mg/dl, are indicated as risk factors for cardiovascular disease. Sources for serum cholesterol are dietary intake of animal fats and production by the liver. Cholesterol is transported in the blood by lipoproteins. The major categories of lipoproteins are very low-density lipoproteins (VLDL), low-density lipoproteins, and high-density lipoproteins (HDL). VLDL and LDL transport fats, primarily triglycerides and cholesterol, from the liver to cells throughout the body, whereas HDL returns fats to the liver. Elevations of either VLDL cholesterol or LDL cholesterol are associated with an increase in risk for developing atherosclerosis, which is a primary cause of heart attacks and strokes. The ratio of total cholesterol to HDL cholesterol and the ratio of LDL cholesterol to HDL cholesterol indicate whether cholesterol is being deposited into tissues or broken down and excreted (Pizzorno and Murray, 1999).

Elevated cholesterol levels can be reduced through changes in diet and/or administration of nutritional supplements or drugs. Three classes of drugs have been used to reduce cholesterol levels: bile acid sequestrants, nicotinic acid (niacin), and statins. The largest reduction in serum cholesterol, 25 to 45 percent, is observed with the statin drugs. Statins inhibit the activity of an enzyme involved in the biosynthesis of cholesterol, namely 3-hydroxy-3-methylglutaryl coenzyme A (HMG-CoA) reductase. The most familiar statin drugs are lovastatin (Mevacor) and simvastatin (Zocor®) (Hardman et al., 1996).

The monacolins present in red yeast rice are also identified as inhibitors of HMG-CoA reductase. Four studies explored the effect of red yeast rice products on lipid levels. Two trials demonstrated significant cholesterol lowering following eight to twelve weeks of treatment with Cholestin. A trial with another red yeast rice product attempted to demonstrate comparable activity to a statin drug, but the trial was performed in a population too small to be significant. Finally, a large trial, in which a third red yeast rice product was compared with placebo, also demonstrated lipid-lowering effects.

Cholestin

Hyperlipidemia (Elevated Blood Lipid Levels)

A double-blind, placebo-controlled, randomized trial included 83 subjects with slightly elevated cholesterol (total serum cholesterol 204 to 338 mg/dl, LDL cholesterol 128 to 277 mg/dl, triacylglycerol 55 to 246 mg/dl, and HDL cholesterol 30 to 95 mg/dl). Participants received either 2.4 g red yeast rice (Cholestin) or placebo for 12 weeks and were put on the American Heart Association's Step I diet. After eight and twelve weeks, total serum cholesterol and LDL cholesterol measurements in the treatment group decreased significantly from baseline and in comparison to placebo. The reduction in total cholesterol in the treatment group after 12 weeks compared with baseline was roughly 40 mg/dl. Triacylglycerol levels also decreased at week 8 in comparison to placebo, and at weeks 8 and 12 in comparison to baseline. HDL cholesterol levels did not alter significantly in either group (Heber et al., 1999).

A multicenter, single-blind trial included 446 subjects with primary hyperlipidemia (serum total cholesterol greater than 230 mg/dl, LDL cholesterol more than 130 mg/dl, or triglycerides of 200 to 400 mg/dl). Subjects received either 1.2 g red yeast rice (Cholestin) or another traditional Chinese medicine (Jiaogulan) with putative hypolipidemic properties. After eight weeks, serum total cholesterol in the red yeast rice group decreased by 23 percent compared with baseline, LDL cholesterol decreased by 30.9 percent, serum triglycerides decreased by 34.1 percent, and HDL cholesterol increased by 19.9 percent. Ninety-three percent of subjects in the Cholestin group bene-fited from treatment compared with 50 percent of the Jiaogulan group (Wang et al., 1997).

Xue-zhi-kang

Hyperlipidemia (Elevated Blood Lipid Levels)

In a drug comparison study conducted in China, 28 hyperlipidemic subjects, with total cholesterol levels of more than 230 mg/dl and tri-glycerides greater than 200 mg/dl, were given either 1.2 g red yeast rice (Xue-zhi-kang) or 10 mg simvastatin (a statin drug) daily for eight weeks. Both treatments decreased total cholesterol and LDL cholesterol after four and eight weeks with no significant differences between the two. Both treatments reduced triglyceride levels, but the reduction with simvastatin was not significant. HDL cholesterol lev-els were not altered (Lu, 1998). This study was limited by the small sample size and the lack of detail in the report.

Zhitai

Hyperlipidemia (Elevated Blood Lipid Levels)

In a double-blind, placebo-controlled trial, 152 hyperlipidemic subjects were given either 5 g red yeast rice (Zhitai tablets) per day or placebo. Subjects initially had serum total cholesterol levels greater than 250 mg/dl and/or triglyceride levels greater than 200 mg/dl. Af-ter two months of treatment, total cholesterol, triglyceride, and LDL cholesterol levels were significantly decreased, and HDL cholesterol levels were significantly increased compared to baseline. Measure-ments in the placebo group did not change, and a significant differ-ence from the treatment group was observed in all of the lipid levels mentioned previously (Zhiwei et al., 1996).

ADVERSE REACTIONS OR SIDE EFFECTS

Side effects reported in the trials discussed in this section consisted of occasional gastrointestinal discomfort. Contrary to studies with other statin drugs, no elevations in liver function tests were observed in any of the studies. David Heber, our reviewer, considered the amounts of monacolin K contained in the red yeast rice products to be too low and the sample sizes too small to expect any adverse effects. The monacolin K content in red yeast rice is approximately 0.2 percent. Therefore, a dose of 2.5 g red yeast rice would be expected to contain 5 mg monacolin K or 10 mg total monacolins. Adverse effects on the liver are noted only with the statin drug lovastatin (Mevacor) at doses of greater than 20 mg per day, and the incidence rate is only 1.5 percent at 80 mg per day (Hardman et al., 1996).

REFERENCES

Hardman JG, Limbird LE, Molinoff PB, Ruddon RW, Gilman AG (1996). *Goodman and Gillman's The Pharmacological Basis of Therapeutics,* Ninth Edition. New York: McGraw-Hill.

Heber D, Yip I, Ashley JM, Elashoff DA, Elashoff RM, Go VLW (1999). Cholesterol-lowering effects of a proprietary Chinese red-yeast-rice dietary supplement. *American Journal of Clinical Nutrition* 69 (2): 231-236.

Lu GP (1998). The comparison of the blood lipids lowering effects of Xue-Zhi-Kang and simvastatin on hypercholesterolemic patients. *Chinese Journal of Internal Medicine* 37 (6): 371-373.

Pizzorno JE, Murray MT, eds. (1999). *Textbook of Natural Medicine,* Second Edition, Volume 2. London: Churchill Livingstone.

Schulz V, Hänsel R, Tyler VE (2001). *Rational Phytotherapy: A Physicians' Guide to Herbal Medicine,* Fourth Edition. Trans. TC Telgar. Berlin: Springer-Verlag.

Wang J, Lu Z, Chi J, Wang W, Su M, Kou W, Yu P, Yu L, Chen L, Zhu J, Chang J (1997). Multicenter clinical trial of the serum lipid-lowering effects of a *Monascus purpureus* (red yeast) rice preparation from traditional Chinese medicine. *Current Therapeutic Research* 58 (12): 964-978.

Zhiwei S, Pulin Y, Meizhen S, Chi J, Zhou Y, Zhu X, Yang C, He C (1996). A prospective study on Zhitai capsule in the treatment of primary hyperlipidemia. *National Medical Journal of China* 76 (2): 156-157.

DETAILS ON RED YEAST PRODUCTS
AND CLINICAL STUDIES

Product and clinical study information is grouped in the same order as in the Summary Table. A profile on an individual product is followed by details of the clinical studies associated with that product. In some instances, a clinical study, or studies, supports several products that contain the same principal ingredient(s). In these instances, those products are grouped together.

Clinical studies that follow each product, or group of products, are grouped by therapeutic indication, in accordance with the order in the Summary Table.

Index to Red Yeast Products

Product Profile: Cholestin™

Manufacturer	**Pharmanex LLC**
U.S. distributor	**Pharmanex Natural Healthcare**
Botanical ingredient	**Red yeast rice extract**
Extract name	**RY-2**
Quantity	600 mg
Processing	Fermented product of rice on which red yeast *(Monascus purpureus)* has been grown
Standardization	0.4% monacolins by weight (0.2% monacolin K)
Formulation	Capsule

Recommended dose: Take two capsules twice daily (morning and evening) with a drink and food to minimize the possibility of digestive discomfort. Must be taken regularly to help maintain healthy cholesterol levels.

DSHEA structure/function: Promotes healthy cholesterol levels.

Cautions: Do not take more than four capsules in a 24-hour period. Immediately discontinue use if you experience any unexplained muscle pain or tenderness, especially if accompanied by flulike symptoms. Do not use if you are pregnant, can become pregnant, or are breast feeding. Consult a physician if you are taking any prescription medication. Cholestin contains several natural HMG-CoA reductase inhibitors, one of which has been associated with rare (in less than 1 to 2 percent of users) but serious side effects. Do not take if: you are at risk of liver disease, have active liver disease, or have any history of liver disease; you consume more than two drinks of alcohol per day; you have a serious infection; you have undergone an organ transplant; you have a serious disease or physical disorder or have undergone major surgery.

Other ingredients: Gelatin.

Comments: This product is no longer available in this form in the United States. Instead of a red yeast rice extract, the product now has policosanol (beeswax extract 5:1) 15 mg per capsule.

Source(s) of information: Product package; Heber et al., 1999; information provided by manufacturer.

Clinical Study: Cholestin

Extract name	RY-2
Manufacturer	Pharmanex LLC
Indication	**Hyperlipidemia** (elevated blood lipid levels)
Level of evidence	**I**
Therapeutic benefit	**Yes**

Bibliographic reference
Heber D, Yip I, Ashley JM, Elashoff DA, Elashoff RM, Go VLW (1999). Cholesterol-lowering effects of a proprietary Chinese red-yeast-rice dietary supplement. *American Journal of Clinical Nutrition* 69 (2): 231-236.

Trial design
Parallel. A one-week placebo run-in phase preceded the trial. Subjects were instructed in the American Heart Association's Step I diet (< 30 percent of energy from fat, < 10 percent of energy from saturated fat, and < 300 mg cholesterol per day).

Study duration	3 months
Dose	4 (600 mg red yeast rice) capsules daily

Route of administration	Oral
Randomized	Yes
Randomization adequate	Yes
Blinding	Double-blind
Blinding adequate	Yes
Placebo	Yes
Drug comparison	No
Site description	University research center
No. of subjects enrolled	88
No. of subjects completed	83
Sex	Male and female
Age	Not given

Inclusion criteria
Subjects with LDL cholesterol > 4.14 mmol/l and triacylglycerol concentrations < 2.94 mmol/l, who had not being treated previously for hypercholesterolemia, and had normal liver and renal function. Subjects came in twice for screening physical examinations and fasting blood samples.

Exclusion criteria
Subjects taking any lipid-regulating drugs, hormone replacement therapy, immunosuppressive agents, drugs known to affect lipid concentrations, or drugs known to be associated with rhabdomyolysis, including erythromycin and cyclosporine, insulin, or oral hypoglycemic agents; or having an endocrine disease known to lead to lipid abnormalities.

End points
Main outcome measures were total cholesterol, total triacylglycerol, and HDL and LDL cholesterol measured twice at baseline and at weeks 8, 9, 11, and 12. The two baseline measurements were averaged, as were the measurements at weeks 8 and 9 and at weeks 11 and 12. At baseline, eight, and twelve weeks, food-frequency questionnaires were given to patients to assess dietary intake.

Results
Eligible subjects had baseline levels of serum cholesterol of 5.28 to 8.74 mmol/l (204 to 338 mg/dl), LDL cholesterol of 3.31 to 7.16 mmol/l (128 to 277 mg/dl), triacylglycerol of 0.62 to 2.78 mmol/l (55 to 246 mg/dl), and HDL cholesterol of 0.78 to 2.46 mmol/l (30 to 95 mg/dl). Total cholesterol and LDL cholesterol concentrations in the treatment group differed significantly from baseline and the placebo group at weeks 8 and 12 (all $p < 0.05$). Triacylglycerol levels differed significantly from the control group at week 8, and from baseline at weeks 8 and 12 (all $p < 0.05$). HDL cholesterol levels

did not change significantly either from baseline or in comparison to placebo.

Side effects
No serious side effects.

Authors' comments
Red yeast rice reduces total cholesterol, LDL cholesterol, and total triacylglycerol concentrations significantly compared with placebo, and provides a novel food-based approach to lowering cholesterol in the general population.

Reviewer's comments
This study is the first U.S. trial of Chinese red yeast rice, and shows definite effects relative to placebo. (5, 6)

Clinical Study: Cholestin3™

Extract name	RY-2
Manufacturer	Pharmanex LLC
Indication	**Hyperlipidemia** (elevated blood lipid levels)
Level of evidence	**II**
Therapeutic benefit	**Yes**

Bibliographic reference
Wang J, Lu Z, Chi J, Wang W, Su M, Kou W, Yu P, Yu L, Chen L, Zhu J, Chang J (1997). Multicenter clinical trial of the serum lipid-lowering effects of a *Monascus purpureus* (red yeast) rice preparation from traditional Chinese medicine. *Current Therapeutic Research* 58 (12): 964-978.

Trial design
Parallel. Patients were divided into four groups: three received red yeast rice and one received a traditional Chinese medicine (Jiaogulan, 1.2 g per day) with putative hypolipidemic properties.

Study duration	2 months
Dose	0.6 g red yeast rice twice daily
Route of administration	Oral
Randomized	Yes
Randomization adequate	Yes
Blinding	Single-Blind

Blinding adequate	No
Placebo	No
Drug comparison	Yes
Drug name	Jiaogulan *(Gynostemma pentaphylla)*
Site description	Multicenter
No. of subjects enrolled	502
No. of subjects completed	446
Sex	Male and female
Age	Mean: 56.2 ± 0.7 years

Inclusion criteria
Clinical diagnosis of primary hyperlipidemia: serum total cholesterol (TC) > 230 mg/dl (5.95 mmol/l), low-density lipoprotein (LDL) cholesterol > 130 mg/dl (3.41 mmol/dl), or triglycerides (TG) of 200 to 400 mg/dl (2.26 to 4.52 mmol/l). In addition, high-density lipoprotein (HDL) cholesterol < 40 mg/dl for men, or < 45 mg/dl for women. Medication for hyperlipidemia was discontinued for more than four weeks.

Exclusion criteria
Patients were excluded from this trial if they had any of the following during the last 6 months: myocardial infarction, stroke, severe trauma or major surgery, nephrotic syndrome, hypothyroidism, acute or chronic hepatobiliary disorders, diabetes mellitus, gout, allergies, or psychosis.

End points
At baseline, and at the end of weeks 4 and 8, patient serum lipids (TC, TG, and HDL cholesterol) were measured after fasting for 12 hours. LDL cholesterol and the ratio of non-HDL to HDL cholesterol were also calculated.

Results
After eight weeks of treatment, TC decreased by 22.7 percent ($p < 0.001$-comparison with baseline) in the red yeast rice patients, and a 7.0 percent reduction was found in the control group ($p < 0.001$-comparison between groups). LDL cholesterol was reduced by 30.9 percent in the red yeast rice group, whereas LDL in the control group was reduced by 8.9 percent. Between-group comparisons were significant ($p < 0.001$). TG followed the same trends as TC and LDL cholesterol, with differences between the groups being highly significant ($p < 0.001$). HDL cholesterol in the red yeast rice group increased by 19.9 percent, and it increased by 8.4 percent in the control group. Differences between the groups were highly significant ($p < 0.001$). The non-HDL cholesterol to HDL cholesterol ratio decreased by 34.5 percent in the red yeast rice group, compared to a decrease of 8.3 percent in the control group ($p < 0.001$-comparison between groups). Treatment with

red yeast rice was effective in 93.2 percent of patients, whereas treatment with control was effective in 50.8 percent of patients.

Side effects
Minor side effects: heartburn, flatulence, dizziness.

Authors' comments
This traditional Chinese rice preparation used as a dietary supplement is extremely effective and well tolerated in reducing elevated serum cholesterol and triglycerides.

Reviewer's comments
Good single-masked study that had clearly defined end points, a large sample, and was well reported. (3, 6)

Product Profile: Xue-zhi-kang

Manufacturer	**Wei-Xin Company, China**
U.S. distributor	None
Botanical ingredient	**Red yeast rice extract**
Extract name	**RY-1**
Quantity	1.2 g contains 13.5 total monacolins
Processing	No information
Standardization	HMG Co-A reductase activity (1.5-1.8%)

Comments: According to personal communication with Pharmanex, this is RY-1, an extract of RY-2 (which is Cholestin). It contains 4 times the quantity of HMG-CoA reductase inhibiting activity (1.5 to 1.8 percent).

Source(s) of information: Lu, 1998; Heber et al., 1999; Pharmanex personal communication, September 2002.

Clinical Study: Xue-zhi-kang

Extract name	RY-1
Manufacturer	Wei-Xin Company, China
Indication	**Hyperlipidemia** (elevated blood lipid levels)
Level of evidence	**III**
Therapeutic benefit	**Trend**

Bibliographic reference

Lu GP (1998). The comparison of the blood lipids lowering effects of Xue-Zhi-Kang and simvastatin on hypercholesterolemic patients. *Chinese Journal of Internal Medicine* 37 (6): 371-373.

Trial design

Parallel. Patients took red yeast rice or simvastatin (10 mg per day) for eight weeks, maintaining food and drink habits throughout the trial. Patients with accompanying hypertension were permitted to continue treatment for these conditions.

Study duration	2 months
Dose	1.2 g red yeast rice daily; 10 mg/day simvastatin
Route of administration	Oral
Randomized	Yes
Randomization adequate	No
Blinding	Not described
Blinding adequate	No
Placebo	No
Drug comparison	Yes
Drug name	Simvastatin (Shu-jiang-zhi)
Site description	Outpatient department
No. of subjects enrolled	28
No. of subjects completed	28
Sex	Male and female
Age	Mean: 57 ± 10 years

Inclusion criteria

Hyperlipidemic (IIa or IIb) subjects with total cholesterol (TC) levels > 230 mg/dl or triglycerides (TG) > 200 mg/dl who were not being treated with other drugs or had stopped treatments more than four weeks before the trial.

Exclusion criteria

Patients with diseases of the liver, kidney, or thyroid gland were excluded.

End points

At baseline, and after four and eight weeks, blood samples were taken from patients after they had fasted for 12 hours. TC, TG, high-density lipoprotein (HDL) cholesterol, and low-density lipoprotein (LDL) cholesterol levels were determined.

Results
Both treatment with red yeast rice and simvastatin decreased TC and LDL cholesterol after four and eight weeks with no significant difference between the groups. Both drugs had a lowering effect on TG, although the decrease with simvastatin was not statistically significant. No obvious effect on HDL cholesterol was indicated. In general, the effect on blood lipids at the end of eight weeks was not different from that at four weeks.

Side effects
Patients experienced no adverse side effects.

Author's comments
Taking 1.2 g daily of red yeast rice significantly lowers serum TC and LDL cholesterol in hypercholesterolemic patients. The lowering degree is nearly the same as that of simvastatin.

Reviewer's comments
This study was limited by several flaws: the inclusion/exclusion criteria were not adequate, the statistical methods were not adequately described or applied, the study was not blinded, and the randomization process was not adequately described. The failure to find significance was due to the small sample size. In addition, bioequivalence of the two drugs was not demonstrated. (0, 3)

Product Profile: Zhitai

Manufacturer	**WBL Peking University Biotech Co. Ltd., China**
U.S. distributor	None
Botanical ingredient	**Red yeast rice extract**
Extract name	None given
Quantity	500 mg
Processing	No information
Standardization	1.0-1.3 mg total monacolins
Formulation	Capsule

Comments: According to personal communication with Pharmanex, this is an earlier version of RY-2 (Cholestin) with much lower potency.

Source(s) of information: Zhiwei et al., 1996; Heber et al., 1999; Pharmanex personal communication, September 2002.

Clinical Study: Zhitai

Extract name	None given
Manufacturer	WBL Peking University Biotech Co. Ltd., China
Indication	**Hyperlipidemia** (elevated blood lipid levels)
Level of evidence	**II**
Therapeutic benefit	**Yes**

Bibliographic reference

Zhiwei S, Pulin Y, Meizhen S, Chi J, Zhou Y, Zhu X, Yang C, He C (1996). A prospective study on Zhitai capsule in the treatment of primary hyperlipidemia. *National Medical Journal of China* 76 (2): 156-157.

Trial design

Parallel. Subjects were divided into three groups: two received active treatment and one received placebo.

Study duration	2 months
Dose	5 tablets Zhitai twice daily (5 g/day)
Route of administration	Oral
Randomized	Yes
Randomization adequate	No
Blinding	Double-blind
Blinding adequate	Yes
Placebo	Yes
Drug comparison	No
Site description	Multicenter
No. of subjects enrolled	152
No. of subjects completed	152
Sex	Male and female
Age	Mean: 55 years

Inclusion criteria

Primary hyperlipidemia: two consecutive blood lipid examinations of one-month interval with serum total cholesterol (TC) > 6.47 mmol/l (250 mg/dl) and/or triglycerides (TG) > 2.26 mmol/l (200 mg/dl). Patients had to have discontinued medications that could affect metabolism of blood lipids at least one month prior to the study. Subjects had a low-fat, low-cholesterol diet for one month before trial.

Exclusion criteria

Patients were excluded if their hyperlipidemia was secondary to other diseases or disease conditions, including diabetes, hypothyroidism, gout, hepatobiliary diseases, pancreatic diseases, or renal diseases. Patients who had in the last six months: acute myocardial infarction, heart surgery, stroke, or other severe diseases.

End points

At baseline, and at one and two months, blood was taken from patients and analyzed for serum TC, TG, high-density lipoprotein (HDL) cholesterol, blood glucose, and serum uric acid. Low-density lipoprotein (LDL) cholesterol was calculated according to the Friedewald formula. Patients also had their body weight, blood pressure, heart rhythm, and heart rate recorded each month.

Results

After treatment for two months with Zhitai, TC, TG, and LDL cholesterol were dramatically decreased, and HDL cholesterol had markedly increased compared to baseline values ($p < 0.01$). Although no significant changes were seen in the control group, very significant differences were found between the two groups for all of these measurements ($p < 0.01$).

Side effects

No patients complained of side effects.

Authors' comments

This dietary supplement is a new type of blood lipid regulator, functioning by reducing blood cholesterol.

Reviewer's comments

This is a well-designed and well-conducted study that demonstrates lipid lowering effects in an adequate study size of Chinese patients. (2, 6)

Saw Palmetto

Other common names: **Sabal palm**
Latin name: *Serenoa repens* **(W. Bartram) Small** [Arecaceae]
Latin synonyms: *Sabal serrulata* **(Michx.) Nutt. ex Schult. &**
  Schult. f.; *Serenoa serrulata* **(Michx.) G. Nichols.**
Plant part: **Fruit**

PREPARATIONS USED
IN REVIEWED CLINICAL STUDIES

Saw palmetto is native to North America and grows wild in Texas, Louisiana, South Carolina, and Florida. Traditionally, Native Americans in this region used the berries for food and as a tonic (USP, 2000). In addition, the berries have been used for more than 100 years to treat benign prostatic hyperplasia. Modern saw palmetto preparations contain lipids extracted from the powdered berries. The primary ingredients include saturated and unsaturated fatty acids (mostly free fatty acids), as well as free and conjugated plant sterols (Schulz, Hänsel, and Tyler, 2001).

Permixon®, manufactured in France by Pierre Fabre Médicament, contains the lipidosterolic extract PA109. PA 109 is a hexane extract whose main components are free (90 percent) and esterified (7 percent) fatty acids, of which about half are unsaturated C_{18} fatty acids. Permixon is also sold as Capistan®, Libeprosta®, and Sereprostat®. Permixon, which is the most clinically studied saw palmetto preparation, is not sold in the United States.

Prostaserene® is a single ingredient product manufactured by Therabel Pharma in Belgium. Prostaserene contains the saw palmetto fruit extract SabalSelect™, which is manufactured by Indena S.p.A in Italy. The extract is made using supercritical carbon dioxide as the solvent, and is characterized as containing 85 to 95 percent fatty acids. Prostaserene is available in 160 mg capsules, but is not sold in the United States. SabalSelect is contained in a product called Serenoa

SAW PALMETTO SUMMARY TABLE

Product Name	Manufacturer/ U.S. Distributor	Product Characteristics	Dose in Trials	Indication	No. of Trials	Benefit (Evidence Level-Trial No.)
Single-Ingredient Products						
Permixon® (EU)	Pierre Fabre Médicament, France/None	Hexane extract (PA 109)	320 mg/day	Benign prostatic hyperplasia	13	Yes (I-1) Trend (I-1, II-3, III-3) No (II-1) Undetermined (III-3) MOA (III-1)
Prostaserene® (EU)*	Therabel Pharma, Belgium (Indena S.p.A., Italy/None	Supercritical carbon dioxide extract (SabalSelect™)	320 mg/day	Benign prostatic hyperplasia	2	Yes (I-1) Undetermined (III-1)
Strogen® uno (EU)	Schaper & Brümmer GmbH & Co. KG, Germany/None	Lipophilic extract (IDS 89)	1,920 mg/day	Benign prostatic hyperplasia	1	MOA (III-1)
ProstActive®	Dr. Willmar Schwabe GmbH & Co., Germany/ Nature's Way Products, Inc.	Ethanolic extract (WS 1473)	300 mg/day	Benign prostatic hyperplasia	1	No (I-1)

Combination Products

Product Name	Manufacturer	Formulation	Dose	Use	Number of Trials	Effective
ProstActive® Plus (US), Prostagutt® forte (EU)	Dr. Willmar Schwabe GmbH & Co., Germany/ Nature's Way Products, Inc.	Saw palmetto (160 mg extract WS 1473), nettle root (120 mg extract WS 1031)	2 capsules per day	Benign prostatic hyperplasia	2	Yes (II-1) Undetermined (I-1)
Nutrilite® Saw Palmetto with Nettle Root	Access Business Group: Home of Nutrilite/Access Business Group: Home of Nutrilite	Saw palmetto (106 mg), nettle root (80 mg), Pumpkin seed oil (160 mg), lemon bioflavonoid extract (33 mg)	1 capsule 3 times daily	Benign prostatic hyperplasia	1	Trend (I-1)

*A single ingredient product that contains the Indena S.p.A Sabal Select™ extract is listed here. The extract has been tested clinically but the final formulation listed below has not.

Product Name	Manufacturer
Serenoa Gelcaps	Thorne Research

Gelcaps, manufactured by Thorne Research, that is sold in the United States.

Strogen® uno is manufactured by Schaper & Brümmer GmbH & Co. KG in Germany. The product contains a lipophilic extract (IDS 89), and is available in 320 mg capsules. Strogen uno is not sold in the United States.

ProstActive® is manufactured in Germany by Dr. Willmar Schwabe GmbH & Co. and contains an ethanolic saw palmetto fruit extract WS 1473 (plant to extract ratio [100:8.5]). ProstActive is available in softgel capsules that contain 320 mg WS 1473, and is sold in the United States by Nature's Way Products, Inc.

ProstActive® Plus contains the nettle (*Urtica dioica* L. spp. *dioica*) root extract WS 1031, in addition to the saw palmetto fruit extract WS 1473. This product is also manufactured by Dr. Willmar Schwabe GmbH & Co. in Germany and sold in the United States by Nature's Way Products, Inc. One softgel capsule of ProstActive Plus contains 160 mg of the ethanolic extract WS 1473 and 120 mg of the ethanolic extract WS 1031. ProstActive Plus is sold in Europe as Prostagutt® forte.

Nutrilite® Saw Palmetto with Nettle Root is manufactured and sold in the United States by the Access Business Group: Home of Nutrilite. Each softgel capsule contains 106 mg saw palmetto fruit extract (characterized as containing > 85 percent fatty acids), 80 mg nettle (*Urtica dioica* L. spp. *dioica*) root extract (characterized as containing > 0.8 percent beta-sitosterol), 160 mg pumpkin (*Cucurbita pepo* L.) seed extract, and 33.3 mg lemon [*Citrus* × *limon* (L.) Osbeck] bioflavonoid concentrate (characterized as containing more than 25 percent total bioflavonoids).

SUMMARY OF REVIEWED CLINICAL STUDIES

Saw palmetto preparations have been assessed in clinical studies for the treatment of symptomatic benign prostatic hyperplasia (BPH), also known as benign prostatic hypertrophy and prostatic adenoma. BPH is a nonmalignant enlargement of the prostate that is common in men over 40 years of age. Symptoms include increased urinary urgency and frequency (diuresis: increased formation and release of urine; and nocturia: frequent and/or excessive urination at night), urinary hesitancy, intermittency, sensation of incomplete voiding, and decreased force of the urine stream. BPH is linked with a normal change in hormone levels that occurs with aging. Testosterone levels decrease while estrogen levels remain constant. This change is implicated in BPH since estrogens induce hyperplasia (cell growth) in laboratory experiments. Further, BPH is associated with an increase in the activity of 5-alpha-reductase, the enzyme that converts testosterone to dihydrotesterone (DHT). The levels of DHT are not increased, but the number of androgen receptors seem to be. DHT has a greater affinity for androgen receptors than testosterone and is thought to stimulate prostatic growth. However, the pathology of BPH is not completely understood. Although BPH is associated with prostate enlargement, the size of the gland is not necessarily indicative of the degree of obstruction of the urethra and the extent of symptoms (Schulz, Hänsel, and Tyler, 2001; Barrett, 1999).

Several different rating systems have been developed to characterize the symptoms of BPH: the International Prostate Symptom Score (IPSS), the American Urological Association (AUA) symptom score, the Vahlensieck classification, and the Alken classification.

The IPSS is derived from a questionnaire regarding urinary urgency, frequency, hesitancy, intermittency, sensation of incomplete voiding, and force of urine stream (Schulz, Hänsel, and Tyler, 2001). The AUA symptom score is also a composite score obtained from seven questions covering frequency, nocturia, weak urinary stream, hesitancy, intermittence, incomplete emptying, and urgency (Barry et al., 1992).

The Vahlensieck classification has four stages based upon symptoms: Stage I is characterized by no voiding difficulties, no residual urine, and a urine flow of more than 15 ml per second; Stage II is characterized by transient voiding difficulties and urine flow between 10 and 15 ml per second; Stage III is characterized by constant voiding dysfunction, urine flow less than 10 ml per second, residual urine greater than 50 ml, and a trabeculated (ridged) bladder; and Stage IV is characterized by residual urine volume of more than 100 ml and bladder dilatation (Schulz, Hänsel, and Tyler, 2001).

The Alken classification has three stages. Stages I to III are similar to Vahlensieck Stages II through IV. Stage I is the irritative stage, characterized by an increase in the frequency of urination, pollakiuria (abnormally frequent urination), nocturia, delayed onset of urination, and weak urinary stream. Stage II is the residual urine stage, characterized by the beginning of the decomposition of the bladder function accompanied by formation of residual urine and the urge to urinate. Stage III is the regressive-obstructive stage, characterized by decomposition of the bladder, vesicular overflowing, continuous drip incontinence, and damage to the urinary system and kidneys due to regressive obstruction (Löbelenz, 1992).

Predominant pharmaceutical treatments of BPH include alphareceptor blockers and 5-alpha-reductase inhibitors. Alpha-adrenergic receptor blockers (e.g., prozosin, terazosin) are thought to relax smooth muscles in the bladder neck and within the prostate and thus reduce symptoms. Five-alpha-reductase inhibitors (e.g., finasteride) prevent the transformation of testosterone to DHT, thus increasing levels of testosterone and reducing levels of DHT (Barrett, 1999).

Suggested pharmacological actions for saw palmetto include antiandrogenic, anti-inflammatory, antiproliferative, and smooth muscle relaxation. Saw palmetto preparations have been shown to inhibit 5-alpha reductase, as well as the binding of DHT to androgen receptors. However, questions remain as to whether these actions, demonstrated in vitro, are clinically relevant (Barrett, 1999).

Permixon

Benign Prostatic Hyperplasia

Thirteen trials were reviewed that studied the use of Permixon as treatment for symptomatic BPH. Included are eight studies controlled with placebo, three controlled with another treatment, one dose-regimen comparison, and one mode of action study. The prevalent dose was 160 mg extract (PA109) twice daily. The benefit of saw palmetto berry (Permixon) in the treatment of BPH appears mostly in terms of symptom relief, which occurred one month to six weeks after beginning treatment.

A large, good-quality, placebo-controlled study of 146 men with BPH showed a statistically significant reduction in symptoms, especially nocturia (30 percent decrease), painful urination (47 percent improvement), and the volume of posturination residue compared to placebo after two to three months (Cukier et al., 1985). Our reviewers, Drs. Elliot Fagelman and Franklin Lowe, commented that this study demonstrated a therapeutic benefit, but that it was short in duration.

Two small studies of good design lasting two months showed statistical benefit compared to placebo. A small trial including 27 men with BPH Stages I or II (rating system not given) reported a reduction in symptoms in 43 percent of the Permixon group and 15 percent of the placebo group after two months (Tasca et al., 1985). Another small study with 22 men with BPH reported a statistical increase in maximal and average urine flow, as well as improvements in daytime and nighttime frequency compared to placebo after two months (Boccafoschi and Annoscia, 1983). Our reviewers rated these two studies as showing merely a trend toward efficacy due to their small sample sizes and short lengths of treatment.

Four trials lasting one month each also showed a trend toward benefit for BPH symptoms. The largest of the four trials, a good-quality study, included 186 men with Stages I or II BPH (rating system not given), as well as a placebo run-in period of a month to eliminate the placebo responders. With Permixon, there was a significant decrease in diuresis (increased formation and release of urine) as well as nocturia (frequent and/or excessive urination at night) compared to placebo. A significant increase in peak urine flow was also observed. However, the global efficacy assessment by both patients and physicians was not significantly different from placebo (Descotes et al., 1995). A trial with 94 men with BPH reported significant improvements in nocturia, flow rate, and postvoiding residue in comparison with placebo. In addition, both the physician and patient self-rating indicated superiority of Permixon in comparison to placebo (Champault, Patel, and Bonnard, 1984). A trial with 59 men with BPH compared Permixon to an extract of *Pygeum africanum* (no details given) and placebo. As a result, a significant difference in improvement in symptoms with Permixon was observed compared to pygeum and placebo. The symptoms with the greatest improvement with Permixon compared to baseline were pain upon voiding (73 percent decrease), urgency (70 percent decrease), tenesmus (spasms of the bladder along with the urge to empty, 82 percent decrease), and nocturia (42 percent decrease) (Mandressi et al., 1983). A small trial with 30 men with BPH reported a reduction in a number of symptoms compared to placebo (Emili, Lo Cigno, and Petrone, 1983). The quality of the smaller three studies was rated as poor due to either the poor trial design or a lack of detail in the trial report.

A good-quality, placebo-controlled study, including 70 men, found a complete lack of benefit beyond the placebo effect. Both groups had a statistical improvement in urinary flow after three months (Reece Smith et al., 1986).

Three drug comparison studies are mentioned later: one compared the activity of Permixon to the 5-alpha reductase inhibitor finasteride, and two compared Permixon to the alpha blockers alfuzosin and prozosin. The largest trial, which included 1,098 men and lasted six months, compared Permixon (320 mg per day) to finasteride (Proscar®, 5 mg per day). Both treatments decreased the IPSS symptom scores, quality-of-life scores, and increased peak urine flow compared to baseline, with no significant difference between the two. Finasteride markedly reduced prostate volume, but Permixon had little effect on volume. Finasteride also reduced levels of PSA (prostate-specific antigen), a serum marker for prostate cancer. Since the potential for confusion exists between the diagnoses of BPH and prostate cancer, the reduction of PSA levels by finasteride is a confounding variable. PSA levels were not altered by Permixon (Carraro et al., 1996). Our reviewers remarked that there was a significant therapeutic benefit compared to baseline for both groups, but that the lack of a placebo group was a limitation. Two small, short studies compared Permixon with two alpha-blockers: alfuzosin and prozosin. Both trials reported the alpha-blockers to be superior to Permixon in reduction of symptoms. A three-week study with 63 men with BPH found alfuzosin (7.5 mg per day) was more effective than Permixon (320 mg per day) in reducing symptoms according to Boyarsky's scale and an obstructive score (Grasso et al., 1995). A three-month study with 41 men with BPH grade I or II (rating system not given), reported that prozosin (4 mg per day) compared to Permixon (320 mg per day) was slightly more effective in reducing frequency of urination and increasing urinary flow. However, this comparison was based upon absolute numbers, and no statistical analysis was completed (Semino et al., 1992). The quality of the last two trials was not good according to the Jadad criteria, and there was no placebo group to act as a benchmark for activity. In addition, the identity of the saw palmetto product was not revealed in the trial report, but gathered from the review by Boyle and colleagues (2000).

A dose-regimen study explored the difference in delivering 320 mg once daily or 160 mg twice daily in a trial including 92 men. After three months, both treatment groups had significantly reduced IPSS scores, with no difference between them (Stepanov et al., 1999). However, the trial did not include a placebo group and therefore the efficacy was rated as undetermined.

A placebo-controlled mode-of-action study with 25 men examined hormone levels in prostate tissue removed after three months of treatment. The results suggested that Permixon may reduce DHT and epidermal growth factor levels and increase testosterone levels (Di Silverio et al., 1998).

Prostaserene

Benign Prostatic Hyperplasia

In a well-conducted trial, 205 men with mild to moderate BPH were given Prostaserene (160 mg twice daily) or placebo for three months. As a result, Prostaserene caused a significant improvement over placebo according to the total symptom score (frequency, nocturia, dysuria, urgency, and hesitancy), as well as the patient and physician quality-of-life scores (Braeckman, Denis et al., 1997). In the same year, another study was published comparing the dose of 160 mg twice daily to 320 mg once daily in a trial lasting for one year. In this study, with 67 men, both treatment regimens improved the IPSS by 60 percent. However, efficacy in general could not be evaluated because the study did not include a placebo (Braeckman, Bruhwyler et al., 1997).

Strogen uno

Benign Prostatic Hyperplasia

A study on Strogen uno evaluated the biochemical changes in prostate tissue removed from men after three months of treatment with either saw palmetto extract (640 mg three times daily) or placebo. The amounts and substrate affinities of enzymes involved in the formation of DHT (5-alpha-reductase) and removal of DHT (3-alpha and 17-beta hydroxysteroid oxidoreductases) were analyzed. Although significant changes were measured in enzyme levels, the alterations were moderate, and the authors of the report concluded that the clinical significance was unknown (Weisser et al., 1997).

ProstActive and ProstActive Plus

Benign Prostatic Hyperplasia

ProstActive failed to show any significant improvement over placebo in a well-conducted small trial with 60 men with BPH Stages I and II, according to Alken, who were given a dose of 100 mg three times daily (Löbelenz, 1992). Two studies were conducted on a combination product containing saw palmetto extract and nettle extract (Prostagutt forte). One study, with 33 men, compared 160 mg saw palmetto extract plus 120 mg nettle extract twice daily for six months to placebo, and reported a beneficial reduction in BPH symptoms compared with placebo, according to the AUA score (Metzker, Kieser, and Holscher, 1996). A large study with 498 men with BPH Stages I and II, according to Alken, compared the combination product to finasteride over one year. The herbal combination appeared to be equivalent to finasteride in causing the reduction in IPSS and improvement to quality of life, but the herbal preparation was better tolerated (Sokeland and Albrecht, 1997). However, due to the lack of a placebo group, the clinical benefit was deemed undetermined.

Nutrilite Saw Palmetto with Nettle Root

Benign Prostatic Hyperplasia

Nutrilite Saw Palmetto with Nettle Root was compared with placebo in a well-designed, six-month trial including 41 men using a dose of one capsule three times daily. No statistical improvement in symptoms was observed in the treatment group compared to the placebo group. However, morphological changes were noted in biopsy samples. A reduction in size of the prostate according to the percentage of atrophied tissue and percentage of epithelium was seen in the treatment group. No change was observed in the placebo group (Marks et al., 2000).

META-ANALYSES AND SYSTEMATIC REVIEWS

Boyle et al. (2000) conducted a meta-analysis on 11 randomized, controlled trials and two open, uncontrolled trials, including a total of

2,859 men with BPH treated with Permixon. The authors concluded that the agent improved urinary peak flow rate significantly and reduced the number of nighttime urinations compared with placebo. The clinical trial size ranged from 22 to 592 subjects and in duration from 21 days to six months. The 11 randomized, controlled trials are reviewed in detail in this section.

A systematic review of 18 randomized, controlled trials involving 2,939 men, using preparations of saw palmetto alone or in combination with other phytotherapeutic agents, concluded that saw palmetto improves urologic symptoms and flow measures in BPH. This improvement was similar to the drug finasteride, and was associated with fewer adverse effects (Wilt et al., 1998).

ADVERSE REACTIONS OR SIDE EFFECTS

In general, saw palmetto was well tolerated with few side effects reported in the trials reviewed. The largest controlled trial with Permixon, which included 1,098 men, reported hypertension as the most frequent adverse event occurring in 3.1 percent, followed by decreased libido in 2.2 percent, and abdominal pain in 1.8 percent (Carraro et al., 1996). A three-year, uncontrolled study with 435 men given IDS 89 (Strogen uno), 320 mg per day, reported good or very good tolerability, as reviewed by both physicians and patients, in 98 percent of subjects. Forty-six adverse events were documented in 34 patients—30 percent were gastrointestinal disturbances (Bach and Ebling, 1996). A review of controlled trials involving 2,939 men concluded that the adverse effects were mild and infrequent, in contrast to finasteride, which was more commonly associated with erectile dysfunction (Wilt et al., 1998).

INFORMATION FROM PHARMACOPOEIAL MONOGRAPHS

Sources of Published Therapeutic Monographs

German Commission E
The United States Pharmacopoeial Convention, Inc.

Indications

The German Commission E monograph approves use of the ripe, dried fruit of saw palmetto and its preparations for urination problems in benign prostatic hyperplasia Stages I and II, according to Alken. The Commission further notes that the medication relieves only the symptoms associated with an enlarged prostate but does not reduce the enlargement (Blumenthal et al., 1998).

Traditionally, saw palmetto has been used to strengthen the male reproductive system, and, more specifically, to treat symptoms of an enlarged prostate. Women have used saw palmetto to treat enlarged ovaries and increase the size of undeveloped mammary glands. For both men and women, it has been used to increase sexual vigor, as a general tonic, as a diuretic, and for genitourinary problems (USP, 2000).

Doses

> Fruit: 1 to 2 g berries or equivalent preparations (Blumenthal et al., 1998; USP, 2000)
>
> Tea: one cup three times a day. Bring one cup water with one-third daily dose of saw palmetto fruit to a boil and then simmer for five minutes (USP, 2000)
>
> Tincture: (fresh fruit 1:2, dried fruit 1:5, 80 percent alcohol) 1 to 2 ml, 3 to 4 times daily (USP, 2000)
>
> Extract:
> * Liquid: (1:1) 0.6 to 1.5 ml per day (USP, 2000)
> * Liposterolic: 320 mg daily lipophilic ingredients extracted with lipophilic solvents (10:1, hexane or ethanol 90 percent v/v) (Blumenthal et al., 1998; USP, 2000)

Contraindications

The Commission E lists no known contraindications (Blumenthal et al., 1998).

Adverse Reactions

The Commission E lists stomach problems in rare cases, and the USP lists mild gastrointestinal complaints, such as diarrhea and nausea (Blumenthal et al., 1998; USP, 2000).

Precautions

The USP states that the use of saw palmetto in pregnant or breast-feeding women and in children cannot be recommended, since it has not been studied (USP, 2000).

Drug Interactions

The Commission E lists no known drug interactions (Blumenthal et al., 1998). The USP suggests that although no interactions have been reported, saw palmetto may have endocrine or alpha-adrenergic blocking effects, although these possible interactions have not been studied (USP, 2000).

REFERENCES

Bach D, Ebling L (1996). Long-term drug treatment of benign prostatic hyperplasia—Results of a prospective 3-year multicenter study using Sabal extract IDS 89. *Phytomedicine* 3 (2): 105-111.

Barrett M (1999). The pharmacology of saw palmetto in treatment of BPH. *Journal of the American Nutraceutical Association* 2 (3): 21-24.

Barry MJ, Fowler FJ Jr, O'Leary MP, Bruskewitz RC, Holtgrewe HL, Mebust WK, Cockett AT (1992). Correlation of the American Urological Association symptom index with the self-administered versions of the Madsen-Iverson, Boyarsky, and Main Medical Assessment Program symptom indexes. Measurement Committee of the American Urological Association. *Journal of Urology* 148 (5): 1549-1557.

Blumenthal M, Busse W, Hall T, Goldberg A, Grünwald J, Riggins C, Rister S, eds. (1998). *The Complete German Commission E Monographs: Therapeutic Guide to Herbal Medicines.* Trans S Klein. Austin: American Botanical Council.

Boccafoschi C, Annoscia S (1983). Comparison between extract of *Serenoa repens* and a placebo in controlled clinical tests on patients with prostate adenomatoses. *Urology* 50: 1257-1268.

Boyle P, Robertson C, Lowe F, Roehrborn C (2000). Meta-analysis of clinical trials of Permixon in the treatment of symptomatic benign prostatic hyperplasia. *Urology* 55 (4): 533-539.

Braeckman J, Bruhwyler J, Vandekerckhove K, Geczy J (1997). Efficacy and safety of the extract of *Serenoa repens* in the treatment of benign prostatic hyperplasia: Therapeutic equivalence between twice and once daily dosage forms. *Phytotherapy Research* 11 (8): 558-563.

Braeckman J, Denis L, de Leval J, Keuppens F, Cornet A, De Bruyne R, De Smedt E, Pacco J, Timmermans L, Van Vliet P, et al. (1997). A double-blind, placebo-controlled study of the plant extract *Serenoa repens* in the treatment of benign hyperplasia of the prostate. *European Journal of Clinical Research* 9: 247-259.

Carraro JC, Raynaud JP, Koch G, Chrisholm GD, Di Silverio F, Teillac P, Calais Da Silva F, Cauquil J, Chopin DK, Hamdy FC (1996). Comparison of phytotherapy (Permixon) with finasteride in the treatment of benign prostate hyperplasia: A randomized international study of 1,098 patients. *The Prostate* 29 (4): 231-240.

Champault G, Patel JC, Bonnard AM (1984). A double-blind trial of an extract of the plant *Serenoa repens* in benign prostatic hyperplasia. *British Journal of Clinical Pharmacology* 18 (3): 461-462.

Cukier, Ducassou, Le Guillou, Leriche, Lobel, Toubol, Doromieux, Grinewald, Pastorini, Raymond, Reziciner, Martinaggi (1985). Permixon versus placebo. *Comptes Rendus de Therapeutique et de Pharmacologie Clinique* 4 (25): 15-21.

Descotes JL, Rambeaud JJ, Deschaseaux P, Faure G (1995). Placebo-controlled evaluation of the efficacy and tolerability of Permixon in benign prostatic hyperplasia after exclusion of placebo responders. *Clinical Drug Investigation* 9 (5): 291-297.

Di Silverio F, Monti S, Sciarra A, Varasano PA, Martini C, Lanzara S, D'Eramo G, Di Nicola S, Toscano V (1998). Effects of long-term treatment with *Serenoa repens* (Permixon) on the concentrations and regional distribution of androgens and epidermal growth factor in benign prostatic hyperplasia. *The Prostate* 37 (2): 77-83.

Emili E, Lo Cigno M, Petrone U (1983). Clinical results on a new drug in the treatment of benign prostatic hyperplasia (Permixon). *Urologia* 50 (5): 1042-1049.

Grasso M, Montesano A, Buonaguidi A, Castelli M, Lania C, Rigatti P, Rocco F, Cesana B, Borghi C (1995). Comparative effects of alfuzosin versus *Serenoa repens* in the treatment of symptomatic benign prostatic hyperplasia. *Archivos Espanoles de Urologia* 48 (1): 97-103.

Löbelenz J (1992). *Extractum sabal fructus* in the therapy of benign prostatic hyperplasia (BPH). *Tpk Therapeutikon* 6 (1/2): 34-37.

Mandressi S, Tarallo U, Maggioni A, Tombolini P, Rocco F, Quadraccia (1983). Medical treatment of benign prostatic hyperplasia: Efficacy of the extract of *Serenoa repens* (Permixon) compared to that of the extract of *Pygeum africanum* and a placebo. *Urologia* 50: 752-758.

Marks LS, Partin AW, Epstein JI, Tyler VE, Simon I, Macairan ML, Chan TL, Dorey FJ, Garris JB, Veltri RW, et al. (2000). Effects of a saw palmetto herbal blend in men with symptomatic benign prastatic hyperplasia. *The Journal of Urology* 163 (5): 1451-1456.

Metzker H, Kieser M, Holscher U (1996). Efficacy of a combined *Sabal-Urtica* preparation in the treatment of benign prostatic hyperplasia (BPH). *Urologe* 36: 292-300.

Reece Smith H, Memon A, Smart CJ, Dewbury K (1986). The value of Permixon in benign prostatic hypertrophy. *British Journal of Urology* 58 (1): 36-40.

Schulz V, Hänsel R, Tyler VE (2001). *Rational Phytotherapy: A Physicians' Guide to Herbal Medicine*, Fourth Edition. Trans. TC Telgar. Berlin: Springer-Verlag.

Semino MA, Ortega JLL, Cobo EG, Banez ET, Rodrigues FR (1992). Symptomatic treatment of benign prostatic hypertrophy: Comparative study of prazosin and *Serenoa repens*. *Archivos Espanoles de Urologia* 45 (3): 211-213.

Sokeland J, Albrecht J (1997). A combination of *Sabal* and *Urtica* extracts versus finasteride in BPH (stage I to II acc. to Alken): A comparison of therapeutic efficacy in a one-year double-blind study. *Urologe (A)* 36 (4): 327-333. (Also published by Sokeland J [2000]. *BJU International* 86 [4]: 439-442.)

Stepanov VN, Siniakova LA, Sarrazin B, Raynaud JP (1999). Efficacy and tolerability of *Serenoa repens* (Permixon) in benign prostatic hyperplasia: A double-blind comparative study of two dosage regimens. *Advances in Therapy* 16 (5): 231-241.

Tasca A, Barulli M, Cavazzana A, Zattoni F, Artibani W, Pagano F (1985). Treatment with *Serenoa repens* extract of the obstructive signs and symptoms caused by prostatic adenoma. *Minerva Urologica e Nefrologica* 37 (1): 87-91.

United States Pharmacopeial Convention, Inc. (USP) (2000). *Saw Palmetto*. <www.usp.org>. Accessed December 3, 2002.

Weisser H, Behnke B, Helpap B, Bach D, Krieg M (1997). Enzyme activities in tissue of human benign prostatic hyperplasia after three months treatment with the *Sabal serrulata* extract IDS 89 (Strogen) or placebo. *European Urology* 31 (1): 97-101.

Wilt TJ, Ishani A, Stark G, MacDonaald R, Lau J, Mulrow C (1998). Saw palmetto extracts for treatment of benign prostatic hyperplasia: A systematic review. *Journal of the American Medical Association* 280 (18): 1604-1609.

DETAILS ON SAW PALMETTO PRODUCTS AND CLINICAL STUDIES

Product and clinical study information is grouped in the same order as in the Summary Table. A profile on an individual product is followed by details of the clinical studies associated with that product. In some instances, a clinical study, or studies, supports several products that contain the same principal ingredient(s). In these instances, those products are grouped together.

Clinical studies that follow each product, or group of products, are grouped by therapeutic indication, in accordance with the order in the Summary Table.

Index to Saw Palmetto Products

Product Profile: Permixon®

Manufacturer	**Pierre Fabre Médicament, France**
U.S. distributor	None
Botanical ingredient	**Saw palmetto fruit extract**
Extract name	**PA 109**
Quantity	80 mg
Processing	*N*-hexane lipidosterolic extract
Standardization	No information
Formulation	Tablet

Recommended dose: Two tablets twice daily.

Comments: Also sold as Capistan®, Libeprosta®, and Sereprostat®.

Source(s) of information: Descotes et al., 1995; Di Silverio et al., 1998; Champault, Patel, and Bonnard, 1984.

Clinical Study: Permixon®

Extract name	PA 109
Manufacturer	Pierre Fabre Médicament, France
Indication	**Benign prostatic hyperplasia**
Level of evidence	I
Therapeutic benefit	**Yes**

Bibliographic reference
Cukier, Ducassou, Le Guillou, Leriche, Lobel, Toubol, Doromieux, Grinewald, Pastorini, Raymond, Reziciner, Martinaggi (1985). Permixon versus placebo. *Comptes Rendus de Therapeutique et de Pharmacologie Clinique* 4 (25): 15-21.

Trial design
Parallel.

Study duration	2 to 3 months
Dose	2 (80 mg) tablets twice daily
Route of administration	Oral
Randomized	Yes
Randomization adequate	Yes
Blinding	Open
Blinding adequate	Yes
Placebo	Yes
Drug comparison	No
Site description	Not described
No. of subjects enrolled	168
No. of subjects completed	146
Sex	Male
Age	60-79 years

Inclusion criteria
Men over 60 years old with prostatic hypertrophy in the "prostatism" stage for whom surgery was not indicated, and with symptoms for at least six months.

Exclusion criteria
Prostatic hypertrophy with mechanical or infectious complications.

End points

Dysuria (painful urination), pollakiuria, and nocturia (nightly urination) were assessed at trial start, day 30, and at the end of the trial. These symptoms were also recorded weekly by the patients. Overall assessment of efficacy and acceptability of the treatment by physician and patient at day 30 and at end of trial.

Results

With Permixon, there was a 30 percent decrease in urination at night, which was significant compared to placebo ($p < 0.001$). The greatest changes were seen with those experiencing more than three visits per night. There was a 47 percent improvement in painful urination compared to placebo ($p < 0.001$). Posturination residue was decreased in the Permixon group, whereas it increased in the placebo group. The difference between the two groups was significant ($p < 0.05$). Assessment of efficacy by the physician was better for Permixon (66.7 percent) than for placebo (26.9 percent).

Side effects

Tolerability was 94.4 percent for Permixon and 91.3 percent for placebo.

Authors' comments

Permixon appears to be a valuable therapeutic solution provided it is used under clearly identified circumstances, in particular in the absence of complications and hence any indication for more aggressive therapeutic measures.

Reviewers' comments

This is a well-run and well-designed trial. The one major drawback of this study is the short duration (two to three months). Also, although the results are statistically significant, the difference may not be clinically significant. (Translation reviewed) (5, 6)

Clinical Study: Permixon®

Extract name	PA 109
Manufacturer	Zambeletti S.p.A, Italy (Pierre Fabre Médicament, France)
Indication	**Benign prostatic hyperplasia**
Level of evidence	**II**
Therapeutic benefit	**Trend**

Bibliographic reference
Tasca A, Barulli M, Cavazzana A, Zattoni F, Artibani W, Pagano F (1985). Treatment with *Serenoa repens* extract of the obstructive signs and symptoms caused by prostatic adenoma. *Minerva Urologica e Nefrologica* 37 (1): 87-91.

Trial design
Parallel. Pretrial washout period of two months.

Study duration	2 months
Dose	160 mg twice daily
Route of administration	Oral
Randomized	Yes
Randomization adequate	No
Blinding	Double-blind
Blinding adequate	Yes
Placebo	Yes
Drug comparison	No
Site description	Not described
No. of subjects enrolled	30
No. of subjects completed	27
Sex	Male
Age	49-81 years

Inclusion criteria
Patients suffering from prostatic adenoma Stages I or II (rating system not given).

Exclusion criteria
Patients having significant hepatic, renal, or cardiac disorders.

End points
Before and after treatment, patients underwent a general physical exam for evaluation of prostate volume, postmicturition bladder residue, uroflowmetrics, urine culture, and a series of clinical chemistry parameters. Subjective aspects were obtained from a questionnaire completed by patients every ten days.

Results
Beneficial results were obtained in 42.9 percent of cases treated with Permixon and in 15.4 percent treated with placebo. A statistical improvement was observed in uroflowmetric recording for Permixon treatment com-

pared to baseline ($p < 0.05$). The placebo group showed no significant change.

Side effects
Tremor, dizziness, and cold sweat in one patient taking Permixon.

Authors' comments
The results obtained with *Serenoa repens* compared with placebo, in homogeneous patient groups, indicate an efficacious action in reducing urinary signs and symptoms and in improving related instrumental parameters.

Reviewers' comments
Overall, this is a good study suggesting a benefit for Permixon versus placebo. However, the number of patients was small, and the treatment duration was short. (Translation reviewed) (3, 4)

Clinical Study: Permixon®

Extract name	PA 109
Manufacturer	Zambeletti S.p.A, Italy (Pierre Fabre Médicament, France)

Indication	**Benign prostatic hyperplasia**
Level of evidence	**II**
Therapeutic benefit	**Trend**

Bibliographic reference
Boccafoschi C, Annoscia S (1983). Comparison between extract of *Serenoa repens* and a placebo in controlled clinical tests on patients with prostate adenomatoses. *Urology* 50: 1257-1268.

Trial design
Parallel.

Study duration	2 months
Dose	2 (160 mg) capsules (morning and night)
Route of administration	Oral

Randomized	Yes
Randomization adequate	No
Blinding	Double-blind
Blinding adequate	No

Placebo	Yes

Drug comparison	No
Site description	Outpatient clinic
No. of subjects enrolled	22
No. of subjects completed	22
Sex	Male
Age	54-80 years

Inclusion criteria
Patients with benign prostatic hypertrophy that could be treated with medication.

Exclusion criteria
Hypertension, cerebral disorders, or chronic bronchopneumopathy.

End points
Tests were performed at baseline and after 30 and 60 days. The clinical symptoms were dysuria, pelvic heaviness, nocturia, and daytime pollakiuria. In some cases, posturination residue and prostate adenoma dimension were established. Urine cultures were performed at baseline and after 30 and 60 days.

Results
The volume of urine, maximum flow, and average flow were increased in the Permixon group compared to placebo ($p < 0.0005$, $p < 0.02$, and $p < 0.05$, respectively). Dysuria and nocturia were also improved ($p < 0.01$ and $p < 0.05$, respectively). Not significant were changes in urination time, urinary residue, and pelvic heaviness. No change was observed in prostate size.

Side effects
None reported.

Authors' comments
The results confirm the usefulness of Permixon in the treatment of specific clinical forms of prostate hyperplasia.

Reviewers' comments
This is a very limited study based on the sample size (only 22 patients). Hypertension alone should not be an exclusion criterion for benign prostatic hyperplasia. Although some statistical benefit is shown, this should be viewed with caution. The treatment length was relatively short. (Translation reviewed) (5, 3)

Clinical Study: Permixon®

Extract name	PA 109
Manufacturer	Pierre Fabre Médicament, France
Indication	**Benign prostatic hyperplasia**
Level of evidence	**II**
Therapeutic benefit	**Trend**

Bibliographic reference

Descotes JL, Rambeaud JJ, Deschaseaux P, Faure G (1995). Placebo-controlled evaluation of the efficacy and tolerability of Permixon in benign prostatic hyperplasia after exclusion of placebo responders. *Clinical Drug Investigation* 9 (5): 291-297.

Trial design

Parallel. Trial preceded by a single-blind placebo run-in period of 30 days. Nonresponders were entered into randomized double-blind, placebo-controlled trial for 30 days.

Study duration	1 month
Dose	160 mg twice daily (morning and evening)
Route of administration	Oral
Randomized	Yes
Randomization adequate	No
Blinding	Double-blind
Blinding adequate	Yes
Placebo	Yes
Drug comparison	No
Site description	Multicenter
No. of subjects enrolled	215
No. of subjects completed	186
Sex	Male
Age	57-75 years

Inclusion criteria

Patients with clinically demonstrated mild to moderate (Stages I or II) benign prostatic hyperplasia, symptoms of dysuria, daytime and nocturnal urinary frequency (> 2 at night excluding bedtime and on awaking) of at least eight weeks duration, and a maximum urinary flow rate > 5 ml/sec. Nonresponders to a 30-day placebo run-in (< 30 percent improvement from baseline in peak urinary flow rate).

Exclusion criteria
Patients with excessively mild symptoms of BPH (nocturnal urinary frequency < 1) of recent onset (< 8 weeks), excessively severe symptoms of BPH (peak urinary flow rate < 5 ml/sec, incontinence, bladder distension, acute urinary retention, or other complications), associated urogenital infection, hematuria, diabetes, neuropathy or pelvic cancer, history of surgery for BPH, or any surgery that could induce dysuria.

End points
Urinary symptoms were assessed at entry into the study, after the placebo run-in, and upon completion. Efficacy was assessed on the basis of changes in symptom scores, peak urinary flow rates, and overall opinions of the response to treatment by both physicians and patients.

Results
Improvement in dysuria severity was seen in a significantly greater proportion of Permixon recipients than placebo recipients (31.3 percent versus 16.1 percent, $p = 0.019$). Daytime urinary frequency fell significantly in Permixon-treated patients compared with placebo recipients ($p = 0.012$). Nocturnal urinary frequency fell to a significantly greater extent with Permixon than with placebo (32.5 percent versus 17.7 percent, $p = 0.028$). Permixon produced a significantly greater increase in mean peak urinary flow rate than did placebo (28.9 percent versus 8.5 percent, $p = 0.038$). The global efficacy of Permixon was not judged significantly different from placebo by the patients or physicians.

Side effects
One patient reported fatigue, depression, and stomach upset.

Authors' comments
Permixon appears to be significantly more effective than placebo and well-tolerated in the short-term treatment of mild to moderate symptomatic BPH.

Reviewers' comments
The study is flawed by leaving out placebo responders, thus eliminating the placebo effect and biasing the study in favor of Permixon. In addition, the randomization process was not adequately described. (3, 6)

Clinical Study: Permixon®

Extract name	PA 109
Manufacturer	Pierre Fabre Médicament, France
Indication	**Benign prostatic hyperplasia**

Level of evidence **III**
Therapeutic benefit **Trend**

Bibliographic reference
Champault G, Patel JC, Bonnard AM (1984). A double-blind trial of an extract of the plant *Serenoa repens* in benign prostatic hyperplasia. *British Journal of Clinical Pharmacology* 18 (3): 461-462.

Trial design
Parallel.

Study duration	1 month
Dose	2 (80 mg) tablets twice daily (320 mg extract/day)
Route of administration	Oral
Randomized	No
Randomization adequate	No
Blinding	Double-blind
Blinding adequate	No
Placebo	Yes
Drug comparison	No
Site description	Outpatient clinic
No. of subjects enrolled	110
No. of subjects completed	94
Sex	Male
Age	Not given

Inclusion criteria
Benign prostatic hyperplasia symptoms of dysuria, nocturia, and frequent and poor urinary flow.

Exclusion criteria
Patients with an acute or unstable episode, adenomas requiring early surgery, carcinomas of the prostate, or prostatic syndromes associated with other genitourinary conditions.

End points
Before and after 30 days of treatment, assessments were made of nocturia, intensity of dysuria, flow rate, and postmicturition residue. In addition, global rating by physicians and self-rating by patients was included.

Results
Permixon improved both objective and subjective signs. Nocturia was de-

creased in both groups, but significantly more so for the Permixon group, $p <$ 0.001. Flow rate was increased by 50.5 percent compared to 5.0 percent for placebo, $p < 0.001$. Postmicturition residue was decreased by 41.9 percent in the Permixon group, and increased by 9.3 percent in the placebo group, $p < 0.001$. Dysuria was greatly improved compared to placebo, $p < 0.001$. Both patient self-rating and physician rating indicated the superiority of Permixon over placebo, both $p < 0.001$.

Side effects
Minor (e.g., headache).

Authors' comments
As predicted by pharmacological and biochemical studies, Permixon appears to be a useful therapeutic tool in the treatment of benign prostatic hyperplasia.

Reviewer's comments
Although a statistical benefit of Permixon was demonstrated in the trial, a lack of randomization limits the usefulness of this study. The duration of treatment, 30 days, is also relatively short, and the blinding was not described adequately. (1, 5)

Clinical Study: Permixon®

Extract name	PA 109
Manufacturer	Pierre Fabre Médicament, France
Indication	**Benign prostatic hyperplasia**
Level of evidence	**III**
Therapeutic benefit	**Trend**

Bibliographic reference
Mandressi S, Tarallo U, Maggioni A, Tombolini P, Rocco F, Quadraccia (1983). Medical treatment of benign prostatic hyperplasia: Efficacy of the extract of *Serenoa repens* (Permixon) compared to that of the extract of *Pygeum africanum* and a placebo. *Urologia* 50: 752-758.

Trial design
Parallel. Three-arm trial. Permixon, extract of *Pygeum africanum* (no details given), and placebo.

Study duration	1 month
Dose	320 mg daily

Route of administration	Oral
Randomized	Yes
Randomization adequate	No
Blinding	Double-blind
Blinding adequate	Yes
Placebo	Yes
Drug comparison	Yes
Drug name	Pygeum extract
Site description	Not described
No. of subjects enrolled	60
No. of subjects completed	59
Sex	Male
Age	50-80 years

Inclusion criteria
Patients complaining of dysuric disorders related to benign prostatic hyperplasia (BPH), confirmed on rectal exam.

Exclusion criteria
Patients treated previously for BPH, or complications secondary to the presence of prostactic hypertrophy.

End points
Subjective and objective parameters were assessed before and after 30 days of treatment. Subjective parameters included pollakiuria, nocturia, dysuria, perineal pain, and nocturnal erections. Objective parameters included rectal examination, urology before and after voiding, and retrograde cystourethrography.

Results
There was a pronounced difference in the efficacy of Permixon compared to placebo ($p < 0.01$) and the *Pygeum africanum* extract ($p < 0.05$). There was no clear difference in the results of patients treated with *Pygeum africanum* and those in the placebo group. The greatest improvements with Permixon compared to baseline were in the following symptoms: pain on voiding (73 percent decrease), urgency (70 percent decrease), tenesmus (spasms and urge to empty the bladder, 82 percent decrease), and nocturia (42 percent decrease).

Side effects
None reported.

Authors' comments
It is thus possible to confirm without any doubt the clinical reliability of the extract of *Serenoa repens* (Permixon) regarding efficacy and tolerance. However, it is not possible to reach any definitive conclusions regarding the comparison of Permixon with *Pygeum africanum* extract.

Reviewers' comments
This trial shows a trend toward symptomatic benefit with Permixon. However, small numbers of patients in each group and lack of a significant description of *Pygeum africanum* limit the utility of this study. The treatment length was short, and the randomization process was not adequately described. (Translation reviewed) (2, 5)

Clinical Study: Permixon®

Extract name	PA 109
Manufacturer	Pierre Fabre Médicament, France
Indication	**Benign prostatic hyperplasia**
Level of evidence	**III**
Therapeutic benefit	**Trend**

Bibliographic reference
Emili E, Lo Cigno M, Petrone U (1983). Clinical results on a new drug in the treatment of benign prostatic hyperplasia (Permixon). *Urologia* 50 (5): 1042-1049.

Trial design
Parallel.

Study duration	1 month
Dose	2 tablets twice daily (morning and evening)
Route of administration	Oral
Randomized	Yes
Randomization adequate	No
Blinding	Double-blind
Blinding adequate	No
Placebo	Yes
Drug comparison	No
Site description	Urology clinic

No. of subjects enrolled   30
No. of subjects completed 30
Sex   Male
Age   44-78 years

Inclusion criteria
Patients with general good health suffering from uncomplicated benign prostatic hyperplasia for whom there is no indication for surgery or immediate endoscopy (due to clinical symptoms and the absence of involvement of the upper urinary tract), and negative urinary cultures.

Exclusion criteria
Patients having a history of surgery of endoscopy on the bladder or urethra.

End points
The number of diurnal or nocturnal urinations, dysuria, the size of the prostate on rectal palpation, and postvoiding residue were evaluated at the start and end of the study.

Results
Permixon decreased the number of diurnal urinations by 32 percent compared with 7.5 percent for placebo. Nocturnal urinations were reduced by 49.8 percent compared with 12.7 percent for placebo. Dysuria (painful urination) was reduced by 88.5 percent compared to 40 percent for placebo. Prostate size was reduced by 26.6 percent compared to no change in the placebo group. Urinary outflow was increased by 32.6 percent, and average urinary output was increased by 28.6 percent (placebo: +2.16 percent and –3 percent, respectively). Postvoiding residue was reduced by 50.9 percent compared with 15.1 percent for placebo.

Side effects
None reported.

Authors' comments
The extract of *Serenoa repens* proved to be an efficacious drug by improving clinical and instrumental parameters in the treated group without causing any side effects.

Reviewers' comments
This is a small study that shows a trend in benefit of saw palmetto fruit. However, the differences may not be clinically significant. Thirty days is also a short duration of therapy. Neither the randomization nor the blinding were described adequately. (Translation reviewed) (1, 4)

Clinical Study: Permixon®

Extract name	PA 109
Manufacturer	Pierre Fabre Médicament, France
Indication	**Benign prostatic hyperplasia**
Level of evidence	**II**
Therapeutic benefit	**No**

Bibliographic reference
Reece Smith H, Memon A, Smart CJ, Dewbury K (1986). The value of Permixon in benign prostatic hypertrophy. *British Journal of Urology* 58 (1): 36-40.

Trial design
Parallel.

Study duration	3 months
Dose	160 mg twice daily
Route of administration	Oral
Randomized	Yes
Randomization adequate	Yes
Blinding	Double-blind
Blinding adequate	No
Placebo	Yes
Drug comparison	No
Site description	One hospital urology department
No. of subjects enrolled	80
No. of subjects completed	70
Sex	Male
Age	55-80 years

Inclusion criteria
Patients with symptom of benign prostatic hyperplasia (BPH).

Exclusion criteria
Malignant prostatic disease.

End points
Measurement of urinary flow rate, midstream specimen of urine, and assessment of residual volume by bladder echography were recorded at baseline and after 2, 4, 8, and 12 weeks. Six months after completion of the trial,

patients were asked via questionnaire whether improvement attained during trial was maintained.

Results
A statistically significant improvement ($p < 0.01$) in urinary flow rate was observed in both treatment and placebo groups, but no significant difference was seen between the two groups. There was no significant difference in bladder residual volume in either group.

Side effects
Two patients stopped taking Permixon because of nausea and vomiting, and withdrew from the trial. One other patient stopped taking Permixon for two to three days due to nausea. One patient developed dizziness and stopped taking Permixon for one day.

Authors' comments
Although the regime of Permixon used in this trial was safe, well tolerated, and associated with considerable symptomatic improvement, no evidence exists that this improvement was due to anything more than the psychosocial value of being involved in the trial and meeting a number sufferers from a similar condition.

Reviewers' comments
Overall, this is a good study demonstrating no difference in efficacy between Permixon and placebo over a 12-week period. The trial duration, however, is short, and a known placebo effect is present in treating BPH. (3, 4)

Clinical Study: Permixon®

Extract name	PA 109
Manufacturer	Pierre Fabre Médicament, France
Indication	**Benign prostatic hyperplasia**
Level of evidence	I
Therapeutic benefit	**Trend**

Bibliographic reference
Carraro JC, Raynaud JP, Koch G, Chrisholm GD, Di Silverio F, Teillac P, Calais Da Silva F, Cauquil J, Chopin DK, Hamdy FC (1996). Comparison of phytotherapy (Permixon) with finasteride in the treatment of benign prostate hyperplasia: A randomized international study of 1,098 patients. *The Prostate* 29 (4): 231-240.

Trial design

Parallel. Permixon or finasteride (Proscar; 5 mg once daily in the morning). Patients took a total of four pills per day (two morning, two evening). The nontreatment pills were placebo.

Study duration	6 months
Dose	160 mg twice daily (morning and night)
Route of administration	Oral
Randomized	Yes
Randomization adequate	Yes
Blinding	Double-blind
Blinding adequate	Yes
Placebo	No
Drug comparison	Yes
Drug name	Finasteride
Site description	87 urology centers
No. of subjects enrolled	1,209
No. of subjects completed	1,098
Sex	Male
Age	49-88 years

Inclusion criteria

Over 50 years old, with benign prostatic hyperplasia diagnosed by digital rectal examination and not requiring surgery, International Prostate Symptom Score (IPSS) > 6, maximum urinary flow between 4 to 15 ml/sec, urine volume > 150 ml, postvoiding residue < 200 ml, prostate > 25 ml, serum prostate-specific antigen (PSA) < 10 ng/ml for prostates < 60 ml and < 15 ng/ml for prostates > 60 ml, good physical and mental condition.

Exclusion criteria

Cancer of the prostate, known history of bladder disease, lower urinary tract pathology or infection, any disease potentially affecting urination, abnormal liver function, administered diuretics or drugs with antiandrogenic or alpha-receptor properties in the preceding three months, or prior treatment with either finasteride or Permixon.

End points

Each patient was evaluated prior to entry and at 6, 13, and 26 weeks. At each visit, peak and mean urinary flow rates were measured, the IPSS was determined, and the patient completed a quality of life and sexual function questionnaire. At weeks 13 and 26, patients underwent transrectal and abdominal ultrasound examinations, as well as blood sampling.

Results
Both Permixon and finasteride decreased the IPSS (−37 percent and −39 percent, respectively), improved quality of life (by 38 percent and 41 percent, respectively), and increased peak urinary flow rate (+25 percent and +30 percent, respectively), with no statistical difference in the percent responders. All improvements were compared to baseline ($p < 0.001$). Finasteride markedly decreased prostate volume (−18 percent) and serum PSA levels (−41 percent). Permixon improved symptoms with little effect on volume (−6 percent), and no change in PSA levels.

Side effects
Side effects were similar in both groups, with hypertension being the most common. Decreased libido and impotence were more common in those taking finasteride.

Authors' comments
Both treatments relieve the symptoms of BPH in about two-thirds of patients. Unlike finasteride, Permixon has little effect on so-called androgen-dependent parameters.

Reviewer's comments
This trial had a good study design. A significant therapeutic benefit was present compared with baseline in both groups. However, the lack of a placebo group prevents a determination whether the improvement is simply the result of a placebo effect. The treatment length is relatively short. If the improvement in those taking Permixon was due to a placebo effect, over a longer period those with finasteride would continue to improve while those on Permixon would not. (5, 6)

Clinical Study: Permixon®

Extract name	PA 109
Manufacturer	Pierre Fabre Médicament, France
Indication	**Benign prostatic hyperplasia**
Level of evidence	**III**
Therapeutic benefit	**Undetermined**

Bibliographic reference
Grasso M, Montesano A, Buonaguidi A, Castelli M, Lania C, Rigatti P, Rocco F, Cesana B, Borghi C (1995). Comparative effects of alfuzosin versus *Serenoa repens* in the treatment of symptomatic benign prostatic hyperplasia. *Archivos Espanoles de Urologia* 48 (1): 97-103.

Trial design

Parallel. Saw palmetto versus alfuzosin 2.5 mg three times daily. Pretrial run-in of seven days. The trial report does not specify the extract or product name. The designation of Permixon came from a review by Boyle and colleages (2000).

Study duration	3 weeks
Dose	160 mg twice daily
Route of administration	Oral
Randomized	Yes
Randomization adequate	No
Blinding	Double-blind
Blinding adequate	No
Placebo	No
Drug comparison	Yes
Drug name	Alfuzosin
Site description	2 urology departments
No. of subjects enrolled	63
No. of subjects completed	63
Sex	Male
Age	Mean: 62 ± 7.5 years

Inclusion criteria

Outpatients ages 50 to 80, diagnosis of symptomatic benign prostatic hyperplasia by digital rectal examination and transrectal ultrasonography, Boyarsky's scale scores for nocturia > 2 and daytime frequency > 1, peak flow rate < 15 ml/sec, and a voided volume > 150 ml.

Exclusion criteria

Concomitant urological disorders; neurologic disturbances; severe cardiac, renal, or hepatic failure; myocardial infarction within the previous six months; taking drugs likely to interfere with the study medication or antihypertensive drugs.

End points

Clinical symptoms (Boyarsky's scale score, visual analog scale, clinical global impression), urinary flow rates (uroflowmetry), and residual urinary volume (transabdominal ultrasound) were recorded. Patients were assessed before pretrial period, at baseline, and after 14 and 21 days.

Results

Statistically significant and clinically relevant differences were found between the two treatments in favor of alfuzosin for Boyarsky's total score (decrease in 38.8 percent for alfuzosin and 26.9 percent for saw palmetto) and obstructive score (decrease of 37.8 percent of alfuzosin and 23.2 percent for saw palmetto, $p = 0.01$ for both). The increase in quality of urination was better with alfuzosin. More responders (increase on day 21 in peak flow rate of at least 25 percent relative to the baseline values) were in the alfuzosin group (71.8 percent) compared to the saw palmetto group (48.4 percent), $p = 0.057$.

Side effects
One complaint of mild pruritus that resolved itself.

Authors' comments
The findings confirm the efficacy and safety of alfuzosin in symptomatic BPH, and indicate the superiority of alfuzosin over saw palmetto in the treatment of urinary signs and symptoms of BPH.

Reviewers' comments
The study is flawed by its limited duration. It is difficult to determine whether saw palmetto offered any real clinical benefit because the study did not include a placebo group. However, there is a definite benefit of alfuzosin over saw palmetto berry in this short-term study. Neither the randomization nor the blinding were adequately described. (1, 4)

Clinical Study: Permixon®

Extract name	PA 109
Manufacturer	Pierre Fabre Médicament, France
Indication	**Benign prostatic hyperplasia**
Level of evidence	**III**
Therapeutic benefit	**Undetermined**

Bibliographic reference
Semino MA, Ortega JLL, Cobo EG, Banez ET, Rodrigues FR (1992). Symptomatic treatment of benign prostatic hypertrophy: Comparative study of prazosin and *Serenoa repens*. *Archivos Espanoles de Urologia* 45 (3): 211-213.

Trial design
Parallel. Patients received saw palmetto or prazosin (0.5 mg every 12 hours for four days, then 1 mg every 12 hours for another four days, and finally 2 mg every 12 hours for the remainder of the 12 weeks). The trial report does

not specify the product. The designation of Permixon comes from Boyle and colleages (2000).

Study duration	3 months
Dose	2 tablets every 12 hours
Route of administration	Oral
Randomized	No
Randomization adequate	No
Blinding	Open
Blinding adequate	No
Placebo	No
Drug comparison	Yes
Drug name	Prazosin
Site description	Not described
No. of subjects enrolled	45
No. of subjects completed	41
Sex	Male
Age	55-81 years

Inclusion criteria
Clinical prostatism, with Grades I or II volume on rectal exam, and no suspicion of prostatic cancer or evidence of an obstructive uropathy.

Exclusion criteria
Patients who had undergone prostatic surgery previously or those suffering from a malignant prostatic disorder, hypertension, habitual hypotension, recent myocardial infarction, liver disease, obstructive uropathy, and Grades III or IV volume prostates.

End points
A rectal exam, urography, and a urodynamic exploration (to determine maximum and mean flow, total volume, and urination time, supplemented by an approximate estimate of residual urine by hypogastric echography) were performed. Patients returned for a follow-up visit after six weeks to evaluate the tolerance of treatment and at the end of twelve weeks to have urodynamic exploration and echographic measurement of residual urine.

Results
Improvement of symptoms was seen in both groups. An overall result shows that 12 percent of patients reported a frequency of less than five times for diurnal urination, compared to 0 percent before treatment. Nocturia decreased, with the number of patients having to get up no more than once increasing from 12 to 24 percent. The number of patients who originally

urinated more than 13 times over the course of the day fell from 14 percent to 2.5 percent. Comparing the two groups, a greater number of patients receiving prazosin improved than those receiving saw palmetto, although the difference was small in terms of both diurnal and nocturnal frequency of urination. An improvement in urodynamic changes in mean flow was observed with both treatments, although a larger number of those receiving prazosin benefited than those receiving saw palmetto. Residual urine was decreased in three patients taking prazosin and one treated with saw palmetto.

Side effects
Prazosin group: hypotension and gastric intolerance; saw palmetto group: none.

Author's comments
It can be concluded form the study that prazosin is slightly more effective in controlling the symptoms of irritation produced by benign prostatic hyperplasia. This remark is made on the basis of absolute figures, in the absence of any statistical analysis.

Reviewers' comments
Although the outcome measures were clearly defined, overall this is a limited study because it was nonrandomized, unblinded, and had no placebo. Although a trend was observed toward a benefit with prazosin over saw palmetto, 12 weeks is a short duration of treatment. (1, 3)

Clinical Study: Permixon®

Extract name	PA 109
Manufacturer	Pierre Fabre Médicament, France
Indication	**Benign prostatic hyperplasia**
Level of evidence	**III**
Therapeutic benefit	**Undetermined**

Bibliographic reference
Stepanov VN, Siniakova LA, Sarrazin B, Raynaud JP (1999). Efficacy and tolerability of *Serenoa repens* (Permixon) in benign prostatic hyperplasia: A double-blind comparative study of two dosage regimens. *Advances in Therapy* 16 (5): 231-241.

Trial design
Parallel. Dose comparison.

Study duration	3 months
Dose	2 (160 mg) capsules once daily or 1 (160 mg) capsule twice daily
Route of administration	Oral
Randomized	Yes
Randomization adequate	No
Blinding	Double-blind
Blinding adequate	No
Placebo	No
Drug comparison	No
Site description	Single center
No. of subjects enrolled	100
No. of subjects completed	92
Sex	Male
Age	Mean: 66.2 ± 5.8 years

Inclusion criteria

Age over 50, symptomatic benign prostatic hyperplasia for more than six months, International Prostate Symptom Score (IPSS) > 13, IPSS quality of life item score > 3, an enlarged prostate of > 25 cm^3, maximum flow rate between 5 and 12 ml/s (with voided volume > 150 ml), postvoiding residual urine < 150 ml, and prostate-specific antigen (PSA) < 15 ng/ml (with prostate size > 60 cm^3) or < 10 ng/ml (prostate size < 60 cm^3).

Exclusion criteria

History of urological disorders; undergone bladder, neck, or prostate surgery, transurethral incision of the prostate, balloon dilatation of the prostate, or thermotherapy; had suspected prostate cancer, progressive prostatitis, or urinary tract infection; or had used drugs within the last two weeks likely to alter the voiding pattern.

End points

Primary efficacy criteria was the change in the IPSS between baseline and end point. Other criteria included IPSS quality-of-life item score, maximum and mean urinary flow rate, and residual urine volume. Assessments were made before treatment and after one and three months.

Results

Both Permixon regimens significantly reduced the IPSS mean total score compared with baseline. This improvement was statistically significant after one month of treatment ($p < 0.0001$), and was maintained after three months. A highly significant decrease in residual urine was observed in both groups ($p < 0.001$). However, no significant differences between the two regimens were seen in any of the measured parameters.

Side effects
None related to treatment.

Authors' comments
Once-daily (2 x 160 mg capsules) and twice-daily (1 x 160 mg capsule) regimens produced marked, comparable, and sustained improvements in the symptoms of BPH, and the drug was well tolerated. The 320 mg once-daily dose might result in better compliance.

Reviewers' comments
Improvement compared with baseline was seen for both doses of Permixon, but the study did not include a placebo group to verify a beneficial effect. Three months is also a relatively short duration of treatment. Neither the randomization nor the blinding were adequately described. (Translation reviewed) (1, 6)

Clinical Study: Permixon®

Extract name	PA 109
Manufacturer	Pierre Fabre Médicament, France
Indication	**Benign prostatic hyperplasia**
Level of evidence	**III**
Therapeutic benefit	**MOA**

Bibliographic reference
Di Silverio F, Monti S, Sciarra A, Varasano PA, Martini C, Lanzara S, D'Eramo G, Di Nicola S, Toscano V (1998). Effects of long-term treatment with *Serenoa repens* (Permixon) on the concentrations and regional distribution of androgens and epidermal growth factor in benign prostatic hyperplasia. *The Prostate* 37 (2): 77-83.

Trial design
Parallel. Patients were split into two groups: one group treated with Permixon and one untreated group.

Study duration	3 months
Dose	320 mg/day
Route of administration	Oral
Randomized	Yes

Randomization adequate   No
Blinding   Not described
Blinding adequate   No

Placebo   No
Drug comparison   No

Site description   Not described

No. of subjects enrolled   25
No. of subjects completed   25
Sex   Male
Age   Mean: 68 ± 6 years

Inclusion criteria

Symptomatic men with established benign prostatic hyperplasia in general good condition, with symptoms of urinary obstruction for one to three years, enlarged prostate (mean volume: 44 ml), mean International Prostate Symptom Score (IPSS) of 15.4, maximum urinary flow rate of less than 15 ml/s, and a voided volume of 150 ml or more.

Exclusion criteria

Patients with residual urinary volume greater than 350 ml if they had a history of previous outlet surgery, histologically diagnosed prostate carcinoma, neurogenic disorders, bacterial prostatis, and other conditions besides BPH known to interfere with normal voiding.

End points

After three months, prostatic specimens were removed, and the tissue was pulverized. In the periurethral, subcapsular, and intermediate regions, testosterone (T), dihydrotestosterone (DHT), and epidermal growth factor (EGF) content was determined.

Results

In the untreated group, T, DHT, and EGF were present in the highest concentrations in the periurethral region compared to the peripheral subcapsular region. In comparison, in the Permixon group, a statistically significant reduction was observed of DHT ($p < 0.001$) and EGF ($p < 0.01$), mainly in the periurethral region. T levels were increased ($p < 0.001$).

Side effects

None mentioned.

Authors' comments

The decrease of DHT and the rise of T in the prostatic tissue of patients treated with Permixon confirms the capacity of this drug to inhibit in vivo 5-alpha-reductase in human pathological prostate. A marked decrease of

EGF associated with DHT reduction was observed. These biochemical effects, similar to those obtained with finasteride, are particularly evident in the periurethral region, whose enlargement is responsible for urinary obstruction. A possible speculation is that the preferential reduction of DHT and EGF content in the periurethral region is involved in the clinical improvement of the obstructive symptoms in BPH during Permixon therapy.

Reviewer's comments
A significant decrease in DHT with increased testosterone was observed in those treated with Permixon, which suggests that inhibition of 5-alpha-reductase is a mechanism of action of Permixon. The sample size was considered small, the randomization process was not adequately described, and the blinding was not described. (1, 5)

Product Profile: Prostaserene®

Manufacturer	**Therabel Pharma, Belgium (Indena S.p.A., Italy)**
U.S. distributor	None
Botanical ingredient	**Saw palmetto fruit extract**
Extract name	**SabalSelect™**
Quantity	160 mg
Processing	Hypercritical carbon dioxide extraction, plant to extract ratio 10:1
Standardization	85-95% fatty acids
Formulation	Capsule

Source(s) of information: Braeckman, Bruhwyler et al., 1997; Indena USA, Inc.

Product Profile: Serenoa Gelcaps

Manufacturer	**Thorne Research (Indena S.p.A., Italy)**
U.S. distributor	**Thorne Research**
Botanical ingredient	**Saw palmetto fruit extract**
Extract name	**SabalSelect™**
Quantity	160 mg
Processing	Plant to extract ratio 10:1
Standardization	Contains 85% liposterols
Formulation	Gelcap

Cautions: If pregnant, consult a health care practitioner before using this, or any other product.

Other ingredients: Gelatin, glycerin, olive oil, and water.

Comments: This product is available only through pharmacies and health care practitioners.

Source(s) of information: Product label; information provided by Indena USA, Inc.

Clinical Study: Prostaserene®

Extract name	SabalSelect™
Manufacturer	Therabel Pharma, Belgium (Indena S.p.A., Italy)

Indication	**Benign prostatic hyperplasia**
Level of evidence	**I**
Therapeutic benefit	**Yes**

Bibliographic reference
Braeckman J, Denis L, de Leval J, Keuppens F, Cornet A, De Bruyne R, De Smedt E, Pacco J, Timmermans L, Van Vliet P, et al. (1997). A double-blind, placebo-controlled study of the plant extract *Serenoa repens* in the treatment of benign hyperplasia of the prostate. *European Journal of Clinical Research* 9: 247-259.

Trial design
Parallel.

Study duration	3 months
Dose	160 mg twice daily
Route of administration	Oral
Randomized	Yes
Randomization adequate	Yes
Blinding	Double-blind
Blinding adequate	Yes
Placebo	Yes
Drug comparison	No
Site description	Multicenter
No. of subjects enrolled	238

No. of subjects completed 205
Sex   Male
Age   Mean: 65 ± 6.8 years

Inclusion criteria
Mild to moderate symptoms of prostatic hyperplasia, maximal flow rate between 5 and 15 ml/sec, no suspicion of cancer upon rectal examination, and no abnormalities in the urinary sediment.

Exclusion criteria
Age over 80; postvoiding residual volume greater than 60 ml; any malformation, tumor, or infection of the genitourinary system; previous endoscopy of the lower urinary tract; or debilitated condition due to any chronic disease.

End points
Patients were evaluated at baseline and after 30, 60, and 90 days of treatment. Assessments were made via questionnaire regarding prostate symptoms, a general physical examination, a rectal palpation, a transrectal echographic prostatic volume determination, urinary flow rate parameters, residual volume measurement, and a cytobacteriological urinary examination.

Results
Saw palmetto offered a significant improvement over placebo in the total symptomatological score (pollakiuria, nocturia, dysuria, urgency, and hesitancy) after 60 days ($p < 0.05$) and 90 days ($p < 0.01$). A nonsignificant tendency was observed for flow rate and prostate volume. Global (quality-of-life) evaluations by patients and physicians rated the saw palmetto group as significantly more improved compared to the placebo group.

Side effects
Side effects probably caused by the medication were seen in 2.5 percent of saw palmetto group (gastrointestinal, sexual, fatigue) and 3.7 percent of placebo group.

Authors' comments
The extract of *Serenoa repens* appears to be an efficacious and well-tolerated therapy in early symptomatic benign prostatic hyperplasia.

Reviewers' comments
This is an excellent study demonstrating a symptomatic improvement in lower urinary tract symptoms with saw palmetto berry, which is the primary goal in treating most men with symptomatic BPH. Ninety days is a relatively short study time, but does not invalidate the study. The drug was well tolerated. (5, 6)

Clinical Study: Prostaserene®

Extract name	SabalSelect™
Manufacturer	Therabel Pharma, Belgium (Indena S.p.A., Italy)

Indication	**Benign prostatic hyperplasia**
Level of evidence	**III**
Therapeutic benefit	**Undetermined**

Bibliographic reference
Braeckman J, Bruhwyler J, Vandekerckhove K, Geczy J (1997). Efficacy and safety of the extract of *Serenoa repens* in the treatment of benign prostatic hyperplasia: Therapeutic equivalence between twice and once daily dosage forms. *Phytotherapy Research* 11 (8): 558-563.

Trial design
Parallel. Dose comparison.

Study duration	1 year
Dose	160 mg capsule twice daily or 320 mg capsule once daily
Route of administration	Oral
Randomized	Yes
Randomization adequate	No
Blinding	Single-blind
Blinding adequate	No
Placebo	No
Drug comparison	No
Site description	Multicenter
No. of subjects enrolled	84
No. of subjects completed	67
Sex	Male
Age	Mean: 65.1 ± 7.3 years

Inclusion criteria
Men at least 75 years old with symptoms of benign prostatic hyperplasia (urgency, nocturia, pollakiuria, dysuria, decrease in flow, and terminal dribbling), maximal urinary flow > 5 ml/s and < 15 ml/s for a mictional volume of 150 ml, IPSS between 12 and 24, residual volume < 100 ml, and serum-specific antigen < 10 ng/ml.

Exclusion criteria
Indication for surgical intervention; any malformation, tumor, or infection of the genitourinary system; previous endoscopy of the lower urinary tract and/or hepatic insufficiency; treatment with other agents for BPH, antibiotics or antiseptics.

End points
Medical evaluations took place at baseline and after 1, 3, 6, 9, and 12 months. The efficacy of treatment was evaluated using the international prostate symptom score (IPSS), quality-of-life score, transrectal echographic prostatic volume determination, urinary flow rates (mean and maximal) for micturition volumes superior or equal to 100 ml, residual volume, and global evaluation of efficacy by the patient and the investigator.

Results
Both dosage forms produced a significant improvement in efficacy variables after one year: IPSS score by 60 percent ($p < 0.0001$), quality-of-life score (85 percent of patients were satisfied), prostatic volume by 12 percent ($p < 0.0001$), maximum flow rate by 22 percent ($p < 0.0001$), mean flow rate by 17 percent ($p < 0.0001$), and residual urinary volume by 16 percent ($p < 0.05$). No significant differences were found between the two groups.

Side effects
The medication was well tolerated with no difference in those with either a once-a-day or twice-a-day dose. Two patients in each group stopped the drug due to side effects.

Authors' comments
The extract of *Serenoa repens* in its two dosage forms is a safe and effective treatment for the micturition problems associated with BPH. Consequently, it appears to offer a potential pharmacologic alternative capable of improving BPH symptoms in patients with mild to moderate disease.

Reviewers' comments
Although the study has some design flaws, it offers a suggestion that a once-a-day dose of Prostaserene is equivalent to a twice-a-day dose. The one-year follow-up is helpful in showing the results over a long time. The study was not double-blind and did not include a placebo arm. (0, 5)

Product Profile: Strogen® uno

Manufacturer	**Schaper & Brümmer GmbH & Co. KG, Germany**

U.S. distributor	None
Botanical ingredient	**Saw palmetto fruit extract**
Extract name	**IDS 89**
Quantity	320 mg
Processing	No information
Standardization	No information
Formulation	Capsule

Source(s) of information: Weisser et al., 1997.

Clinical Study: Strogen® uno

Extract name	IDS 89
Manufacturer	Schaper & Brümmer GmbH & Co. KG, Germany
Indication	**Benign prostatic hyperplasia**
Level of evidence	**III**
Therapeutic benefit	**MOA**

Bibliographic reference
Weisser H, Behnke B, Helpap B, Bach D, Krieg M (1997). Enzyme activities in tissue of human benign prostatic hyperplasia after three months treatment with the *Sabal serrulata* extract IDS 89 (Strogen) or placebo. *European Urology* 31 (1): 97-101.

Trial design
Parallel.

Study duration	3 months
Dose	2 (320 mg) capsules 3 times daily
Route of administration	Oral
Randomized	Yes
Randomization adequate	No
Blinding	Double-blind
Blinding adequate	No
Placebo	Yes
Drug comparison	No
Site description	Single center
No. of subjects enrolled	18

No. of subjects completed 16
Sex   Male
Age   Not given

Inclusion criteria
Ages 45 to 75 years with symptoms of urinary obstruction, reduced maximum urinary flow < 15 ml/s, voided volume > 50 ml, enlarged prostate (> 60 g), and indication for benign prostatic hyperplasia surgery.

Exclusion criteria
Concomitant urological diseases (neurogenic bladder, acute or chronic prostatitis, acute or recurrent urinary tract infection, urethral stenosis, urinary tract stones, prostate cancer, severe hematuria), cardiogenic nocturia, peptic ulcer, severe hepatic impairment, renal insufficiency, abuse of alcohol, or taking any other drugs for BPH during the two months prior to the trial.

End points
After three months of treatment, the prostate was removed, and the amounts and substrate affinities of enzymes involved in both the formulation of dihydrotestosterone (DHT) (5-alpha-reductase) and the removal of DHT (3-alpha- and 3-beta-hydroxysteroid oxidoreductase [$HSOR_{red}$]) were measured, along with amounts of creatine kinase (an indication of cellular energy demand). These measurements were taken in the stroma and epithelium of the removed prostate.

Results
In epithelium, the substrate affinity (K_m) of the 5-alpha reductase decreased slightly. In stroma, the amount (V_{max}) value of the 3-alpha-$HSOR_{red}$ increased statistically, leading to a moderate increase in V_{max}/K_m. In stroma, the Vmax value of the 3-beta-$HSOR_{red}$ increased moderately, but not statistically. In stoma, the V_{max} value of creative kinase increased significantly, leading to a statistically distinct increase of V_{max}/K_m.

Side effects
None mentioned.

Authors' comments
This trial revealed significant biochemical changes at the cellular level of BPH tissue. However, the alterations are merely moderate, and their biochemical causes and consequences regarding the pathophysiology of BPH are rather uncertain.

Reviewers' comments
This study was done to evaluate biochemical change after treatment with saw palmetto extract in those for whom surgery was indicated. The authors excluded those with prostates less than or equal to 60 gm—a potential flaw,

since one can have symptomatic BPH with a small prostate. The sample size was small, and 3 months is also a short duration of treatment. Neither the randomization nor the blinding were adequately described. (1, 4)

Product Profile: ProstActive®

Manufacturer	**Dr. Willmar Schwabe GmbH & Co., Germany**
U.S. distributor	**Nature's Way Products, Inc.**
Botanical ingredient	**Saw palmetto fruit extract**
Extract name	**WS 1473**
Quantity	320 mg
Processing	Plant to extract ratio 100:8.5, ethanol (w/w) 90%
Standardization	No information
Formulation	Softgel capsule

Recommended dose: Take one softgel daily with water at mealtimes. Allow two to eight weeks of use before noticeable results.

DSHEA structure/function: Promotes prostate health, maintains normal urine flow, and supports normal 5-alpha-reductase activity within the prostate gland.

Other ingredients: Gelatin, glycerin, caramel, carmine, titanium dioxide.

Source(s) of information: Product package (© 2002 Nature's Way Products, Inc.); information provided by distributor.

Clinical Study: ProstActive®

Extract name	WS 1473
Manufacturer	Dr. Willmar Schwabe GmbH & Co., Germany
Indication	**Benign prostatic hyperplasia**
Level of evidence	**I**
Therapeutic benefit	**No**

Bibliographic reference
Löbelenz J (1992). *Extractum sabal fructus* in the therapy of benign prostatic hyperplasia (BPH). *Tpk Therapeutikon* 6 (1/2): 34-37.

Trial design
Parallel. Pretrial run-in phase of seven days.

Study duration	6 weeks
Dose	1 (100 mg) capsule 3 times daily
Route of administration	Oral
Randomized	Yes
Randomization adequate	Yes
Blinding	Double-blind
Blinding adequate	Yes
Placebo	Yes
Drug comparison	No
Site description	Not described
No. of subjects enrolled	60
No. of subjects completed	Not given
Sex	Male
Age	40-82 years

Inclusion criteria
Benign prostatic hypertrophy in Stages I and II (according to Alken) with a maximum micturition volume of 20 ml/s. During the trial, patients were only allowed to take medication that would not interfere with the assessment of efficacy, and the dosage was to remain constant.

Exclusion criteria
None mentioned.

End points
Patients were evaluated at the beginning of the seven-day run-in phase and at the start of therapy, as well as on the fifteenth, twenty-ninth, and forty-third days (termination of study). The target parameter was maximum micturitional volume per second. Secondary parameters were residual volume of urine, sonographic evaluation, the force of urine, postmicturitional drip, incontinence, and prostate-specific antigen.

Results
Maximum micturitional volume per second increased by 67 percent in the saw palmetto group compared to baseline, and by 53 percent in the placebo group. Mean urine flow increased in the saw palmetto group by 0.6 ml/s, whereas it increased by 0.3 ml/s in the placebo group. No statistically significant difference was observed for any outcome measure.

Side effects
None mentioned.

Author's comments
The investigation shows that a conservative treatment of patients suffering from benign prostatic hyperplasia in Stages I and II with phytopharmaceuticals can result in an improvement of symptoms.

Reviewers' comments
This was a well-designed study, although it was of short duration and had a relatively small numbers of patients. No statistically significant benefit was seen in the treatment arm, and the differences described were not clinically significant either. (Translation reviewed) (5, 5)

Product Profile: ProstActive® Plus

Manufacturer	**Dr. Willmar Schwabe GmbH & Co., Germany**
U.S. distributor	**Nature's Way Products, Inc.**
Botanical ingredient	**Saw palmetto fruit extract**
Extract name	**WS 1473**
Quantity	160 mg
Processing	Plant to extract ratio 12:1, ethanol (w/w) 90%
Standardization	No information
Botanical ingredient	**Nettle root extract**
Extract name	**WS 1031**
Quantity	120 mg
Processing	Plant to extract ratio 10:1, ethanol (w/w) 60%
Standardization	No information
Formulation	Softgel capsules

Recommended dose: Take one capsule twice daily with water. Best results are obtained with continuous use.

DSHEA structure/function: Promotes prostate health, maintains proper urinary flow.

Comments: Sold as Prostagutt® forte in Europe.

Source(s) of information: Product label (© 1998 Nature's Way Products, Inc.); information provided by distributor.

Clinical Study: Prostagutt® forte

Extract name	Saw palmetto WS 1473; Nettle WS 1031
Manufacturer	Dr. Willmar Schwabe GmbH & Co., Germany
Indication	**Benign prostatic hyperplasia**
Level of evidence	**II**
Therapeutic benefit	**Yes**

Bibliographic reference
Metzker H, Kieser M, Holscher U (1996). Efficacy of a combined *Sabal-Urtica* preparation in the treatment of benign prostatic hyperplasia (BPH). *Urologe* 36: 292-300.

Trial design
Parallel. Placebo run-in phase of two weeks. Trial of 24 weeks followed by a another 24 weeks of a therapy phase (single-blind phase during which all patients received active treatment).

Study duration	6 months
Dose	1 (160 mg saw palmetto extract and 120 mg nettle extract) capsule twice daily
Route of administration	Oral
Randomized	Yes
Randomization adequate	·Yes
Blinding	Double-blind
Blinding adequate	Yes
Placebo	Yes
Drug comparison	No
Site description	One urology practice
No. of subjects enrolled	40
No. of subjects completed	33
Sex	Male
Age	52-84 years

Inclusion criteria
Symptomatic benign prostatic hyperplasia Stages I to II according to Alken, maximum urinary volume > 150 ml and < 20ml/s, with a maximum change of 3 ml/s between inclusion and the end of the run-in phase.

Exclusion criteria
Patients younger than 50 years, necessity of surgical intervention, infection

of the urinary tract, concomitant medication that might interfere, cardiac insufficiency, or severe organic complaint requiring additional therapy.

End points
Evaluations were carried out at inclusion, after run-in, and after 8, 16, 24, and 48 weeks. They included a uroflowmetric test, transabdominal sonographic determination of residual urine and prostate size, and subjective symptoms and life quality (AUA symptom score).

Results
After 24 weeks of therapy, an improvement of 3.3 ml/s in maximal urine volume per second was seen following treatment with the saw palmetto-nettle combination. In comparison, an improvement of only 0.55 ml/s ($p < 0.001$) was seen in the placebo group. Only marginal changes in residual urine quantity and prostate size occurred in both groups. The AUA symptom score, corresponding to the International Prostate Symptom Score, showed a continuous and noticeable decrease in score due to treatment (after 8, 16, and 24 weeks, $p < 0.001$) but only an insignificant change in the placebo group. Patients in the placebo group who gained only slight improvement during the trial showed a clear improvement once they were given active treatment. Nevertheless, there was a clear advantage for those patients who had been receiving the active treatment from the beginning of the study.

Side effects
No adverse events.

Authors' comments
The present study confirms the efficacy of a combined saw palmetto-nettle preparation in the context of objective and subjective parameters, showing a very good tolerance at the same time.

Reviewers' comments
This is a well-designed study. However, the limited number of patients is a significant flaw. A significant benefit was observed in the treatment group, but these differences may not be clinically significant. Although six months is a relatively short duration, it does not invalidate the results. (5, 5)

Clinical Study: PRO 160/120 (Prostagutt® forte)

Extract name	Saw palmetto WS 1473; Nettle WS 1031
Manufacturer	Dr. Willmar Schwabe GmbH & Co.
Indication	**Benign prostatic hyperplasia**
Level of evidence	I
Therapeutic benefit	**Undetermined**

Bibliographic reference
Sokeland J, Albrecht J (1997). A combination of *Sabal* and *Urtica* extracts versus finasteride in BPH (stage I to II acc. to Alken): A comparison of therapeutic efficacy in a one-year double-blind study. *Urologe (A)* 36 (4): 327-333. (Also published by Sokeland J [2000]. *BJU International* 86 [4]: 439-442.)

Trial design
Parallel, drug comparison, double dummy design. PRO 160/120 versus finasteride (one 5 mg capsule daily). Pretrial run-in with placebo for two weeks.

Study duration	1 year
Dose	1 (160 mg saw palmetto extract and 120 mg nettle extract) capsule twice daily
Route of administration	Oral
Randomized	No
Randomization adequate	Yes
Blinding	Double-blind
Blinding adequate	Yes
Placebo	No
Drug comparison	Yes
Drug name	Finasteride
Site description	Multicenter
No. of subjects enrolled	543
No. of subjects completed	489
Sex	Male
Age	50-88 years

Inclusion criteria
Diagnosis of benign symptomatic prostatic hyperplasia in Stages I to II according to Alken; maximum urinary flow < 20 ml/s; micturition volume > 150 ml; change in maximum urinary flow between inclusion and the end of the run-in phase < 3 ml/s.

Exclusion criteria
Age younger than 50 years; need for surgical intervention in the lower urinary tract during trial; symptomatic infections of urinary tract; cardiac insufficiency; severe organic diseases; simultaneous participation in other trials; carcinoma of the prostate; prostate-specific antigen > 10ng/l; or benign prostatic hyperplasia in Stage III according to Alken.

End points
Clinical exams were conducted at the beginning and end of the run-in phase, at six-week intervals, and finally at week 48. The primary variable was maximum urinary flow after 24 weeks of treatment. Secondary endpoints were average urinary flow, micturition volume, and micturition time. Urinary symptoms were recorded by the International Prostate Symptom Score (IPSS) and quality of life was assessed via questionnaire.

Results
An increase of the urinary flow rate could be observed in both treatment groups (1.9 ml/s with PRO 160/120; 2.4 ml/s with finasteride). During the trial, the average urinary flow increased, whereas the micturition time decreased, in both groups. The micturition volume did not show any relevant differences after treatment with either agent. The IPSS decreased from 11.3 at the baseline to 8.2 after 24 weeks and 6.5 after 48 weeks with PRO 160/120, and from 11.8 to 8.0 and 6.2 with finasteride, respectively. Quality of life improved between the start and end of therapy from 7.5 to 4.3 with PRO 160/120 and from 7.7 to 4.1 with finasteride.

Side effects
Seventy-four adverse events occured in 48 patients in the PRO 160/120 group compared to 96 events in 54 patients treated with finasteride. Reduced ejaculation, erectile dysfunction, and pain in joints were more common with finasteride.

Authors' comments
The analysis showed that the efficacy of both PRO 160/120 and finasteride was equivalent and unrelated to prostate volume. PRO 160/120 was better tolerated than finasteride.

Reviewers' comments
Overall, this is a good study demonstrating equivalent benefit of Prostagutt forte and finasteride. However, without a placebo control one cannot tell wjetjer either agent is beneficial over placebo. The treatment length was adequate. (4, 6)

Product Profile: Nutrilite® Saw Palmetto with Nettle Root

Manufacturer	**Access Business Group: Home of Nutrilite**
U.S. distributor	**Access Business Group: Home of Nutrilite**
Botanical ingredient	**Saw palmetto fruit extract**
Extract name	None given
Quantity	106 mg

Processing	Liposterolic (oil) extract
Standardization	> 85% fatty acids
Botanical ingredient	**Lemon fruit concentrate**
Extract name	N/A
Quantity	33.3 mg
Processing	No information
Standardization	> 25% total bioflavonoids
Botanical ingredient	**Pumpkin seed extract**
Extract name	None given
Quantity	160 mg
Processing	Seed oil extract
Standardization	No information
Botanical ingredient	**Stinging nettle root extract**
Extract name	None given
Quantity	80 mg
Processing	Powdered extract
Standardization	> 0.8% beta-sitosterol
Formulation	Capsule (softgel)

Recommended dose: Take one softgel three times per day, preferably with meals.

DSHEA structure/function: For men, saw palmetto and pumpkin seed oil support normal prostate function. Nettle root supports normal urinary flow.

Cautions: Children under 12 years of age, pregnant or lactating women, or anyone with a medical condition should consult with a physician before using this product.

Other ingredients: Vitamin A (100 percent as beta-carotene) 100 IU, gelatin, glycerin, yellow beeswax, soybean oil, lecithin, corn oil, natural caramel color.

Source(s) of information: Product label (© 1997 Amway Corp.); information provided by distributor.

Clinical Study: Nutrilite® Saw Palmetto with Nettle Root

Extract name	None given
Manufacturer	Access Business Group: Home of Nutrilite
Indication	**Benign prostatic hyperplasia**

Level of evidence   I
Therapeutic benefit   **Trend**

Bibliographic reference
Marks LS, Partin AW, Epstein JI, Tyler VE, Simon I, Macairan ML, Chan TL, Dorey FJ, Garris JB, Veltri RW, et al. (2000). Effects of a saw palmetto herbal blend in men with symptomatic benign prostatic hyperplasia. *The Journal of Urology* 163 (5): 1451-1456.

Trial design
Parallel.

Study duration	6 months
Dose	1 capsule (including 106 mg saw palmetto extract) 3 times daily
Route of administration	Oral
Randomized	Yes
Randomization adequate	Yes
Blinding	Double-blind
Blinding adequate	Yes
Placebo	Yes
Drug comparison	No
Site description	One urology practice
No. of subjects enrolled	44
No. of subjects completed	41
Sex	Male
Age	Mean: 64 ± 8.7 years

Inclusion criteria
Ages 45 to 80 years in general good health with clinical diagnosis of benign prostatic hyperplasia based on moderate to severe symptoms and palpation of an enlarged prostate gland on rectal exam; International Prostate Symptom Score > 9, question 5 >1, 2 of any questions 1-4, 6 or 7 must be > 3; prostate-specific antigen (PSA) < 15 ng/ml; prostate volume > 30 cm^3.

Exclusion criteria
History of allergy to saw palmetto, history of any illness or condition that may interfere with the study, significant abnormalities on prestudy screening, treatment with an investigational drug within one month of screening, drug or alcohol abuse or dependence, urethral stricture, previous radiotherapy to pelvis, chronic prostatitis, previous bladder surgery, prostatectomy, or other invasive procedure for BPH, neurogenic bladder, or history of recurrent acute urinary retention.

End points
Routine clinical measures (symptom score, uroflowmetry, and postvoid residual urine volume), blood chemistry studies (PSA, sex hormones, and multiphasic analysis), prostate volumetrics by magnetic resonance imaging, and prostate biopsy for zonal morphometry and semiquantitative histology studies.

Results
Saw palmetto herbal blend and placebo groups had improved clinical parameters with a statistically insignificant advantage for the saw palmetto group. Neither PSA nor prostate volume changed from baseline. Morphological examination of the biopsy samples revealed that the percent epithelium in the transition zone decreased from 17.8 percent at baseline to 10.7 percent after six months of treatment with saw palmetto ($p < 0.01$). The percent atrophic glands increased from 25.2 percent to 40.9 percent after treatment with saw palmetto ($p < 0.01$). These changes were not observed in the placebo group.

Side effects
No adverse effects.

Author's comments
Saw palmetto herbal blend appears to be a safe, highly desirable option for men with moderately symptomatic BPH. Therapy resulted in a contraction of prostatic epithelial tissues, apparently via a nonhormonal mechanism.

Reviewers' comments
This is a well-designed study showing a trend toward improvement in clinical parameters. The small number of patients limited the ability to detect slight clinical changes as noted by the authors. Six months is a reasonable length of time. However, if the study was of longer duration, an increased improvement with treatment may be noted since those with a placebo effect fail to improve. (5, 5)

St. John's Wort

Latin name: *Hypericum perforatum* **L.** [Clusiaceae]
Plant parts: **Flower, leaf**

PREPARATIONS USED
IN REVIEWED CLINICAL STUDIES

St. John's wort is an herb with bright yellow flowers, whose benefit in treating psychiatric disorders may have been recognized by Paracelsus during the Renaissance. St. John's wort is native to Europe, North America, South America, and Asia. Most contemporary preparations of St. John's wort are aqueous alcoholic extracts with plant/extract ratios of 4 to 7:1. St. John's wort products have been characterized and standardized to the content of hypericin and hyperforin. The dried buds, flowers, and distal leaves contain 0.2 to 0.3 percent and 1 to 4 percent of these constituents, respectively (Schulz, Hänsel, and Tyler, 2001).

Hypericin content is often measured using ultraviolet (UV) spectroscopy using a method described by the German Pharmaceutical Codex (Deutscher Arzneimittel-Codex [DAC]) that determines the total quantity of a class of compounds called dianthrones, which includes hypericin, psuedohypericin, protohypericin, and protopseudohypericin. The UV spectroscopy results are quoted as total hypericin. These constituents are also analyzed using high performance liquid chromatography (HPLC), a system that allows for measurement of individual constituents. Measurements generated from UV and HPLC analysis are not interchangeable and should not be confused. The other ingredient commonly used to characterize St. John's wort products, hyperforin, is quantified using HPLC analysis.

Kira® tablets contain 300 mg of the St. John's wort extract LI 160 and are distributed in the United States by Lichtwer Pharma U.S., Inc. The product is manufactuered by Lichtwer Pharma AG, Germany, and sold in Europe under the name of Jarsin® 300. The LI 160 extract

ST. JOHN'S WORT SUMMARY TABLE

Product Name	Manufacturer/ U.S. Distributor	Product Characteristics	Dose in Trials	Indication	No. of Trials	Benefit (Evidence Level-Trial No.)
Kira®* (US); Jarsin® (EU)	Lichtwer Pharma AG, Germany (Indena S.p.A., Italy/Lichtwer Pharma US, Inc.	Extract (LI 160/St. John Select™) containing 0.3% hypericin, > 3% hyperforin	3 × 300 mg daily	Depression	13	Yes (I-2, II-3, III-1) Trend (II-3, III-1) Undetermined (III-1) No (I-2)
				Electro-physiological effects	1	MOA (II-1)
				Neuroendo-crine effects	1	MOA (II-1)
Perika™; Movana™ (US); Neuroplant® (EU)	Dr. Willmar Schwabe GmbH & Co., Germany/ Nature's Way Products, Inc..; Pharmaton Natural Health Products	Ethanolic extract (WS 5572) con-taining 5% hyperforin, 0.14% total hypericin	3 × 300 mg	Depression	5	Yes (I-2, II-1) Trend (II-1) Undetermined (III-1)
				Electro-physiologi-cal effects	1	MOA (II-1)
				Neuroendo-crine effects	1	MOA (III-1)
St. John's Wort Ze 117™-Remotiv® (EU)	Zeller AG, Switzer-land/General Nutri-tion Corp.; Rexall Sundown	Ethanolic extract (Ze 117™) con-taining 0.2% hypericin	2 × 250 mg	Depression	3	Yes (I-2, II-1)

Hyperiforce (EU)	Bioforce AG, Switzerland/None	Fresh plant alcoholic extract, 0.33 mg hypericin per tablet	3 × 60 mg	Depression	1	Undetermined (II-1)
STEI 300 (EU)	Steiner Arzneimittel, Germany/None	Ethanolic extract containing 0.2%-0.3% hypericins and 2%-3% hyperforin	1,050 mg	Depression	1	Yes (II-1)
Dysto-lux® (EU)	Dr Loges & Co. GmbH, Germany/None	Ethanolic extract (LoHyp-57), plant/extract ratio 5-7:1	4 × 200 mg	Depression	1	Yes (II-1)

*Products sold in the United States that contain the Indena extract in the Lichtwer Pharma product (St. John Select) are listed following. The extract in these products has been tested clinically but the final formulation has not. The exception is the HBC Protocols, Inc. product, which was studied in two drug interaction studies described in the Drug Interactions section (Piscitelli et al., 2000; Burstein et al., 2000).

Product Name
St. John's Wort Extract
Hypericum Perforatum II
Hyper-Ex®

Manufacturer
Enzymatic Therapy
HBC Protocols, Inc.
Thorne Research

(aqueous methanol; 4-7:1) is manufactured by Indena S.p.A. in Italy, and is standardized to contain 0.24 to 0.32 percent total hypericins and a minimum of 3 percent hyperforin. The Indena extract is also known as St. John Select™, and is the basis of several other products available in the United States, namely, St. John's Wort Extract by Enzymatic Therapy, Hyper-Ex® by Thorne Research, and Hypericum Perforatum II by HBC Protocols, Inc.

WS 5572 is an extract of the aerial parts of St. John's wort with a plant to extract ratio of 2.5-5:1 (60 percent ethanol w/w). It is manufactured in Germany by Dr. Willmar Schwabe GmbH & Co. and is characterized as containing a minimum of 3 percent hyperforin. WS 5572 is sold in the United States in the products called Perika™, distributed by Nature's Way Products, Inc., and Movana™, distributed by Pharmaton Natural Health Products. Both of these products are available in 300 mg tablets. WS 5572 is sold in Europe in products such as Neuroplant, Neuroplant 300, and Neuroplant forte. A very similar extract, WS 5570, was used in two of the studies we reviewed (Lecrubier et al., 2002; Schüle et al., 2001). Although WS 5570 contains the same hyperforin and hypericin content as the WS 5572 extract, the specifications are slightly different: 80 percent ethanol v/v with a plant to extract ratio of 3-7:1. The WS 5570 extract is not included in any of products described previously. WS 5573 contains a low level of hyperforin (0.5 percent) and was used to delineate the importance of this constituent. It was compared with WS 5572 in two trials (Laakmann et al., 1998; Schellenberg, Sauer, and Dimpfel, 1998), and is not included in any of products described earlier.

Ze 117™ is manufactured in Switzerland by Zeller AG, and is an aqueous ethanolic (50 percent w/w) extract of the flowering tops of St. John's wort (4-7:1). The extract is standardized to contain 0.2 percent hypericin and less than or equal to 0.2 percent hyperforin. Ze 117 is sold in the United States as St. John's Wort Ze 117™, distributed by General Nutrition Corporation, and as St. John's Wort (Ze 117™), distributed by Rexall Sundown. Both of these products are available in 500 mg caplets.

Hyperiforce tablets contain a fresh plant extract of the shoot tips (60 percent alcohol, ratio 3.9-5.0:1) that is standardized to contain 0.33 mg total hypericin per tablet. This product is sold in Europe as Hyperiforce, manufactured by Bioforce AG in Switzerland, but is not available in the United States as a single ingredient product. Bioforce

USA distributes a product called St. John's Wort Complex that contains the St. John's wort extract in addition to extracts of hops flowers and the aerial parts of lemon balm. This formula has not been tested clinically.

STEI 300 is an extract of St. John's wort, and is manufactured by Steiner Arzneimittel in Germany. This extract (60 percent ethanol w/w) is characterized as containing 0.2 to 0.3 percent hypericin and pseudohypericin and 2 to 3 percent hyperforin. STEI 300 is not sold in the United States.

Dysto-lux® is manufactured in Germany by Dr. Loges & Co. GmbH. It contains LoHyp-57, an ethanolic extract (60 percent ethanol w/w) with a plant to extract ratio of 5-7:1. Dyxto-lux is not available in the United States.

SUMMARY OF REVIEWED CLINICAL STUDIES

The most common indication treated with St. John's wort is mild to moderate major depression. The essential feature of a major depressive episode, as defined in the DSM-IV (*Diagnostic and Statistical Manual of Mental Disorders,* Fourth Edition), is a period of at least two weeks during which depressed mood or the loss of interest in nearly all activities is observed (American Psychiatric Association, 1994). Additional symptoms of depression include changes in appetite or weight, sleep, and psychomotor activity, decreased energy, feelings of worthlessness or guilt, difficulty concentrating, or recurrent thoughts of death or suicidal ideation. Major depressive episodes can be mild, moderate, or severe. Depressive disorders are also defined in the World Health Organization's (WHO) *International Classification of Diseases,* Tenth Revision (ICD-10) (WHO, 1992). Some of the reviewed trials had inclusion criteria according to earlier versions of these manuals: DSM-III and ICD-9.

The Hamilton Depression Rating Scale (HAM-D) is an observer rating scale used to evaluate the degree of depression, and is often used to evaluate the success of treatment. The physician interviews the patient and assigns a score based on the severity of 17 or 21 items. The definition of therapeutic success is usually a 50 percent reduction in the total HAM-D score or a total score less than ten.

The usual treatment for depression includes psychotherapy and antidepressant medication, which includes selective serotonin reuptake inhibitors (SSRI), tricyclic antidepressants, and, more rarely, monoamine oxidase inhibitors.

The majority of the reviewed studies indicate that St. John's wort extracts may be a viable treatment option for patients with mild to moderate depression. However, some recent trials have not shown any efficacy compared to placebo, casting doubt upon the benefit for depression. However, we must keep in mind that at least one-third of published clinical trials of approved antidepressants are negative for efficacy (Thase, 1999). Nevertheless additional studies are required to explore treatment for longer than eight weeks.

Two mode-of-action studies explored the effect of LI 160 and WS 5570 on pituitary hormone secretion as a means of exploring the effects on neurotransmitters. The theory is that antidepressants that act via noradrenaline reuptake inhibition pathways stimulate growth hormone secretion, whereas those that act via serotonin reuptake inhibitors stimulate prolactin. Cortisol secretion is increased by both noradrenaline and serotonin reuptake inhibitors. In addition, plasma levels of growth hormone can be elevated by dopamine reuptake inhibitors. A small, one-day study with eight healthy males exploring the mode of action of LI 160 found that administration of one dose of 2,700 mg LI 160 extract caused an increase in plasma concentrations of growth hormone, a decrease in prolactin levels, and no effect on cortisol levels compared to placebo. The authors of this study interpreted the results to be due to an increase in the dopamine function (Franklin et al., 1999). In contrast, another study found that administration of 300 or 600 mg WS 5570 had no effect on prolactin levels, only a minimal, inconsistent effect on growth factor levels, and a significant effect on cortisol levels. The authors of this study suggested an effect on noradrenaline and serotonin reuptake inhibitors due mainly to the constituent hyperforin. Further, they suggested that the discrepancies between the two studies might be a function of dose (Schüle et al., 2001).

LI 160

Depression

We reviewed 13 studies that explored the effect of LI 160 on depression. The usual dose was 900 mg extract per day for a period of one to two months. Four placebo-controlled studies reported a therapeutic benefit in comparison to placebo, one was undetermined, and two showed no benefit in comparison to placebo. We also reviewed six randomized, controlled, double-blind studies comparing LI 160 with other antidepressants. Four of the trials used tricyclic antidepressants (maprotiline, imipramine, amitriptyline), and two used sertraline, an SSRI. All six studies showed a comparable benefit with both treatments, although in one study both treatments were negative in comparison to placebo. Two studies explored the mode of action of the extract, one measuring brain electroencephalograph (EEG) traces and the other measuring plasma levels of pituitary hormones.

Four trials showed LI 160 to have significant antidepressant activity in comparison to placebo after one month of treatment with 300 mg LI 160 extract three times daily. In a good-quality study with 101 subjects with mild to moderate depression as defined in the DSM-III-R, HAM-D scores fell from 21 to 8.9 in the St. John's wort group (Hänsgen and Vesper, 1996). In another good-quality study with 67 adults with major depression according to the DSM-III-R, the HAM-D score of the treatment group fell from 21.8 to 9.2. In the placebo group, the HAM-D scores fell from 20.4 to 14.7 (Hänsgen, Vesper, and Ploch, 1994). Two smaller studies included participants rated according to the ICD-9 scale. The first study, including a total of 89 subjects, reported that the initial HAM-D score of 15.8 in the treatment group fell to 7.2 (Sommer and Harrer, 1994). The second study, with 39 subjects, reported an HAM-D responder rate of 70 percent for the St. John's wort group and 47 percent for the placebo group (Hübner, Lande, and Podzuweit, 1994).

A six-week study of 60 subjects with mild to moderate depression as defined by the ICD-9 also reported a higher HAM-D responder rate than placebo (66.6 percent compared to 26.7 percent) (Schmidt and Sommer, 1993). However, a lack of detail in the analysis of the results prohibited our reviewers, Drs. Hannah Kim and Debbie

Goebert, from forming any conclusion regarding therapeutic efficacy for depression.

In contrast, a recent, large, well-conducted, placebo-controlled study of 167 patients with initial HAM-D scores of at least 20 who were treated for two months, reported that LI 160 was not more effective than placebo in the treatment of major depression as defined by the DSM-IV (Shelton et al., 2001). It has been suggested that the reason this study was negative was that it used more severely depressed patients than the other studies (mean baseline HAM-D score of 23). However, it is not uncommon for trials with approved antidepressants to be negative, and this phenomenon might be due to the difficulty in measuring depression. Another study of 48 subjects with depression as defined by the ICD-9 scale and an initial HAM-D mean score of 23.7 in the treatment group also reported no significant difference from placebo after four weeks of the standard dose of LI 160 (Lehrl et al., 1993).

Four drug comparison trials compared the effectiveness of LI 160 with tricyclic antidepressants. The first trial compared 900 mg LI 160 extract with 75 mg maprotiline daily for one month in 86 subjects diagnosed as depressed according to the ICD-10, and with an initial HAM-D score greater than 15 (mean of 21). With both treatments, the HAM-D scores fell by approximately 50 percent after one month (Harrer, Hübner, and Podzuweit, 1994). Another trial examined the effectiveness of 900 mg LI 160 and 75 mg amitriptyline on 120 subjects with a current major depressive episode according to the DSM-IV, and with an initial HAM-D score between 17 and 24. After six weeks of treatment, both groups improved with no significant difference in the response to one treatment compared to the other (Wheatley, 1997). A third study compared 900 mg LI 160 extract to 75 mg imipramine in 130 subjects with depression according to DSM-III-R. Again, after six weeks, a significant reduction in HAM-D scores was seen in both groups: from 20.2 to 8.8 in the LI 160 group and from 19.4 to 10.7 in the imipramine group (Vorbach, Hübner, and Arnoldt, 1994). Our reviewers criticized these trials because they all used low, or what is considered subtherapeutic, doses of the tricyclic antidepressant drugs. A fourth trial used twice the dose of imipramine (150 mg rather than 75 mg per day) along with a higher dose of LI 160 (1,800 mg per day) on 186 adults with depression according to the ICD-10. After six weeks, mean HAM-D scores decreased similarly in both groups according to intent-to-treat analysis (Vorbach, Arnoldt, and Hübner, 1997). The authors of the studies suggested the possibility that St. John's wort could be a more attractive option for treatment of mild to moderate depression due to fewer side effects with LI 160 compared to the tricyclic antidepressant drugs.

Two drug comparison trials compared the effectiveness of LI 160 with the SSRI sertraline (Zoloft). A small trial, which included 20 subjects diagnosed with depression according to DSM-IV, and having an initial HAM-D score of at least 17, compared sertraline, 75 mg per day, with LI 160, 900 mg per day. After seven weeks, both groups improved with no significant difference between treatments (Brenner et al., 2000). A large trial with 245 adults diagnosed with major depression according to DSM-IV criteria, and a minimum HAM-D score of 20, compared sertraline to LI 160, and also included a placebo group. During the two-month trial, the dose of either treatment could be increased if benefit was not apparent. The dose of sertraline ranged from 50 to 100 mg per day, and the dose for LI 160 ranged from 900 to 1,500 mg per day. Assessments of HAM-D scores at the end of the trial revealed that neither LI 160 nor sertraline provided a statistically significant benefit compared to placebo (Hypericum Depression Trial Study Group, 2002). By the authors' own admission, up to 35 percent of trials with approved antidepressants do not show a benefit when compared with placebo.

Electrophysiological Effects

A trial including 24 healthy subjects compared the effect of administration of LI 160 (900 mg per day) to the tricyclic antidepressant maprotiline (30 mg per day) on EEG traces. After one month of treatment, changes in the visually evoked potentials in the beta region were similar for both agents. The authors of the study stated that this finding was in agreement with clinical studies reporting similar antidepressant activity (Johnson et al., 1994).

Neuroendocrine Effects

A small, one-day study of eight healthy males exploring the mode of action of LI 160 found an increase in plasma concentrations of growth hormone, a decrease in prolactin levels, and no effect on cortisol levels compared to placebo. The authors interpreted these results as an increase in the neurotransmitter dopamine function. The amount given (2,700 mg extract) was three times the usual therapeutic dose (Franklin et al., 1999).

WS 5572

Depression

We reviewed five studies that explored the activity of WS 5572 or WS 5570 for depression. The usual dose was 900 mg extract per day for a period of one to two months. Three placebo-controlled studies reported a therapeutic benefit, and one was undetermined. We also reviewed one study comparing WS 5572 to the tricyclic antidepressant trimipramine. Two studies explored the mode of action of the extract: one measuring brain EEG traces and the other measuring plasma levels of pituitary hormones.

In a landmark trial, Laakmann and colleagues (1998) compared a St. John's wort extract containing 5 percent hyperforin (WS 5572) with one that contained 0.5 percent hyperforin (WS 5573). Previous characterization of products had emphasized another ingredient, hypericin. This trial indicated that hyperforin might be more important in treating depression than hypericin. The trial included 138 mild to moderately depressed subjects as defined by DSM-IV criteria, with a minimum HAM-D score of 17. The three-arm design included the two different extracts containing different amounts of hyperforin and identical amounts of hypericin: Both extracts were given in doses of 900 mg and were compared to placebo. After six weeks, a statistically significant HAM-D score reduction was observed in the group given the extract containing 5 percent hyperforin compared with the placebo group, whereas the activity reported with the extract containing 0.5 percent hyperforin was not different from placebo.

A placebo-controlled phase III trial included 332 subjects with mild to moderate depression (DSM-IV) and a HAM-D total score between 18 and 25 who were given either 900 mg WS 5570 per day or placebo for six weeks. Treatment with WS 5570 caused a significantly greater decrease in the HAM-D score compared to placebo, from a baseline of 21.9 (all subjects) to 12.0, or 13.8, respectively. In addition, there were significantly more treatment responders, as defined by a 50 percent reduction in the total HAM-D score, in the WS

5570 group (52.7 percent compared to 42.3 percent) (Lecrubier et al., 2002). Another trial with WS 5572 included 65 mild to moderately depressed subjects as defined by DSM-IV criteria, with a minimum HAM-D score of 16. After six weeks, there was a significantly greater reduction in HAM-D scores in the treatment group compared to placebo (Kalb, Trautmann-Sponsel, and Kieser, 2001). An earlier placebo-controlled study of 50 subjects with mild to moderate depression according to ICD classification (edition not given) also reported significant reductions in the HAM-D scoring with WS 5572 compared to placebo. The study was rated as having undetermined efficacy due to poor methodology (Reh, Laux, and Schenk, 1992).

A study of 48 mild to moderately depressed subjects according to DSM-III-R compared Neuroplant forte (WS 5572 extract) to a low dose (25 mg/day) of trimipramine, a tricyclic antidepressant. Similar reductions in HAM-D scores were observed, with initial scores of 13.0 (trimipramine) and 11.2 (Neuroplant forte) dropping to 7.9 and 7.7, respectively, after six weeks. A placebo arm was not included in this trial. Neuroplant forte decreased alpha activity as measured by EEG both with resting and while performing a recognition task. Trimipramine produced an increase in alpha activity under these conditions along with a decrease in delta and gamma activity. The authors concluded that these results indicated a sedative effect with trimipramine that was not seen with Neuroplant forte (Woelk et al., 1996).

Electrophysiological Effects

A mode-of-action study compared the extracts containing 5 percent hyperforin (WS 5572) and 0.5 percent hyperforin (WS 5573) with placebo on quantitative topographic electroencephalography (qEEG) in 53 healthy volunteers. QEEG-measured frequency spectra have been used as a tool to study the action of drugs. The spectrum is divided into frequency bands, namely delta, theta, alpha, and beta. After eight days of 900 mg extract per day, both extracts produced power increases in the delta, theta, and alpha-1 bands that could be distinguished from placebo. This effect was greater with the extract containing 5 percent hyperforin. Although changes in the qEEG were consistent with effects by noradrenergic (theta bands) and serotonergic (alpha-1 bands) neurotransmitters, the authors admitted that the relationship between acute EEG effects of antidepressant drugs and clinical therapeutic efficacy is far from understood (Schellenberg, Sauer, and Dimpfel, 1998).

Neuroendocrine Effects

A mode-of-action study explored the effect of WS 5570 on pituitary hormone secretion as a means of exploring the effects on neurotransmitters. The effects of WS 5570 on cortisol, growth hormone, and prolactin were examined in 12 healthy subjects. Blood samples were taken one hour prior to and up to five hours after oral administration of 300 mg WS 5570, 600 mg WS 5570, or placebo. As a result, a significant increase in cortisol levels with the 600 mg dose compared to placebo occurred 30 to 90 minutes after oral consumption. The lower dose did not affect cortisol levels. No consistent effect on growth hormone levels was observed, and neither dose affected prolactin levels. The authors suggested that WS 5570, at high doses, acts as a noradrenaline and serotonin reuptake inhibitor, thereby increasing the levels of these neurotransmitters, and, in turn, increasing cortical release (Schüle et al., 2001).

Ze 117

Depression

Three large, well-conducted studies found Ze 117 to be better than placebo and equivalent to therapeutic doses of the tricyclic antidepressant imipramine and the SSRI fluoxetine in treating mild to moderate depression. A placebo-controlled study included 136 subjects with mild to moderate depression according to the ICD-10 and HAM-D scores between 16 and 24. The group given 500 mg Ze 117 per day for six weeks showed significant improvement compared to the placebo group, according to both intention-to-treat and protocol-compliant analysis of HAM-D scores (Schrader, Meier, and Brattstrom, 1998). Another study compared the efficacy of 500 mg Ze 117 per day to 150 mg per day of the tricyclic antidepressant imipramine. This study included 277 participants with mild to moderate depression according to ICD-10 criteria, and an initial HAM-D score of at least 18. Both Ze 117 and imipramine were therapeutically equivalent according to the HAM-D ratings (Woelk, 2000). A third study compared the efficacy of 500 mg Ze 117 per day to 20 mg per day of the SSRI fluoxetine (Prozac). This six-week study included 238 patients with mild to moderate depression according to ICD-10 criteria, and an initial HAM-D score between 16 and 24. According to HAM-D scores, the two treatments were equivalent (Schrader, 2000).

Hyperiforce

Depression

Hyperiforce was tested in a dose-comparison study using tablets containing one-sixth, one-third, and the usual amount of the same crude extract (subjects were given the equivalent of 0.16, 0.33, and 1.0 mg hypericin per day, respectively) over a period of six weeks. The trial included 260 subjects with mild to moderate depression according to ICD-10 criteria. An initial average HAM-D score of approximately 16 was reduced significantly in all three groups. The highest dose showed a trend toward better efficacy, but this difference was not significant (Lenoir, Degenring, and Saller, 1997). Because this trial did not include a placebo group, it is difficult to evaluate the effectiveness of any of these doses.

STEI 300

Depression

St. John's wort extract STEI 300 (1050 mg daily) was compared with the tricyclic antidepressant imipramine (100 mg daily) in an eight-week study including 251 moderately depressed patients as defined by the ICD-10, and with an initial HAM-D minimum score of 18. STEI 300 was more effective than placebo and comparable to imipramine in reducing HAM-D scores (Philipp, Kohnen, and Hiller, 1999).

Dysto-lux (LoHyp-57)

Depression

Another St. John's wort extract, LoHyp-57 (800 mg daily), was compared to the SSRI fluoxetine (Prozac, 20 mg per day) for six weeks in a trial that included 137 subjects ages 60 to 80 years with mild to moderate depression according to the ICD-10. Similar response rates were demonstrated for these patients, who had initial average HAM-D scores of 14 to 17 (Harrer et al., 1999).

SYSTEMATIC REVIEWS AND META-ANALYSES

A recent meta-analysis of 22 randomized, controlled trials, with a total of 2,517 patients, found that St. John's wort was more effective than placebo and not different in activity from other antidepressants. Numerous St. John's wort products were included (e.g., Jarsin, Neuroplant, Ze 117, and STEI 300). Only two trials tested treatment in severe depression (Vorbach, Arnoldt, and Hübner, 1997; Shelton et al., 2001); the majority tested treatment in mild to moderate depression. An initial analysis was conducted on 14 placebo-controlled studies that met the general criteria of including Hamilton Depression Rating Scale (HAM-D) scores. A secondary analysis was conducted on six placebo-controlled studies that met the stricter criteria of including intention-to-treat analysis (ITTA) and adherence to predefined inclusion and exclusion criteria in addition to HAM-D scores. Both of these analyses came to the conclusion that St. John's wort was significantly better than placebo, with the effect size being smaller in the second analysis. The relative risk (RR) was 1.98 (95 percent confidence interval [CI] 1.49 to 2.62) in the general analysis and 1.77 (1.16 to 2.70) in the stricter analysis. St. John's wort compared to other antidepressants were also analyzed twice—once with nine studies meeting general criteria, and again with four studies meeting the more stringent criteria mentioned earlier. Both comparisons found that the activity of St. John's wort was not significantly different from active antidepressants: RR 1.0 (0.90 to 1.11) and RR 1.04 (0.94 to 1.15), respectively. Most trials compared St. John's wort with tricyclic antidepressants, and only two used an SSRI. There was no publication bias in the trials according to a funnel plot analysis (Whiskey, Werneke, and Taylor, 2001).

Earlier meta-analyses came to similar conclusions. Linde and colleagues (1996) reviewed 23 randomized, controlled trials including 1,757 patients with mild to moderate depression. Analysis of 15 placebo-controlled trials yielded that St. John's wort preparations were significantly better than placebo, with an RR of 2.67 (95 percent CI 1.78 to 4.01). Analysis of eight trials comparing the activity of St. John's wort to tricyclic antidepressants found their activity to be similar: RR 1.10 (0.93 to 1.31). Kim, Streltzer, and Goebert (1999) conducted an analysis on blinded, controlled studies with well-defined depressive disorders (ICD-10, DSM-III-R or DSM-IV) and outcome measures, including HAM-D scores. Six controlled, double-blind, clinical studies with a total of 651 patients with mild to moderate depression met the entry requirements, including two placebo-controlled studies and four drug comparison studies. In reviewing the placebo-controlled trials, Kim, Streltzer, and Goebert reported that St. John's wort was 1.5 times more likely than placebo to cause an antidepressant response. In reviewing the four comparison trials with tricyclic antidepressants (maprotiline, amitriptyline, imipramine), they found the two treatments to be equivalent.

POSTMARKETING SURVEILLANCE STUDIES

A multicenter postmarketing surveillance study was carried out with 101 children ages 1 through 12 years with depression and psychovegetative disorders. The dose ranged from 300 to 1,800 mg LI 160 extract per day with the median dose being 300 mg. With no standardized measure available to assess depression in children, physicians and parents filled out a questionnaire covering 12 typical symptoms. The number of physicians rating treatment effectiveness as good or excellent was 72 percent after two weeks and 97 percent after four weeks. Although 90 percent of children completed four weeks of treatment, only 75 percent extended their treatment for an additional two weeks. All of those remaining in the study were rated as good or excellent after six weeks (Hübner and Kirste, 2001).

A multicenter postmarketing surveillance study was conducted on 2,166 patients diagnosed with mild to moderate depression who took either one or two (600 mg) WS 5572 tablets (Neuroplant) per day. Patients with more severe depression were given the higher dose, and both groups were followed for six weeks. At that time, the physicians and patients evaluated the efficacy of both doses and found them to be mostly good or very good with no significant difference between the two (Rychlik et al., 2001). An earlier study had administered the customary dosage of 300 mg three times daily to 5,546 patients (Lemmer, von den Driesch, and Klieser, 1999). Because the same standard methods were used for both studies, Rychlik and colleagues (2001) compared them and concluded that there was no relevant therapeutic disadvantage with the administration of 600 mg once daily compared to 300 mg three time daily.

ADVERSE REACTIONS OR SIDE EFFECTS

The most common side effects of *Hypericum* in the trials reviewed earlier were generally mild and consisted of gastrointestinal disturbances, dry mouth, sleep disturbances, headaches, pruritis, and possible photosensitivity. A meta-analysis of 22 randomized, controlled trials reported that side effects were mild, and those occurring in more than 1 percent of the study population included nausea and vomiting, dry mouth, headaches, fatigue, abdominal pain, dizziness, and restlessness (Whiskey, Werneke, and Taylor, 2001). In a large, prospective, open-label study in which data were systematically gathered from 3,250 patients, only 2.4 percent of patients reported an adverse effect. The most common effects were gastrointestinal complaints, allergic rash, tiredness, anxiety, and confusion (Woelk, Burkard, and Grunwald, 1994).

A multicenter, postmarketing surveillance study carried out with 101 children ages one through twelve years treated with 300 to 1,800 mg LI 160 extract per day for four to six weeks reported good tolerability with no adverse events (Hübner and Kirste, 2001). Another multicenter, postmarketing surveillance study conducted on 2,166 patients given one or two (600 mg) WS 5572 tablets (Neuroplant) per day reported the incidence of adverse drug reactions to be less than 1 percent. The reactions included skin irritation and itching of the area around the eyelids, allergic exanthema, nervousness and unrest, stomach problems, diarrhea, and sleep disorders (Rychlik et al., 2001).

A crossover trial with 12 older women found no effect on rapid eye movement (REM) sleep after a month of administration of 900 mg extract (LI 160). This was in contrast to effects of tricyclic antidepressants, which do interfere with REM sleep (Schulz and Jobert, 1994). A drug comparison study with 160 depressed patients reported no pathological effect on cardiac function as measured via electrocardiogram (ECG) following administration of a high dose of Jarsin 300 (1,800 mg per day) for six weeks compared with 150 mg of the tricyclic antidepressant imipramine. The rationale for this study is that patients suffering from depression with a preexisting conductive dysfunction are at increased risk for ventricular arrhythmia when taking tricyclic antidepressants. As expected, in susceptible individuals, imipramine caused a prolongation of conduction intervals. In contrast, St. John's wort extract caused a small increase in conduction in those individuals. The authors of the study concluded that in the treatment of patients with a preexisting conductive dysfunction, or elderly patients, a high dose of LI 160 is safer with regard to cardiac function than tricyclic antidepressants (Czekalla et al., 1997).

Although few study participants in clinical trials reported photosensitivity as an adverse effect, photosensitivity has been reported following intravenous administration of hypericin, one of the constituents of St. John's wort. Studies were therefore designed to measure this effect following an oral dose of extract LI 160. In a single-dose trial, 48 volunteers received either six or twelve tablets of LI 160 containing 5.4 or 10.8 mg total hypericins. In a steady-state trial reported in the same publication, 24 volunteers received an initial dose of six tablets (5.4 mg hypericins) and subsequently three tablets per day (2.7 mg hypericins) for seven days. There was no effect from either the single dose or multiple doses on thresholds for producing skin erythema (redness/inflammation) following exposure to ultraviolet light, visible light, or solar-simulated radiation (Schempp et al., 2001). In an earlier study, 50 healthy volunteers were given twice the usual dose of extract, 600 mg three times daily (5.4 mg total hypericins per day), and the minimum dose of UV light required to produce erythema on the skin was measured. At the end of 15 days of administration of the extract, the time required to cause a burn decreased by 21 percent ($p < 0.01$) (Brockmöller et al., 1997). It appears from these studies that photosensitivity is not a major concern following oral administration of the usual dose of 900 mg per day of St. John's wort extract.

DRUG INTERACTIONS

Evidence suggests that St. John's wort preparations can interact with drugs, namely anticoagulants (e.g., phenprocoumon, warfarin), cyclosporin, digoxin, and protease inhibitors used for HIV therapy (e.g., indinavir). Data also suggests that St. John's wort may interact with antidepressants, such as the tricyclic antidepressants (e.g., amitriptyline) and the serotonin reuptake inhibitors (e.g., sertraline, nefazodone, paroxetine). A few cases have been reported of breakthrough bleeding with women on low-dose estrogen oral contraceptives while also taking St. John's wort. The basis for these interactions appears to be stimulation of drug-metabolizing enzymes in the P450 family and possible induction of the P-glycoprotein transport mechanism (Schulz, 2001). St. John's wort preparations do not appear to interact with alcohol or carbamazepine, an anticonvulsant drug used to treat epilepsy (Schmidt et al., 1993; Burstein et al., 2000).

In vitro tests have suggested that the St. John's wort constituent responsible for, at least some of, these drug interactions is hyperforin. A study compared the interactions of LI 160 (high hyperforin content, daily dose 25 to 30 mg in 900 mg extract) with digoxin to the interaction between Ze 117 (very low hyperforin content; daily dose approximately 1 mg in 500 mg extract) and digoxin. The study found that whereas administration of LI 160 decreased digoxin plasma levels, Ze 117 did not (Brattström, 2002). More details of this study are given later.

Anticoagulants

Indication for the interaction between St. John's wort and the anticoagulant phenprocoumon comes from a randomized, placebo-controlled, double-blind, crossover study in which ten healthy subjects were given three (300 mg) tablets per day of LI 160 for 11 days. On the last day, subjects were given a single dose of 12 mg phenprocoumon. After a two-week washout period, the same subjects were given a placebo for 11 days and again a single dose of phenprocoumon. Compared to values with placebo, the plasma concentrations of phenprocoumon (area under the curve, 0 to 72 hours) were significantly lower (17.4 percent) with St. John's wort (Maurer et al., 1999). In addition, there have been seven case reports suggesting that St. John's wort reduces the anticoagulant activity of warfarin, causing a decreased International Normalized Ratio (INR) (Yue, Bergquist, and Gerden, 2000).

Immunosuppressants

Indication for the interaction between St. John's wort and cyclosporine comes from reports of acute rejection in two heart transplant patients who were taking cyclosporine to suppress their immune systems. Previously stable cyclosporine plasma levels were decreased by the addition of St. John's wort. This situation was reversed upon cessation of the herb (Ruschitzka et al., 2000). A similar situation was reported in kidney transplant patients (Breidenbach et al., 2000).

Cardiac Glycosides

The interaction between digoxin and St. John's wort LI 160 extract was investigated in a single-blind, placebo-controlled, parallel study with 25 healthy volunteers. Volunteers received digoxin (0.25 mg/day) for five days, then digoxin with either placebo or 900 mg LI 160 per day for another ten days. As a result, no statistically significant change in plasma digoxin levels was observed after the first dose of LI 160. However, after ten days of treatment, a 25 percent decrease in plasma digoxin levels (24 hours area under the curve) was observed compared to the placebo group. The effect on plasma digoxin levels increased over time with the days of coadministration of LI 160 (Johne et al., 1999).

Another study compared the interaction of LI 160 and digoxin with the interaction between another St. John's wort preparation, Ze 117, and digoxin. Twenty-two volunteers were given digoxin for seven days, and their dose was adjusted to achieve a constant plasma level (1 ng per ml). For the next 14 days the volunteers additionally received placebo, Ze 177 (500 mg per day), or LI 160 (900 mg per day). The doses of St. John's wort preparations were different, but they were consistent with those used in their respective clinical efficacy studies. Digoxin plasma measurements were taken over the 14-day period. The results confirmed the interaction between LI 160 and digoxin: digoxin levels were reduced by 27 percent (24 hours area under the curve) after 14 days coadministration. However, the extract Ze 117 had no such effect. The author of the study concluded that the differences in the activity of the two extract was due to differences in hyperforin concentrations. Ze 117 contains a very low quantity of hyperforin (approximately 1 mg in 500 mg extract) compared to LI

160 (25 to 30 mg in 900 mg extract). The differences in total extract quantities may have also played a role (Brattström, 2002).

HIV Protease Inhibitors

An open-label study with eight volunteers found that St. John's wort decreased the plasma levels (area under the curve, 0 to 5 hours) of the protease inhibitor indinavir by 57 percent. Pharmacokinetic profiles of indinavir were measured before and after 14 days of administration of St. John's wort (300 mg three times daily; HBC Protocols, Inc.) (Piscitelli et al., 2000).

Antidepressants

An interaction between the tricyclic antidepressant amitriptyline and St. John's wort was demonstrated in an open study with 12 depressed patients treated with 150 mg amitriptyline-hydrochloride for 12 days, with or without 12 days of pretreatment with 900 mg LI 160. The plasma level (area under the curve [AUC], 1 to 12 hours) of amitriptyline was reduced by 22 percent, and the AUC of its metabolite, nortriptyline, was reduced by 42 percent (Roots, 1999). There may also be an interaction with other classes of antidepressants. Six cases of serotonergic syndrome have been reported following concomitant ingestion of St. John's wort and serotonin reuptake inhibitors sertraline, nefazodone, and paroxetine (Gordon, 1998; Lantz, Buchalter, and Giambanco, 1999).

Birth Control Tablets

Possible interaction of St. John's wort with oral contraceptives was indicated by reports of breakthrough bleeding in five women taking low-dose estrogen preparations (30 microg ethinyloestradiol) (Ernst, 1999). A study with the extract Ze 117 did not find any effect on plasma levels of the hormones ethinylestradiol or desogestrel. In this study, 16 women took the pill (0.02 mg ethinylestradiol and 0.15 mg desogestrel) daily for at least three months. They were then given 500 mg Ze 117 from day 7 through day 22 of their cycle. No decrease was found in plasma levels of the hormones when day 21 was compared to day seven. No spotting or irregular bleeding was reported, and the levels of the enzyme responsible for metabolizing desogestrel to 3-keto desogestrel, CYP 2C19, was not altered (Brattström, 2002).

Alcohol

A crossover trial, with 32 normal volunteers given 900 mg LI 160 extract or placebo for seven days explored a possible interaction between St. John's wort and alcohol. When the volunteers were given sufficient alcohol to establish blood levels between 0.45 and 0.8 percent, they were subjected to a battery of tests covering cognitive capacities required for operation of machines and for driving. The St. John's wort extract did not have any effect on the action of the alcohol (Schmidt et al., 1993).

Anticonvulsants

St. John's wort does not appear to affect plasma levels of the anticonvulsant drug carbamazepine, which is used to treat epilepsy. In a study of eight healthy men, carbamazepine was administered for 14 days, reaching a steady state with 400 mg once daily. St. John's wort, 300 mg extract (HBC Protocols, Inc.) taken three times daily for 14 days concurrently, did not alter the plasma levels of carbamazepine (Burstein et al., 2000). This finding is somewhat unexpected, since carbamazepine is thought to be primarily metabolized via CYP3A4, a P450 isoenzyme whose activity is thought to be stimulated by St. John's wort (Roby et al., 2000).

INFORMATION FROM PHARMACOPOEIAL MONOGRAPHS

Sources of Published Therapeutic Monographs

American Herbal Pharmacopoeia
European Scientific Cooperative on Phytotherapy
German Commission E
United States Pharmacopeia—Drug Information

Indications

The German Commission E approves the use of dried, aboveground parts of St. John's wort, taken internally, to treat psychovegetative disturbances, depressive moods, anxiety and/or nervous unrest (Blumenthal et al., 1998). The European Scientific Cooperative on Phytotherapy (ESCOP) states that St. John's wort can be used to treat mild to moderate depressive states (ICD-10 categories F32.0 and F32.1) and somatoformic disturbances, including symptoms such as restlessness, anxiety, and irritability (ESCOP, 1996). The *American Herbal Pharmacopoeia (AHP)* states that, in addition to treating mild to moderate depressions, St. John's wort is used for the treatment of several neurological conditions, including anxiety, insomnia due to restlessness, irritability, neuralgia, trigeminal neuralgia, neuroses, migraine headaches, fibrositis, and sciatica (Upton et al., 1997). According to the *United States Pharmacopeia—Drug Information (USP-DI)* botanical monograph series, St. John's wort extract has been used to treat mild to moderate depression (*USP-DI*, 1998).

Both the Commission E and the *AHP* suggest that oily hypericum preparations be used internally for dyspeptic complaints and externally for treatment and posttherapy of acute and contused injuries, myalgia, and first-degree burns (Blumenthal et al., 1998; Upton et al., 1997).

Other uses listed by the *AHP* include to treat pain and inflammation of nerve origin (painful tooth socket following tooth extraction; shingles; herpes communis; chronic neuralgia stemming from fractures, spinal injuries, musculoskeletal trauma, and surgical trauma; nerve injury resulting in lancinating, burning, or tingling pains; and twitching or spasm following a traumatic injury), gastric conditions (ulcer and functional gastritis, nervous dyspepsia, inflammatory bowel syndrome, and internal hemorrhoids), enuresis due to nervous anxiety or nerve irritation in the bladder, and as an antiviral agent (Upton et al., 1997).

Doses

Preparations containing: 0.2 to 1 mg of total hypericin daily (Blumenthal et al., 1998; ESCOP, 1996); 0.5 to 3 mg total hypericin daily (Upton et al., 1997)

Dried aboveground parts: 2 to 4 g daily (Blumenthal et al., 1998; ESCOP, 1996; Upton et al., 1997).
Infusion: 1 to 2 cups twice daily corresponding to 2 to 4 g herb (Upton et al., 1997; ESCOP, 1996)
Tincture: (1:5) 2 to 4 ml three times daily (Upton et al., 1997); equivalent to 0.2 to 1 mg total hypericin daily (ESCOP, 1996)
Extract: fluid extracts, aqueous alcoholic extracts, equivalent to 0.2 to 1 mg total hypericin daily (ESCOP, 1996)
Oil: (gastric complaints) 1 tsp on an empty stomach morning and evening (Upton et al., 1997)

Treatment Period

ESCOP states there is usually no treatment length restriction. However, an antidepressant effect is not expected before 10 to 14 days of treatment, and if no response is apparent after four to six weeks, treatment should be discontinued (ESCOP, 1996).

Contraindications

The Commission E and ESCOP list no known contraindications for St. John's wort (Blumenthal et al., 1998; ESCOP, 1996). The *USP-DI* suggests that using St. John's wort to treat suicidal and psychotic patients may be inappropriate (*USP-DI, 1998*).

Adverse Reactions

The Commission E states that photosensitization is possible, especially in fair-skinned individuals (Blumenthal et al., 1998). ESCOP adds that photosensitization may occur at higher dosages (ESCOP, 1996). The *USP-DI* states that the following adverse reactions have been reported: phototoxicity, gastrointestinal symptoms, allergic reaction, dizziness, constipation, dry mouth, restlessness, sleep disturbances, and fatigue (*USP-DI, 1998*).

Precautions

The AHP recommends that care should be taken when using external preparations in conjunction with therapies utilizing ultrasound or ultraviolet light. St. John's wort should also be used with caution in pregnancy (Upton et al., 1997). The *USP-DI* states that the use of St. John's wort is not recommended for children and pregnant or breast-feeding women, and that individuals at risk of phototoxic reactions should use caution when exposed to the sun (*USP-DI,* 1998).

Drug Interactions

The Commission E and ESCOP list no known drug interactions (Blumenthal et al., 1998; ESCOP, 1996). The *USP-DI* warns that although no interactions have been reported, St. John's wort may interact with selective serotonin reuptake inhibitors and monoamine oxidase (MAO) inhibitors (*USP-DI,* 1998).

REFERENCES

American Psychiatric Association (1994). *Diagnostic and Statistical Manual of Mental Disorders,* Fourth Edition. Washington, DC: American Psychiatric Association.

Blumenthal M, Busse W, Hall T, Goldberg A, Grümwald J, Riggins C, Rister S, eds. (1998). *The Complete German Commission E Monographs: Therapeutic Guide to Herbal Medicines.* Trans. S Klein. Austin: American Botanical Council.

Brattström A (2002). Der johanniskrautextrakt Ze 117 (Saint John's wort extract Ze 117). *Deutsche Apothekar Zeitung* 142 (30): 97-101.

Breidenbach T, Kliem V, Burg M, Radermacher J, Hoffmann MW, Klempnauer J (2000). Profound drop of cyclosporin A whole blood trough levels caused by St. John's wort *(Hypericum perforatum). Transplantation* 69 (10): 2229-2230.

Brenner R, Azbel V, Madhusoodanan S, Pawlowska M (2000). Comparison of an extract of *Hypericum* (LI 160) and sertraline in the treatment of depression: A double-blind, randomized pilot study. *Clinical Therapeutics* 22 (4): 411-419.

Brockmöller J, Reum T, Bauer S, Kerb R, Hübner WD, Roots I (1997). Hypericin and pseudohypericin: Pharmacokinetics and effects on photosensitivity in humans. *Pharmacopsychiatry* 30 (Suppl. 2): 94-101.

Burstein AH, Horton RL, Dunn T, Alfaro RM, Piscitelli SC, Theodore W (2000). Lack of effect of St. John's wort on carbamazepine pharmacokinetics in healthy volunteers. *Clinical Pharmacology and Therapeutics* 68 (6): 605-612.

Czekalla J, Gastpar M, Hübner WD, Jager D (1997). The effect of hypericum extract on cardiac conduction as seen in the electrocardiogram compared to that of imipramine. *Pharmacopsychiatry* 30 (Suppl. 2): 86-88.

Ernst E (1999). Second thoughts about safety of St. John's wort. *The Lancet* 354 (9195): 2014-2015.

European Scientific Cooperative on Phytotherapy (ESCOP) (1996). Hyperici Herba: St. John's Wort. In *Monographs on the Medicinal Uses of Plant Drugs* (Fascicle 1: p. 10). Exeter, UK: European Scientific Cooperative on Phytotherapy.

Franklin M, Chi J, McGavin C, Hockney R, Reed A, Campling G, Whale RWR, Cowen PJ (1999). Neuroendocrine evidence for dopaminergic actions of *Hypericum* extract (LI 160) in healthy volunteers. *Biological Psychiatry* 46 (4): 581-584.

Gordon J (1998). SSRIs and St. John's wort: Possible toxicity? *American Family Physician* 57 (5): 950- 953.

Hänsgen KD, Vesper J (1996). Antidepressant efficacy of a high-dose extract of St. John's wort. *Münchener Medizinische Wochenschrift* 138 (3): 35-39.

Hänsgen K, Vesper J, Ploch M (1994). Multicenter double-blind study examining the antidepressant effectiveness of the *Hypericum* extract LI 160. *Journal of Geriatric Psychiatry and Neurology* 7 (Suppl. 1): S15-S18. (Also published in Hänsgen K, Vesper J, Ploch M [1993] Multizentrische doppelblindstudie zur antidepressiven wirchsamkeit des *Hypericum*-extraktes LI 160. *Nervenheilkunde* 12: 285-289.)

Harrer G, Hübner W, Podzuweit H (1994). Effectiveness and tolerance of the hypericum extract LI 160 compared to maprotiline: A multicenter double-blind study. *Journal of Geriatric Psychiatry and Neurology* 7 (Suppl. 1): S24-S28. (Also published in Harrer G, Hübner W, Podzuweit H [1993]. Wirsamkeit und verträglichkeit des *Hypericum*-präparates LI 160 im vergleich mit Maprotilin. *Nervenheilkunde* 12: 297-301.)

Harrer G, Schmidt U, Kuhn U, Biller A (1999). Comparison of equivalence between the St. John's wort extract LoHyp-57 and fluoxetine. *Arzneimittel-Forschung/Drug Research* 49 (4): 289-296.

Hübner WD, Kirste T (2001). Experience with St. John's wort *(Hypericum perforatum)* in children under 12 years with symptoms of depression and psychovegetative disturbances. *Phytotherapy Research* 15 (4): 367-370.

Hübner W, Lande S, Podzuweit H (1994). *Hypericum* treatment of mild depressions with somatic symptoms. *Journal of Geriatric Psychiatry and Neurology* 7 (Suppl. 1): S12-S14. (Also published in Hübner W, Lande S, Podzuweit H [1993]. Behandlung larvierter depressionen mit Johanniskraut. *Nervenkeilkunde* 12: 278-280.)

Hypericum Depression Trial Study Group (2002). Effect of *Hypericum perforatum* (St. John's Wort) in major depressive disorder: A randomized controlled trial. *Journal of the American Medical Association* 287 (14): 1807-1814.

Johne A, Brockmoller J, Bauer S, Maurer A, Langheinrich M, Roots I (1999). Pharmacokinetic interaction of digoxin with an herbal extract from St. John's wort *(Hypericum perforatum)*. *Clinical Pharmacology and Therapeutics* 66 (4): 338-345.

Johnson D, Ksciuk H, Woelk H, Sauerwein-Giese E, Frauendorf A (1994). Effects of *Hypericum* extract LI 160 compared with maprotiline on resting EEG and evoked potentials in 24 volunteers. *Journal of Geriatric Psychiatry and Neurology* 7 (Suppl. 1): S44-S46. (Also published in Johnson D, Ksciuk H, Woelk H, Sauerwein-Giese E, Frauendorf A [1993]. Wirkungen von Johanniskraut-extrakt LI 160 im vergleich Maprolitin auf Ruhe-EEG und evozierte potentiale bei 24 probanden. *Nervenheilkunde* 12: 328-330.)

Kalb R, Trautmann-Sponsel RD, Kieser M (2001). Efficacy and tolerability of hypericum extract WS 5572 versus placebo in mildly to moderately depressed patients: A randomized, double-blind, multicenter clinical trial. *Pharmacopsychiatry* 34 (3): 96-103.

Kim HL, Streltzer J, Goebert D (1999). St. John's Wort for depression: A meta-analysis of well-defined clinical trials. *The Journal of Nervous and Mental Disease* 187 (9): 532-539.

Laakmann G, Schüle C, Baghai T, Kieser M (1998). St. John's wort in mild to moderate depression: The relevance of hyperforin for the clinical efficacy. *Pharmacopsychiatry* 31 (Suppl. 1): 54-59. (Also published in Laakmann G, Dienel A, Kieser M [1998]. Clinical significance of hyperforin for the efficacy of *Hyperium* extracts on depressive disorders of different severities. *Phytomedicine* 5 [6]: 435-442.)

Lantz MS, Buchalter E, Giambanco V (1999). St. John's wort and antidepressant drug interactions in the elderly. *Journal of Geriatric Psychiatry and Neurology* 12 (1): 7-10.

Lecrubier Y, Clerc G, Didi R, Kieser M (2002). Efficacy of St. John's wort extract WS 5570 in major depression: A double-blind, placebo-controlled trial. *The American Journal of Psychiatry* 159 (8): 1361-1366.

Lehrl S, Willemsen A, Papp R, Woelk H (1993). Results of measurements of the cognitive capacity in patients treated with hypericum extract. *Nervenheilkunde* 12: 281-284.

Lemmer W, von den Driesch V, Klieser E (1999). Johanniskraut Spezialextract WS 5572 bei leichen bis mittelschwerer depression. *Fortschritte der Medizin* 117 (3): 143-154. Cited in Rychlik R, Siedentop H, von den Driesch V, Kasper S (2001). St. John's wort extract WS 5572 in mild to moderate depression: Efficacy and tolerability of 600 and 1200 mg active ingredient/day. *Fortschritte der Medizin* 119 (3/4): 119-128.

Lenoir S, Degenring FH, Saller R (1997). Hyperiforce tablets for the treatment of mild to moderate depression. *Schweizerische Zeitschrift für Ganzheits Medizin* 9 (5): 226-232.

Linde K, Ramirez G, Mulrow C, Pauls A, Weidenhammer W, Melchart D (1996). St. John's wort for depression—An overview and meta-analysis of randomized clinical trials. *British Medical Journal* 313 (7052): 253-257.

Maurer A, Johne A, Bauer S, Brockmoller J, Donath F, Roots I, Langheinrich M, Hübner WD (1999). Interaction of St. John's wort extract with phenprocoumon. In Abstracts of the First Joint Meeting of the German Clinical Pharmacologists. *European Journal of Clinical Pharmacology* June 10-12: A22 (abstract 79).

Philipp M, Kohnen R, Hiller KO (1999). *Hypericum* extract versus imipramine or placebo in patients with moderate depression: Randomised multicenter study of treatment for eight weeks. *British Medical Journal* 319 (7224): 1534-1538.

Piscitelli SC, Burstein AH, Chaitt D, Alfaro RM, Falloon J (2000). Indinavir concentrations and St. John's wort. *The Lancet* 355 (9203): 547-548.

Reh C, Laux P, Schenk N (1992). *Hypericum* extract in depressions—An effective alternative. *Therapiewoche* 42: 1576-1581.

Roby CA, Anderson GD, Kantor E, Dryer DA, Burstein AH (2000). St. John's wort: Effect on CYP3A4 activity. *Clinical Pharmacology and Therapeutics* 67 (5): 451-457.

Roots I (1999). Drug interactions with St. John's Wort: Expert report for the BfArM. *Federal Institute for Drugs and Medical Devices,* Germany, January 12.

Ruschitzka F, Meier PJ, Turina M, Luscher TF, Noll G (2000). Acute heart transplant rejection due to Saint John's wort. *The Lancet* 355 (9203): 548-549.

Rychlik R, Siedentop H, von den Driesch V, Kasper S (2001). St. John's wort extract WS 5572 in mild to moderate depression: Efficacy and tolerability of 600 and 1200 mg active ingredient/day. *Fortschritte der Medizin* 119 (3/4): 119-128.

Schellenberg R, Sauer S, Dimpfel W (1998). Pharmacodynamic effects of two different hypericum extracts in healthy volunteers measured by quantitative EEG. *Pharmacopsychiatry* 31 (Suppl. 1): 44-53.

Schempp CM, Müller K, Winghofer B, Schulte-Mönting J, Simon JC (2001). Single-dose and steady-state administration of *Hypericum perforatum* extract (St. John's wort) does not influence skin sensitivity to UV radiation, visible light, and solar simulated radiation. *Archives of Dermatology* 137 (4): 512-513.

Schmidt U, Harrer G, Kuhn U, Berger-Deinert W, Luther D (1993). Interaction of *Hypericum* extract with alcohol. *Nervenheilkunde* 6: 314-319.

Schmidt U, Sommer H (1993). Extract of St. John's Wort in the outpatient therapy of depressions with unimpaired attention and reaction faculties. *Fortschritte der Medizin* 111 (19): 339-342.

Schrader E (2000). Equivalence of St. John's wort extract (Ze 117) and fluoxetine: A randomized, controlled study in mild-moderate depression. *International Clinical Psychopharmacology* 15 (2): 61-68.

Schrader E, Meier B, Brattström A (1998). *Hypericum* treatment of mild-moderate depression in a placebo-controlled study: A prospective, double-blind, randomized, placebo-controlled, multicenter study. *Human Psychopharmacology* 13 (3): 163-169.

Schüle C, Baghai T, Ferrera A, Laakmann G (2001). Neuroendocrine effects of *Hypericum* extract WS 5570 in 12 healthy male volunteers. *Pharmacopsychiatry* 34 (Suppl. 1): S127-S133.

Schulz H, Jobert M (1994). Effects of *Hypericum* extract on the sleep EEG in older volunteers. *Journal of Geriatric Psychiatry and Neurology* 7 (Suppl. 1): S39-S43. (Published previously in Schulz H, Jobert M [1993]. Der einfluss von Johanniskrautextrakt auf das schlaf-EEG bei älteren probandinen. *Nervenkeilkunde* 12: 323-327).

Schulz V (2001). Incidence and clinical relevance of the interactions and side effects of *Hypericum* preparations. *Phytomedicine* 8 (2): 152-160.

Schulz V, Hänsel R, Tyler VE (2001). *Rational Phytotherapy: A Physicians' Guide to Herbal Medicine,* Fourth Edition. Trans. TC Telgar. Berlin: Springer-Verlag.

Shelton RC, Keller MB, Gelenberg A, Dunner DL, Hirschfeld R, Thase ME, Russell J, Lydiard RB, Crits-Cristoph P, Gallop R, et al. (2001). Effectiveness of St. John's wort in major depression: A randomized trial. *Journal of the American Medical Association* 285 (15): 1978-1986.

Sommer H, Harrer G (1994). Placebo-controlled double-blind study examining the effectiveness of an *Hypericum* preparation in 105 mildly depressed patients. *Journal of Geriatric Psychiatry and Neurology* 7 (Suppl. 1): S9-S11.

Thase ME (1999). How should efficacy be evaluated in randomized clinical trials of treatments for depression? *Journal of Clinical Psychiatry* 60 (Suppl. 4): 23-31.

United States Pharmacopeia-Drug Information (USP-DI) (1998). Botanical Monograph Series: *Hypericum* (St. John's Wort). Rockville, MD: The United States Pharmacopeial Convention, Inc.

Upton R, Graff A, Williamson E, Bunting D, Gatherum DM, Walker EB, Butterweck V, Liefländer-Wulf U, Nahrstedt A, Wall A, et al. (1997). *St. John's Wort,* Hypericum perforatum. *Quality Control, Analytical and Therapeutic Monograph. American Herbal Pharmacopoeia and Therapeutic Compendium.* Ed. R Upton. Santa Cruz: American Herbal Pharmacopoeia.

Vorbach EU, Arnoldt KH, Hübner WD (1997). Efficacy and tolerability of St. John's wort extract LI 160 versus imipramine in patients with severe depressive episodes according to ICD-10. *Pharmacopsychiatry* 30 (Suppl. 2): 81-85.

Vorbach EU, Hübner WD, Arnoldt KH (1994). Effectiveness and tolerance of the hypericum extract LI 160 in comparison with imipramine: Randomized double-blind study with 135 outpatients. *Journal of Geriatric Psychiatry and Neurology* 7 (Suppl. 1): S19-S-23. (Also published in Vorbach EU, Hübner WD, Arnoldt KH [1993]. Wirksamkeit und verträglichkeit des *Hypericum*-extraktes LI 160 im vergleich mit imipramin: Randomisierte doppleblindstudie mit 135 ambulanten patienten. *Nervenkeilkunde* 12: 290-296.)

Wheatley D (1997). LI 160, an extract of St. John's wort, versus amitriptyline in mildly to moderate depressed outpatients—A controlled 6-week clinical trial. *Pharmacopsychiatry* 30 (Suppl. 2): S77-S80.

Whiskey E, Werneke U, Taylor D (2001). A systematic review and meta-analysis of *Hypericum perforatum* in depression: A comprehensive clinical review. *International Clinical Psychopharmacology* 16 (5): 239-252.

Woelk H (2000). Comparison of St. John's wort and imipramine for treating depression: Randomised controlled trial. *British Medical Journal* 321 (7260): 536-539.

Woelk H, Burkard G, Grunwald J (1994). Benefits and risks of the *Hypericum* extract LI 160: Drug monitoring study with 3,250 patients. *Journal of Geriatric Psychiatry and Neurology* 7 (Suppl. 1): S34-S38.

Woelk H, Johnson D, Frauendorf A, Ksciuk H, Sauerwein-Geisse E (1996). Study to evaluate the effects of Neuroplant forte (extr. *Hypericum perforatum* L., St. John's wort) compared to trimipramine on cerebral activity in depressed patients. Internal report.

World Health Organization (WHO) (1992). *International Statistical Classification of Diseases and Related Health Problems,* Tenth Revision. Geneva: World Health Organization.

Yue QY, Bergquist C, Gerden B (2000). Safety of St. John's wort *(Hypericum perforatum). The Lancet* 355 (9203): 576-577.

DETAILS ON ST. JOHN'S WORT PRODUCTS AND CLINICAL STUDIES

Product and clinical study information is grouped in the same order as in the Summary Table. A profile on an individual product is followed by details of the clinical studies associated with that product. In some instances, a clinical study, or studies, supports several products that contain the same principal ingredient(s). In these instances, those products are grouped together.

Clinical studies that follow each product, or group of products, are grouped by therapeutic indication, in accordance with the order in the Summary Table.

Index to St. John's Wort Products

Product Profile: Kira®

Manufacturer	**Lichtwer Pharma AG, Germany (Indena S.p.A., Italy)**
U.S. distributor	**Lichtwer Pharma U.S., Inc.**
Botanical ingredient	**St. John's wort flower and leaf extract**
Extract name	**LI 160 (St. John Select™)**
Quantity	300 mg
Processing	Plant to extract ratio 4-7:1; aqueous methanolic extract
Standardization	0.24-0.32% total hypericin
Formulation	Tablet

Recommended dose: Take one tablet three times daily with water at mealtimes. Results observed after two to four weeks of usage. Kira's safety profile also supports longer-term use.

DSHEA structure/function: Maintain a healthy emotional balance. Supports emotional well-being. Supports a healthy balance among the brain's chemical messengers to promote a feeling of well-being.

Cautions: If you are pregnant, nursing a baby, or giving to children under age of 12, consult a healthcare professional before using this product. Recent data suggest that if you are taking any drug product, and in particular a blood-thinner or anti-organ rejection medicine, you should consult with your health care professional to avoid any interactions with St. John's Wort. St. John's Wort, and certain other food/herbal products, may affect Cytochrome P-450 enzyme activity within the body, a normal metabolic pathway that is also affected by certain drug products. When taking this product, use caution in exposure to excessive sunlight.

Other ingredients: Lactose, powdered cellulose, hydroxypropyl methylcellulose, silicon dioxide, titanium dioxide (mineral based whitening pigment), magnesium stearate, talc (natural tableting aid), triethyl citrate, vanillin.

Comments: Sold as Jarsin® 300 in Europe.

Source(s) of information: Product package; Kira product information (www.lichtwer.com/kira/kira_prod_info.html); Jarsin® 300 product information, Lichtwer Pharma GmbH, 1996; information provided by Indena USA.

Product Profile: St. John's Wort Extract

Manufacturer	**Enzymatic Therapy (Indena S.p.A., Italy)**
U.S. distributor	**Enzymatic Therapy**
Botanical ingredient	**St. John's wort aerial parts extract**
Extract name	**St. John Select™**
Quantity	300 mg
Processing	Plant to extract ratio 3-4:1, aqueous methanolic extract
Standardization	A minimum of 0.3% hypericin and 3% hyperforin
Formulation	Capsule

Recommended dose: One capsule three times daily.

DSHEA structure/function: Dietary supplement to promote mental well-being.

Cautions: Due to the St. John's wort extract, in extremely rare cases light-skinned people may experience a sensitivity to excessive sun exposure. If taking a prescription drug, consult a physician prior to use.

Other ingredients: Gelatin, magnesium stearate, silicon dioxide, titanium dioxide.

Source(s) of information: Product label; information provided by Indena USA, Inc.

Product Profile: Hypericum Perforatum II

Manufacturer	**HBC Protocols, Inc. (Indena S.p.A., Italy)**
U.S. distributor	**HBC Protocols, Inc.**
Botanical ingredient	**St. John's wort flowering tops extract**
Extract name	**St. John Select™**
Quantity	300 mg
Processing	Plant/extract ratio 3-4:1, aqueous methanolic extract
Standardization	0.3% hypericin and 4% hyperforin
Botanical ingredient	**Grape seed extract**
Extract name	**LeucoSelect®**
Quantity	1 mg
Processing	Plant/extract ratio 100:1
Standardization	95% polyphenols (80-85% oligomeric proanthocyanidins)
Formulation	Tablet

Recommended dose: Take one tablet three times daily.

DSHEA structure/function: Promotes a balanced emotional outlook.

Cautions: Not to be used by people taking MAO inhibitors. May cause hypersensitivity to sunlight. Not to be taken by pregnant women. Talk to your doctor if you are on prescription medication.

Other ingredients: Calcium phosphate dibasic, microcrystalline cellulose, vegetable oil, croscarmelose sodium, magnesium stearate, silicon dioxide.

Source(s) of information: Product label; information provided by Indena USA, Inc.

Product Profile: Hyper-Ex®

Manufacturer	**Thorne Research (Indena S.p.A., Italy)**
U.S. distributor	**Thorne Research**
Botanical ingredient	**St. John's wort flower extract**
Extract name	**St. John Select™**
Quantity	300 mg
Processing	Plant to extract ratio 3-4:1, aqueous methanolic extract
Standardization	0.3% hypericin
Formulation	Capsule

Cautions: If pregnant, consult your health care practitioner before using this, or any other product.

Other ingredients: Cellulose capsule.

Comments: This product is available only through pharmacies and health care practitioners.

Source(s) of information: Product label; information from Indena USA, Inc.

Clinical Study: Jarsin® 300

Extract name	LI 160
Manufacturer	Lichtwer Pharma AG, Germany
Indication	**Depression**
Level of evidence	**I**
Therapeutic benefit	**Yes**

Bibliographic reference
Hänsgen KD, Vesper J (1996). Antidepressant efficacy of a high-dose extract of St. John's wort. *Münchener Medizinische Wochenschrift* 138 (3): 35-39.

Trial design
Parallel. Patients received either *Hypericum* extract or placebo for four weeks, then both groups received LI 160 for the last two weeks of the trial. All patients were informed that they would receive the active treatment for at least two weeks.

Study duration	1 month
Dose	3 (300 mg) tablets daily
Route of administration	Oral
Randomized	Yes
Randomization adequate	Yes
Blinding	Double-blind
Blinding adequate	Yes
Placebo	Yes
Drug comparison	No
Site description	17 practices (neurology and psychiatry)
No. of subjects enrolled	108
No. of subjects completed	101
Sex	Male and female
Age	18-70 years (mean: 52)

Inclusion criteria
Outpatients of specialist neurology and psychiatry clinics with mild to moderate major depression as defined in the DSM-III-R; a total score of 16 or more on the Hamilton Depression Scale (HAM-D); and patients who had suffered from their current depression for between two weeks and six months. Psychoactive medication was discontinued at least a week prior to the start of the study.

Exclusion criteria
Patients who had psychotic features or severe systemic diseases, patients who were dependent on alcohol, medication, or drugs of abuse, and patients who were at risk of suicide.

End points
Efficacy was assessed by the HAM-D, the von Zerssen Depression Scale (D-S), the Kasielke and Hänsgen Symptom Rating Scale (BEB), and the Clinical Global Impressions scale (CGI). Response to the HAM-D scale was defined as a total score of less than 10 or a reduction in score by at least 50 percent. Patients were assessed at baseline and at two, four, and six weeks.

Results
In the first four weeks, the response rate on the HAM-D was 70 percent in

the LI 160 group and 24 percent for the placebo group. Scores fell from 21.0 to 8.9 for the LI 160 group and from 20.4 to 14.4 for the placebo group. Differences were highly significant ($p < 0.001$) after both two and four weeks. Scores on the D-S fell from 21.2 to 9.3 for the *Hypericum* group—levels within the range for normal healthy subjects. In the placebo group, mean scores decreased from 19.6 to 14.6. Again, differences were highly significant ($p < 0.001$) after both two and four weeks. Differences between the two groups on the BEB were also significant ($p < 0.01$) after two and four weeks, with marked improvements in the *Hypericum* group in general well-being, cardiovascular symptoms, and anxiety/phobia symptoms. When both groups were given the active treatment, the scores in the original *Hypericum* group fell to 6.3 on the D-S scale, whereas the score reduction in the original placebo group was very similar to that obtained in the active treatment group during the first two weeks of treatment.

Side effects
One patient in the *Hypericum* group reported mild sleep disturbances.

Authors' comments
Over the first four weeks of the study, the changes detected by the self-rating methods were judged to be consistent with the changes detected with the observer-rating method. The degree of improvement was unequivocally greater than that which could be expected from spontaneous remission or statistical regression. St. John's wort extract LI 160 markedly reduces depressive symptoms in mild to moderate depression. In view of its efficacy and lack, or virtual lack, of side effects, it can be recommended as the antidepressant of choice, especially for outpatients.

Reviewers' comments
This is a good, well-designed, and well-conducted study. A minor flaw was the short washout period for pretreatment medications. Also, the authors did not state who administered HAM-D scales and whether a coexisting treatment was allowed. (5, 6)

Clinical Study: Jarsin® 300

Extract name	LI 160
Manufacturer	Lichtwer Pharma AG, Germany
Indication	**Depression**
Level of evidence	I
Therapeutic benefit	**Yes**

Bibliographic reference
Hänsgen K, Vesper J, Ploch M (1994). Multicenter double-blind study examining the antidepressant effectiveness of the *Hypericum* extract LI 160. *Journal of Geriatric Psychiatry and Neurology* 7 (Suppl. 1): S15-S18. (Also published in Hänsgen K, Vesper J, Ploch M [1993]. Multizentrische doppelblindstudie zur antidepressiven wirchsamkeit des *Hypericum*-extraktes LI 160. *Nervenheilkunde* 12: 285-289.)

Trial design
Parallel. During the first four weeks of the trial, patients received either LI 160 or placebo. During the last two weeks of the study, all patients received LI 160. All patients were informed that every participant in the study would receive the active treatment for at least two weeks during the course of the study, but were not told which weeks.

Study duration	1 month
Dose	3 (300 mg) tablets daily
Route of administration	Oral
Randomized	Yes
Randomization adequate	Yes
Blinding	Double-blind
Blinding adequate	Yes
Placebo	Yes
Drug comparison	No
Site description	11 practices (neurology, psychiatry, and general)
No. of subjects enrolled	72
No. of subjects completed	67
Sex	Male and female
Age	18-70 years (mean: 53)

Inclusion criteria
Ages 18 to 70 years with major depression according to the DSM-III-R, Hamilton Depression Scale (HAM-D) > 15, duration of depressive episode for a minimum of two weeks and a maximum of six months.

Exclusion criteria
Psychotic episodes, suicide risk, severe mental illness, drug use, or pregnancy.

End points
Efficacy and safety were monitored by the HAM-D, depression scale of Von Zerssen (D-S), complaint inventory (BEB), and by the Clinical Global Im-

pressions Scale (CGI). Patients were monitored at baseline and during treatment at weeks 2, 4, and 6.

Results

HAM-D fell from 21.8 to 9.2 after four weeks for the LI 160 group, and from 20.4 to 14.7 for the placebo group. There was a significant difference from placebo after two and four weeks ($p < 0.001$). Levels further declined at the six-week end point, particularly in the original placebo group, which was now taking *Hypericum* extract. D-S registered the treatment group within the normal range after four weeks, with a significant difference from placebo ($p < 0.001$). The level of symptoms according to the BEB fell significantly more in the LI 160 group than in the placebo group ($p = 0.01$). The CGI scale showed the severity of illness much reduced after four weeks of treatment with *Hypericum* compared with placebo. The CGI also showed a noticeable improvement in the placebo group in the last two weeks after switching to LI 160.

Side effects

One subject in treatment group reported a sleep disturbance.

Authors' comments

Because of its potent and specific efficacy with few or no side effects, *Hypericum* extract LI 160 can be recommended as an antidepressant for treatment of depressed outpatients.

Reviewers' comments

This was a multisite and multidiscipline (neurology, psychiatry, and general practices) study, but the trial report did not describe who and how many subjects were recruited from each site and whether the observer was trained to administer the scales used. (5, 6)

Clinical Study: Jarsin® 300

Extract name	LI 160
Manufacturer	Lichtwer Pharma AG, Germany
Indication	**Depression**
Level of evidence	**II**
Therapeutic benefit	**Yes**

Bibliographic reference

Sommer H, Harrer G (1994). Placebo-controlled double-blind study examining the effectiveness of an *Hypericum* preparation in 105 mildly depressed patients. *Journal of Geriatric Psychiatry and Neurology* 7 (Suppl. 1): S9-S11.

Trial design
Parallel.

Study duration	1 month
Dose	3 (300 mg) tablets daily
Route of administration	Oral
Randomized	Yes
Randomization adequate	Yes
Blinding	Double-blind
Blinding adequate	No
Placebo	Yes
Drug comparison	No
Site description	3 medical practices
No. of subjects enrolled	105
No. of subjects completed	89
Sex	Male and female
Age	24-68 years (mean: 45)

Inclusion criteria
Depressive symptoms according to ICD-9: 300.4 (neurotic depression) and 309.0 (brief depressive reaction).

Exclusion criteria
Severe renal or hepatic dysfunction; heart failure; Parkinson's disease; endocrine or CNS tumors; alcohol, drug, or medication dependency; pregnancy, breast feeding, and inadequate contraceptive measures. Any prior treatment with psychoactive drugs must have been discontinued for at least four weeks.

End points
Patients were evaluated at baseline and at two and four weeks. Depressive symptoms were estimated using the Hamilton Depression Scale (HAM-D). Responders were those whose total score fell to a value below 10 or by at least 50 percent of the baseline value.

Results
The values of the mean basic HAM-D scores fell from 15.8 to 9.6 and 7.2 after two and four weeks, respectively, in the hypericum group. In the placebo group, scores fell from 15.8 to 12.3 and 11.3 after two and four weeks, respectively. The differences between the groups were statistically significant

at two weeks, increasing after four weeks ($p < 0.05$ and $p < 0.01$, respectively). Clinical improvement was noted in depressive mood, difficulty initiating sleep, and psychological anxiety. At the end of four weeks, according to the HAM-D, 67 percent of the *Hypericum* group could be classified as responders, compared to 28 percent receiving placebo.

Side effects
Two patients in the *Hypericum* group experienced skin reddening, itching, and tiredness.

Authors' comments
Hypericum preparations have therapeutic effects that are very similar to those of traditional antidepressants, but they are not burdened with side effects. *Hypericum* is, therefore, a low-risk antidepressant for treatment of mild and moderate depression.

Reviewers' comments
This trial is greatly limited by its poor statistics. The report did not clarify how many men and women were in the sample, and no standard deviations or indication of variability (range) were given. It is unclear why the authors used nonparametric tests. They also did not use intent-to-treat analysis. (3, 3)

Clinical Study: Jarsin 300®

Extract name	LI 160
Manufacturer	Lichtwer Pharma AG, Germany
Indication	**Depression**
Level of evidence	**III**
Therapeutic benefit	**Yes**

Bibliographic reference
Hübner W, Lande S, Podzuweit H (1994). *Hypericum* treatment of mild depressions with somatic symptoms. *Journal of Geriatric Psychiatry and Neurology* 7 (Suppl. 1): S12-S14. (Also published in Hübner W, Lande S, Podzuweit H [1993]. Behandlung larvierter depressionen mit Johanniskraut. *Nervenkeilkunde* 12: 278-280.)

Trial design
Parallel. Pretrial washout period of two weeks.

Study duration	1 month
Dose	3 (300 mg) tablets daily

Route of administration   Oral

Randomized   Yes
Randomization adequate   Yes
Blinding   Double-blind
Blinding adequate   Yes

Placebo   Yes
Drug comparison   No

Site description   1 internal medicine practice

No. of subjects enrolled   40
No. of subjects completed   39
Sex   Male and female
Age   20-64 years (mean: 51)

Inclusion criteria

Neurotic depression (300.4) and temporary depressive neurosis (309.0) according to the ICD-9.

Exclusion criteria

No other neurotic or psychiatric illness, and no other psychiatric substances two weeks prior to trial.

End points

Outcome was measured by the Hamilton Depression Scale (HAM-D), the von Zerssen Health Complaint Survey (B-L), the Clinical Global Impressions (CGI), and questions on typical somatic symptoms. Patients were examined at baseline and at the end of weeks 2 and 4. Baseline values on the HAM-D tests were compared to final scores. The responder rate (decrease of 50 percent or below 10 points on final HAM-D) was calculated and compared for the two treatment groups.

Results

Treatment and placebo groups began with a HAM-D score of 12.55 ± 1.28 and 12.37 ± 1.34, respectively. The *Hypericum* group showed a responder rate of 70 percent, compared to 47 percent for the placebo group. (Actual HAM-D scores were displayed in a graph and not given numerically.) A significant difference of 5 percent was observed between the two groups at the end of four weeks ($p < 0.05$). The CGI scale showed change in condition as "very much better" in nine of the *Hypericum* patients and "unchanged" or "slightly worse" in another seven. In the placebo group, four cases were "very much better," whereas 14 were "unchanged" or "slightly/very much worse."

Side effects
None reported by patients.

Authors' comments
The results of the present study show that these patients benefited from taking the investigational product in contrast to placebo. Because of good tolerability, and thus high compliance, LI 160 may be helpful for patients with masked depressions.

Reviewers' comments
The authors did not state exclusion/inclusion criteria clearly, and the sample size was very small. The clinical generalizability of the results is therefore unclear. The authors also used the ICD-9, an outdated reference, to rate patients' depression. They did not state clearly who administered the instruments and whether they were trained. Also, the washout period for previous medication was short. (5, 3)

Clinical Study: Jarsin®

Extract name	LI 160
Manufacturer	Lichtwer Pharma AG, Germany
Indication	**Depression**
Level of evidence	**III**
Therapeutic benefit	**Undetermined**

Bibliographic reference
Schmidt U, Sommer H (1993). Extract of St. John's Wort in the outpatient therapy of depressions with unimpaired attention and reaction faculties. *Fortschritte der Medizin* 111 (19): 339-342.

Trial design
Parallel.

Study duration	6 weeks
Dose	300 mg 3 times daily
Route of administration	Oral
Randomized	Yes
Randomization adequate	No
Blinding	Double-blind
Blinding adequate	Yes
Placebo	Yes

Drug comparison	No
Site description	Multicenter
No. of subjects enrolled	65
No. of subjects completed	60
Sex	Male and female
Age	24-68 years

Inclusion criteria

Mild to moderately severe depression; outpatients; a short-duration depressive condition classified by the ICD-9: neurotic depression; total score on the Hamilton Depression Scale (HAM-D) between 16 and 20 points; no medical treatment within two weeks of study; possession of a valid driver's license for at least four years; and several years experience in driving a motor vehicle

Exclusion criteria

Depression resulting from organic causes; HAM-D over 20, indicating severe depression; chronic depressive clinical pictures; attempted suicide; accompanying medical treatment with verified cognitative influences; and abuse of narcotics, alcohol, or medical drugs.

End points

The HAM-D test was administered to patients prior to the study and at the end of the study; response to treatment was defined as a total score of less than 10 on the HAM-D after treatment, or at least a 50 percent decrease in HAM-D score. Patients were given the Vienna Determination Unit test, which measures reactions necessary for driving in traffic. Patients also took the d_2 Brickenkamp attention load test to measure concentration ability.

Results

In the St. John's Wort group, the HAM-D response rate was 66.6 percent, whereas it was 26.7 percent in the placebo group. None of the psychomotor tests or the d2 attention load test indicated impaired cognitive performance due to treatment.

Side effects

Two patients experienced redness, itching, and fatigue; overall tolerability was good to very good.

Authors' comments

The recommended daily dose of Jarsin did not influence attention, concentration, or reaction. This herbal antidepressant can thus be recommended for continued long-term treatment, especially in cases where the use of chemical substances produces distressing side effects.

Reviewers' comments
This was a descriptive study only. Insufficient data/statistical results were given for depression results. The data emphasized the driving reaction time results, which have nothing to do with depression effectiveness ratings. The authors also do not give enough data information to replicate for antidepressant effects. Due to the lack of results regarding depression, no clear conclusions could be made regarding this treatment. (Translation reviewed) (2, 3)

Clinical Study: LI 160

Extract name	LI 160
Manufacturer	Lichtwer Pharma AG, Germany
Indication	**Depression**
Level of evidence	I
Therapeutic benefit	**No**

Bibliographic reference
Shelton RC, Keller MB, Gelenberg A, Dunner DL, Hirschfeld R, Thase ME, Russell J, Lydiard RB, Crits-Cristoph P, Gallop R, et al. (2001). Effectiveness of St. John's wort in major depression: A randomized trial. *Journal of the American Medical Association* 285 (15): 1978-1986.

Trial design
Parallel. Single-blind pretrial washout period of one week with placebo. If insufficient improvement was seen by week 4, the dose of 300 mg three times daily was increased to 300 mg four times daily for the remainder of the trial.

Study duration	2 months
Dose	1 (300 mg) tablet 3-4 times daily
Route of administration	Oral
Randomized	Yes
Randomization adequate	Yes
Blinding	Double-blind
Blinding adequate	Yes
Placebo	Yes
Drug comparison	No
Site description	11 academic medical centers
No. of subjects enrolled	200
No. of subjects completed	167
Sex	Male and female
Age	Mean: 42 years

Inclusion criteria

Physically healthy outpatients, 18 years or older, diagnosed as having major depressive disorder (single episode or recurrent), without psychotic features according to DSM-IV, of at least four weeks' duration, and a score of at least 20 on the 17-item Hamilton Rating Scale for Depression (HAM-D). Patients in psychotherapy were allowed to continue treatment if they had been in therapy for at least three months prior to baseline, and if the frequency of sessions remained the same during the study.

Exclusion criteria

DSM-IV diagnosis of a current cognitive disorder, post-traumatic stress disorder, eating disorder, or a substance use disorder in the last six months; panic disorder in the last year; current or past history of bipolar disorder, any psychotic disorder, or borderline, antisocial, or schizotypal personality disorder; HAM-D suicide score greater than 2 or significant risk of suicide; prior trial of St. John's wort (at least 450 mg/day) for the treatment of depression or those who had taken St. John's wort in the last month; failure to respond to a trial of fluoxetine hydrochloride (20 mg/day) for at least four weeks (or equivalent) in the current episode, or failure to respond to more than one adequate trial of antidepressants in a previous episode; improvement greater than 25 percent or score of less than 20 on the 17-item HAM-D after the washout period. No other psychotropic medications were allowed, with the exception of zolpidem tartrate, up to 10 mg/day for sleep for the first three weeks of the trial.

End points

Efficacy and safety assessments were performed at screening, baseline, and at the end of weeks 1, 2, 4, 6, and 8. The primary outcome measure was the rate of change of the HAM-D over the treatment period. Secondary outcome measures included the physician-rated Clinical Global Impression-Improvement (CGI-I) and -Severity (CGI-S) scales, vital signs, and a review of adverse events. The Beck Depression Inventory (BDI) (self-rated) and the Global Assessment of Function scale were performed at screening, baseline, and at week 8. The Hamilton Anxiety (HAM-A) scale was performed at weeks 2 and 8. Laboratory assessments and an EEG were completed at screening and at the end of the trial. Response was defined as a HAM-D score of 12 or less (at least 50 percent improvement from baseline) and a CGI-I score of 1 or 2. Remission was defined as an HAM-D score of 7 or less with a CGI score of 1 or 2.

Results

In terms of the change in HAM-D scores during the trial, the intent-to-treat sample revealed a significant time effect ($p < 0.001$), but no significant treatment effect or time-by-treatment interaction. In addition, no significant difference in the response rates was seen in the ITT sample by week 8. There was, however, a significantly higher remission rate for St. John's wort compared to placebo (p = 0.02). A nonsignificant difference in both response rate and remission rate between St. John's wort and placebo (p = 0.07 for both) was seen in those who completed the trial. Analysis of HAM-A scores revealed a significant time effect (p < 0.001) and a significant treatment effect (p = 0.02), but did not find a significant treatment-by-time interaction. Similar results to the primary efficacy analysis of the HAM-D scores were obtained for the CGI scales (significant time effects, but no significant treatment effect or treatment-by-time interactions). In the ITT sample, nonsignificant treatment effects were seen for the BDI and the Global Assessment of Function scale. To address the possibility that St. John's wort could be effective for less severely depressed patients, patients with HAM-D scores of 22 (median) or less (20 to 22) were evaluated separately. However, no significant different in the rate of change in HAM-D scores were seen between St. John's wort and placebo, nor were there any significant differences in responder rates or remission rates.

Side effects
Abdominal discomfort, insomnia, and headaches occurred in 10 percent or more of patients in one or both treatment groups, with a greater proportion of St. John's wort patients reporting headaches. One patient in each group withdrew due to adverse events.

Authors' comments
These results do not support significant antidepressant or antianxiety effects for St. John's wort when contrasted with placebo in a clinical sample of depressed patients. The results of this study suggest that persons with significant major depression should not be treated with St. John's wort. Although the primary data analyses were negative, St. John's wort did produce a significantly greater proportion of remission in the ITT analysis compared with placebo.

Reviewers' comments
This is a very good study that addressed many previous studies' flaws. It was multisite and used trained evaluators (for DSM-IV). The trial length was adequate, and the dose of St. John's wort was increased if no improvement was observed by week 4. Good statistics! (5, 6)

Clinical Study: Jarsin® 300

Extract name	LI 160
Manufacturer	Lichtwer Pharma AG, Germany

Indication   **Depression**
Level of evidence **III**
Therapeutic benefit **Trend**

Bibliographic reference
Lehrl S, Willemsen A, Papp R, Woelk H (1993). Results of measurements of the cognitive capacity in patients treated with hypericum extract. *Nervenheilkunde* 12: 281-284.

Trial design
Parallel. Pretrial run-in with placebo for two weeks.

Study duration	1 month
Dose	3 (300 mg) tablets daily
Route of administration	Oral
Randomized	Yes
Randomization adequate	No
Blinding	Double-blind
Blinding adequate	Yes
Placebo	Yes
Drug comparison	No
Site description	4 general practices
No. of subjects enrolled	50
No. of subjects completed	48
Sex	Male and female
Age	Mean: 49 years

Inclusion criteria
Subjects between 20 and 64 years of age with a diagnosis of "neurotic depression" (ICD-9: 300.4) and "short-term depressive reaction" (ICD-9: 309.0) with an initial score of 16 to 26 on the Hamilton Depression Scale (HAM-D), and an initial score of more than 16 points in the Multiple-Choice Vocabulary test A (MWT-A).

Exclusion criteria
Serious organic diseases or a history of drug and alcohol abuse and suicidal tendencies. Those who had an increase in HAM-D scores by about 20 percent or more during the two-week pretreatment period.

End points
End points were: HAM-D, the Hamilton Anxiety Scale (HAM-A), the subjective complaints scale (SB-S), the short general information processing test (KAI), and the Clinical Global Impression scale (CGI).

Results
During the treatment period, the mean HAM-D of the active treatment group fell from 23.7 to 17.4. In the placebo group, the HAM-D fell from 21.6 to 16.8. No significant difference was observed between the two groups. Evaluation using the HAM-A revealed a drop from 28.5 to 21.9 in the St John's wort group, and from 30.1 to 20.9 in the placebo group. On the subjective complaints scale, under the active substance, the score fell from 39.7 to 34.5, and in the placebo group, from 41.2 to 37.7. Under the active treatment, IQ increased from 92.6 to 95.9 (by 3.2 points), and in the placebo group, IQ increased from 95.8 to 96.7 (by 0.9 points)—the difference is not significant ($p < 0.10$)

Side effects
None mentioned.

Authors' comments
The results suggest that under treatment with *Hypericum* extract, cognitive capacity not only does not decline further, but even starts to increase again. An increase in cognitive capacity, indicated here by the KAI results, would have considerable positive effects on many aspects of career and everyday activities. However, from this viewpoint, the study reported here is a pilot study.

Reviewers' comments
There was a trend toward an increase in cognitive capacity in depressed patients. The outcome measures are clearly defined, and the sample size is appropriate. However, the botanical preparation was not described adequately. (Translation reviewed) (3, 4) (*Note:* the product information was obtained from a literature review citing this study and from correspondence with the manufacturer.)

Clinical Study: LI 160

Extract name	LI 160
Manufacturer	Lichtwer Pharma AG, Germany
Indication	**Depression**
Level of evidence	**II**
Therapeutic benefit	**Trend**

Bibliographic reference
Harrer G, Hübner W, Podzuweit H (1994). Effectiveness and tolerance of the hypericum extract LI 160 compared to maprotiline: A multicenter double-

blind study. *Journal of Geriatric Psychiatry and Neurology* 7 (Suppl. 1): S24-S28. (Also published in Harrer G, Hübner W, Podzuweit H [1993]. Wirsamkeit und verträglichkeit des *Hypericum*-präparates LI 160 im vergleich mit Maprotilin. *Nervenheilkunde* 12: 297-301.)

Trial design
Parallel. Patients received either LI 160 extract or maprotiline (75 mg daily).

Study duration	1 month
Dose	3 (300 mg) tablets daily
Route of administration	Oral
Randomized	Yes
Randomization adequate	No
Blinding	Double-blind
Blinding adequate	No
Placebo	No
Drug comparison	Yes
Drug name	Maprotiline
Site description	6 practices (neurology and psychiatry)
No. of subjects enrolled	102
No. of subjects completed	86
Sex	Male and female
Age	24-65 years

Inclusion criteria
Depressed according to ICD-10, F32.1 (single, moderately depressive episode for at least two weeks), and Hamilton Depression Scale (HAM-D) > 15.

Exclusion criteria
Treatment with other drug therapies within four weeks.

End points
At baseline, and at weeks 2 and 4, antidepressant efficacy was assessed using the HAM-D, the von Zerssen's Depression Scale (D-S), and the Clinical Global Impressions scale (CGI). Response to the HAM-D scale was defined as a score of less than 10 or a decrease in score of at least 50 percent. Twenty-two symptoms were also assessed according to four grades of severity. At the end of the trial, physicians and patients judged the efficacy and tolerance of the medications.

Results
Under both treatments, HAM-D scores fell by approximately 50 percent after four weeks. Although maprotiline appeared more effective after two weeks,

no significant difference was observed at the end of four weeks. The mean score with LI 160 decreased 49.3 percent, from 20.5 to 12.2, and with maprotiline the score decreased 50.7 percent, from 21.5 to 10.5. Similar results were measured using the D-S.

Side effects
Side effects reported for 25 percent of subjects treated with LI 160 , with gastrointestinal symptoms, dizziness, and confusion accounting for more than half. Side effects reported for 35 percent of subjects receiving maprotiline included tiredness, gastrointestinal symptoms, dizziness, confusion, and dryness of mouth.

Authors' comments
The action of maprotiline begins more rapidly than that of *Hypericum,* and the D-S scale actually showed a significant difference between the two groups after two weeks of treatment. This difference had disappeared after four weeks, however.

Reviewers' comments
This was a relatively well-designed study. A subtherapeutic dose of maprotiline was used, which the authors acknowledge and explain. The treatment period was also short. (5, 6)

Clinical Study: LI 160

Extract name	LI 160
Manufacturer	Lichtwer Pharma AG, Germany
Indication	**Depression**
Level of evidence	**II**
Therapeutic benefit	**Yes**

Bibliographic reference
Wheatley D (1997). LI 160, an extract of St. John's wort, versus amitriptyline in mildly to moderate depressed outpatients—A controlled 6-week clinical trial. *Pharmacopsychiatry* 30 (Suppl. 2): S77-S80.

Trial design
Parallel. Pretrial single-blind placebo run-in phase of three to seven days. Patients then received either LI 160 or amitriptyline (75 mg daily).

Study duration	6 weeks
Dose	3 (300 mg) tablets daily

Route of administration   Oral

Randomized   Yes
Randomization adequate   No
Blinding   Double-blind
Blinding adequate   No

Placebo   No
Drug comparison   Yes
Drug name   Amitriptyline

Site description   Multicenter

No. of subjects enrolled   165
No. of subjects completed   120
Sex   Male and female
Age   20-65 years (mean: 40)

Inclusion criteria

Mildly to moderately depressed outpatients ages 20 to 65 years, with a current major depressive episode according to DSM-IV criteria and an initial Hamilton Depression Scale (HAM-D) score between 17 and 24. Antidepressants had to be omitted at least 14 days before the placebo run-in period; for fluoxetine, 42 days were required.

Exclusion criteria

Major exclusion criteria included pregnancy or lactation; known history or presence of serious renal, hepatic, or cardiovascular diseases; blood dyscrasia or anemia; organic brain diseases; and the established exclusion criteria for the use of tricyclic antidepressants. Patients who improved during the placebo run-in phase to a HAM-D total score of less than 16, or with a reduction of more than 25 percent. The use of psychoactive medication was contraindicated, with the exception of temazepam, zopiclone, or zolpidem as hypnotics.

End points

Six visits were performed: pretreatment screening (day −7 to −3), baseline visit (day 0), safety visit (day 7), two maintenance visits (days 14 and 28), and final evaluation (day 42). Depression was rated on visits 1, 2, 4, and 6. The primary outcome was response to treatment, defined as an HAM-D total score of less than 10 at the end of the treatment period, or a reduction in HAM-D score of at least 50 percent compared to baseline. Secondary efficacy parameters were the Montgomery-Asberg Rating Scale for Depression (MADRS) and the Clinical Global Impressions (CGI). The main tolerability parameter was the number of adverse events. At visits 1 and 6, blood samples were taken for routine hematology and biochemistry screens. Adverse events were recorded at baseline and at visits 3 through 6.

Results
No statistically significant difference between the two groups was shown in response rate to treatment. 59.7 percent in the LI 160 group and 77.8 percent in the amitriptyline group were classified as responders ($p = 0.064$). A significantly better result was seen in the amitriptyline group in total HAM-D and MADRS scores ($p < 0.05$ for both rating scales). No significant difference between the two groups could be shown in CGI severity-of-illness scores ($p = 0.73$). The same applies to the CGI global improvement scores ($p = 0.49$). In terms of the HAM-D sleep factor, the amitriptyline group was significantly more improved at week 2 compared to the LI 160 group ($p = 0.004$). The trend still existed at the end of the study ($p = 0.053$).

Side effects
Thirty-seven percent of the patients in the LI 160 group and 64 percent of patients in the amitriptyline group reported adverse events ($p < 0.05$). The most common side effects in the LI 160 group were headache, nausea/vomiting, dry mouth, and constipation.

Author's comments
LI 160 possesses a comparable efficacy to amitriptyline with a clear tolerability advantage. The reported trial may have one major limitation: the dose of 75 mg of amitriptyline per day is about half of the maximally recommended dose of this drug in outpatient settings. However, 75 mg/day is the dose that most depressed patients receive, and is regarded as sufficiently effective in this context. Since side effects are the most important limiting factor for patient compliance, *Hypericum* extract offers the possibility to treat patients more adequately with antidepressant pharmacotherapy. Patient information concerning possible adverse events specifically associated with tricyclics may have biased the incidence of these in the LI 160 group.

Reviewers' comments
This was a good study overall. However, a subtherapeutic dose of amitriptyline (one-half the usual dose) was used. Also, no statements/descriptions of the outpatient sites were provided. The doctors were trained on HAM-D. (5, 6)

Clinical Study: Jarsin® 300

Extract name	LI 160
Manufacturer	Lichtwer Pharma AG, Germany
Indication	**Depression**
Level of evidence	**II**
Therapeutic benefit	**Yes**

Bibliographic reference
Vorbach EU, Hübner WD, Arnoldt KH (1994). Effectiveness and tolerance of the hypericum extract LI 160 in comparison with imipramine: Randomized double-blind study with 135 outpatients. *Journal of Geriatric Psychiatry and Neurology* 7 (Suppl. 1): S19-S-23. (Also published in Vorbach EU, Hübner WD, Arnoldt KH [1993]. Wirksamkeit und verträglichkeit des *Hypericum*-extraktes LI 160 im vergleich mit imipramin: Randomisierte doppleblind-studie mit 135 ambulanten patienten. *Nervenkeilkunde* 12: 290-296.)

Trial design
Parallel. Pretrial washout phase of at least two weeks. Subjects received either LI 160 or imipramine (75 mg daily).

Study duration	6 weeks
Dose	3 (300 mg) tablets daily
Route of administration	Oral
Randomized	Yes
Randomization adequate	Yes
Blinding	Double-blind
Blinding adequate	Yes
Placebo	No
Drug comparison	Yes
Drug name	Imipramine
Site description	20 centers
No. of subjects enrolled	135
No. of subjects completed	130
Sex	Male and female
Age	Mean: 53.4 ± 12.6 years

Inclusion criteria
Ages 18 to 75 with typical depression according to DSM-III-R, with a single episode (296.2) or recurrent episodes (296.3), neurotic depression (300.4), and adjustment disorder with depressed mood (309.0).

Exclusion criteria
Severe depression requiring inpatient treatment; schizophrenia or marked agitation requiring additional medication; a known history of attempted suicide or acute suicidal state; chronic alcohol or drug dependency; acute confusional state; use of drugs with cerebral effects; use of monoamine oxidase (MAO) inhibitors within the previous two weeks; and use of drugs taken for research purposes within the previous three months.

End points

At baseline and at the end of the study, patients were examined clinically, including neurologic and psychiatric assessment, and various blood tests. Main assessment criteria were the Hamilton Depressive Scale (HAM-D), the Depression Scale according to von Zerssen (D-S), and the Clinical Global Impressions (CGI).

Results

A significant reduction in HAM-D scores was observed in both groups ($p <$ 0.001), from 20.2 to 8.8 in the *Hypericum* group, and from 19.4 to 10.7 in the imipramine group. Group comparisons showed no significant differences. Similar therapeutic effects were also shown by the D-S, and by three criteria in the CGI scale (therapeutic effect, alteration in status at the end of treatment, and change in severity of the illness). Improvement was seen in 81.8 percent of patients on LI 160 versus 62.5 percent of patients on imipramine. No patients on *Hypericum* and two patients on imipramine experienced worsening of their condition. The rest of the patients were unchanged. In the group of patients with HAM-D scores of 21 or more at baseline, LI 160 efficacy was significantly better than imipramine with regard to HAM-D score and CGI ($p < 0.05$). No clinically relevant changes were seen in either group with regard to safety parameters or blood parameters measured at the start of the trial.

Side effects

Eleven symptoms were reported in *Hypericum* group. The most common were dry mouth (four) and dizziness (two).

Authors' comments

The difference between the two groups was statistically significant in favor of LI 160 in patients with a HAM-D score greater than 21. However, no statistically significant differences in efficacy were observed between the two treatment groups. It is significant that side effects occurred less frequently and were less severe in the LI 160 group than in the imipramine group.

Reviewers' comments

This is a good study, but a subtherapeutic dose of imipramine was used. It is not clear, therefore, whether this was more of a placebo comparison study for St. John's wort. (5, 6)

Clinical Study: Jarsin®

Extract name	LI 160
Manufacturer	Lichtwer Pharma AG, Germany

Indication	**Depression**
Level of evidence	**II**
Therapeutic benefit	**Trend**

Bibliographic reference
Vorbach EU, Arnoldt KH, Hübner WD (1997). Efficacy and tolerability of St. John's wort extract LI 160 versus imipramine in patients with severe depressive episodes according to ICD-10. *Pharmacopsychiatry* 30 (Suppl. 2): 81-85.

Trial design
Parallel. Pretrial, single-blind, placebo washout phase of three to five days. Dose was increased step-wise within one week until the final dose of 1,800 mg LI 160 or 150 mg imipramine per day was reached.

Study duration	6 weeks
Dose	3 × 600 mg LI 160 daily
Route of administration	Oral
Randomized	Yes
Randomization adequate	Yes
Blinding	Double-blind
Blinding adequate	Yes
Placebo	No
Drug comparison	Yes
Drug name	Imipramine
Site description	20 centers
No. of subjects enrolled	209
No. of subjects completed	186
Sex	Male and female
Age	Mean: 49.5 ± 11.9 years

Inclusion criteria
Subjects ages 18-70 years diagnosed in accordance with ICD-10 F 33.2 (severe episode of a major depressive disorder, recurrent, without psychotic symptoms); at least two prior episodes of two-weeks or longer duration were required. Lithium was allowed if prescribed at least three months before the trial and continued unchanged. Any treatment with MAO inhibitors had to be discontinued at least 14 days before the start of the trial.

Exclusion criteria
Patients with suicidal tendency, hallucinations, and depressive delusional content were not included. Likewise, patients with possible preexisting schizophrenic disorders or pronounced agitation, chronic alcohol or drug dependency, as well as acute confusional state were excluded. Patients with

an improvement of more than 20 percent on the HAM-D scale during the three- to five-day washout phase before the study were also excluded. No psychotropic medication (excluding chloralhydrate in cases of sleep disturbance) was allowed.

End points

Patients were assessed at days −3, 0, 7, 14, 28, and 42 using the Hamilton Depression Scale (HAM-D), the Clinical Global Impressions (CGI) scale and the Depression Scale according to von Zerssen (D-S). Adverse events were also recorded. Tolerability and safety measures were performed at days 0 and 42. Response to the HAM-D was defined as a reduction of at least 50 percent of the HAM-D total score. Patients and investigators rated improvement following treatment as very good, good, moderate, or unsatisfactory.

Results

Mean HAM-D values decreased similarly in the two study groups: from 25.3 to 14.4 in the LI 160 group, and from 26.1 to 13.4 in the imipramine group. No statistically significant difference was seen between the two groups in the D-S scale ($p = 0.36$). The CGI showed a trend in favor of imipramine ($p = 0.079$). Response rate, defined by a 50 percent decrease in HAM-D score, was 35.3 percent in the LI 160 group, and 41.2 percent in the imipramine group. Post hoc analysis of a subgroup with a reduction of at least 33 percent in the total HAM-D score resulted in 62.7 percent responders with imipramine and 57.9 percent with LI 160, confirming the equivalent efficacy of the two treatments.

Side effects

Statistically fewer (25 percent interval) adverse events were reported with LI 160 (23 percent compared to 41 percent of those on imipramine). The most frequent side effects with hypericum included restlessness, dizziness, tiredness/sedation, and gastric symptoms.

Authors' comments

LI 160 can be used to treat severely depressed patients, provided that the dose is adjusted from 900 to 1800 mg per day. LI 160 provides treatment with a considerably reduced side effect profile compared to tricyclics.

Reviewers' comments

Impressive study that replicated previous work on mild major depression and treated patients with higher (but still subtherapeutic) doses of imipramine. The authors used intent-to-treat analysis. (5, 6)

Clinical Study: LI 160

Extract name	LI 160
Manufacturer	Lichtwer Pharma AG, Germany
Indication	**Depression**
Level of evidence	**II**
Therapeutic benefit	**Trend**

Bibliographic reference
Brenner R, Azbel V, Madhusoodanan S, Pawlowska M (2000). Comparison of an extract of *Hypericum* (LI 160) and sertraline in the treatment of depression: A double-blind, randomized pilot study. *Clinical Therapeutics* 22 (4): 411-419.

Trial design
Parallel. Patients in the hypericum group received 600 mg/day during week 1, followed by 900 mg/day for the remainder of the trial. Patients in the sertraline group received 50 mg/day during week 1, followed by 75 mg/day for the remainder of the trial. Doses of either drug could be reduced to the week 1 amount if patients experienced adverse effects.

Study duration	7 weeks
Dose	900 mg hypericum daily
Route of administration	Oral
Randomized	Yes
Randomization adequate	No
Blinding	Double-blind
Blinding adequate	Yes
Placebo	No
Drug comparison	Yes
Drug name	Sertraline (an SSRI)
Site description	Community hospital
No. of subjects enrolled	30
No. of subjects completed	20
Sex	Male and female
Age	Mean: 45.5 ± 12.6 years

Inclusion criteria
Outpatients ages 18 to 65 years with a score of at least 17 on the Hamilton Rating Scale for Depression (HAM-D) and a DSM-IV diagnosis of major depressive disorder (single or recurrent episodes), dysthymic disorder, adjustment disorder with depressed mood, or depressive disorder not otherwise

specified. All patients had discontinued selective seratonin reuptake inhibitor (SSRI) or tricyclic antidepressant (TCA) therapy for seven days before randomization.

Exclusion criteria

Pregnant women or women not using medically accepted birth control; patients with severe depression and a history of attempted suicide or acute suicidal state; schizophrenia or marked agitation requiring additional medication; chronic alcohol or drug dependency; failure to respond to adequate trials of an antidepressant drug; patients who had received an investigational drug within four weeks of the study, or who had been treated with hypericum or sertraline previously; patients with mental retardation or emotional or intellectual difficulties hindering consent or compliance; patients whose HAM-D scores improved by more than 20 percent between screening and baseline.

End points

Primary outcome: changes in the HAM-D and Clinical Global Impressions (CGI) global severity scores. Treatment response was defined as a reduction of at least 50 percent in total HAM-D score from baseline to end of trial. At the baseline visit, each patient completed the Depression Scale (D-S) before seeing the investigator. Weekly for the next seven weeks, the investigator obtained HAM-D and CGI scores, and recorded adverse events and concomitant medications. Patients again completed the D-S at weeks 3 and 7.

Results

In both treatment groups, symptoms of depression were significantly improved ($p < 0.05$), with no significant differences between patients receiving hypericum and those receiving sertraline. A clinical response (at least 50 percent reduction in HAM-D scores) was seen in a similar proportion of patients in the hypericum group (47 percent) and sertraline group (40 percent). The between-group difference was not statistically significant. At week 2, mean HAM-D scores were reduced 29 percent and 30 percent in the hypericum and sertraline groups, respectively. At week 4, the respective reductions were 54 percent and 46 percent, and at the end point they were 40 percent and 42 percent.

Side effects

In hypericum group, one patient complained of headache and numbness of hands, and another complained of headache and dizziness.

Authors' comments

The results demonstrate that hypericum is at least as efficacious as the SSRI sertraline. The failure to reach statistical significance between treatments appears to be attributable primarily to the lack of a clinically significant difference rather than the small sample size. Both drugs were well tolerated.

Reviewers' comments

Good study, but the sample size was small. The authors also used an inappropriate statistical method (analysis of covariance [ANCOVA]), which was not optimal because of the small sample size. The lack of difference between the two groups may be due to the small sample size. (3, 4)

Clinical Study: LI 160

Extract name	LI 160
Manufacturer	Lichtwer Pharma AG, Germany
Indication	**Depression**
Level of evidence	**I**
Therapeutic benefit	**No**

Bibliographic reference

Hypericum Depression Trial Study Group (2002). Effect of *Hypericum perforatum* (St. John's Wort) in major depressive disorder: A randomized controlled trial. *Journal of the American Medical Association* 287 (14): 1807-1814.

Trial design

Parallel. One week, single-blind, placebo run-in phase before baseline. Patients then received either hypericum (900 mg/d), sertraline (50 mg/day), or placebo. Daily doses of the three treatments could be increased to 1,200 mg (hypericum), 75 mg (sertraline), or placebo equivalent after three or four weeks, and to 1,500 mg (hypericum), 100 mg (sertraline), or placebo equivalent at week 6 if the Clinical Global Impression Scale for severity (CGI-S) was 4 or more at week 3, or 3 or more at weeks 4 or 6.

Study duration	2 months
Dose	900 mg *Hypericum* daily (in three doses)
Route of administration	Oral
Randomized	Yes
Randomization adequate	Yes
Blinding	Double-blind
Blinding adequate	Yes
Placebo	Yes
Drug comparison	Yes

Drug name	Sertraline
Site description	Multicenter

No. of subjects enrolled   340
No. of subjects completed 245
Sex   Male and female
Age   Mean: 42 years

Inclusion criteria
At least 18 years of age; current diagnosis of major depression (meeting DSM-IV criteria for major depressive disorder); minimum total score of 20 on the 17-item Hamilton Depression (HAM-D) scale and a maximum score of 60 on the Global Assessment of Functioning (GAF) at screening and baseline following a one-week, single-blind, placebo run-in; no more than a 25 percent decrease in HAM-D total score between screening and baseline; capacity to give informed consent and follow study procedures; and identification of personal contact to be notified if warranted by clinical concerns.

Exclusion criteria
Score above 2 on the HAM-D suicide item; attempted suicide in the past year or current suicide or homicide risk; being pregnant, planning pregnancy, breastfeeding, or not using medically acceptable birth control; clinically significant liver disease or liver enzyme levels elevated to at least twice the normal upper limit; serious unstable medical illness; history of seizure disorder; severe combined immunodeficiency (SCID) diagnoses indicating alcohol or other substance-abuse disorder, bipolar disorder, panic disorder, or obsessive-compulsive disorder; history of psychotic features of affective disorder; evidence of untreated or unstable thyroid disorder; no response to at least two adequate trials of antidepressants in any depressive episode; daily use of hypericum or sertraline for at least four weeks within the past six months; current use of other psychotropic drugs, other medicines, dietary supplements, natural remedies, or botanical preparations with psychoactive properties; use of investigational drugs within 30 days of baseline or of other psychotropic drugs within 21 days of baseline (within six weeks for fluoxetine); allergy or hypersensitivity to study medications; positive urine drug screen; introduction of psychotherapy within two months of enrollment or any ongoing psychotherapy specifically designed to treat depression; and mental retardation or cognitive impairment.

End points
The primary end points were the change in HAM-D total scores from baseline to week 8, and the incidence of full response (defined as a CGI-I score of 1 or 2 and a HAM-D score of 8 or less). Secondary end points included GAF, CGI, Beck Depression Inventory (BDI), and the Sheehan Disability Scale (SDS). Patients were assessed either weekly or biweekly for the eight

weeks of the study. All tests were assessed at each visit, except the SDS, which was assessed only at baseline and week 8.

Results
Neither hypericum nor sertraline preformed significantly different from placebo on either of the two primary outcome measures. The mean differences in HAM-D scores were −8.68 for hypericum, −10.53 for sertraline, and −9.20 for placebo. Full response occurred in 23.9 percent of hypericum patients, 24.8 percent of sertraline patients, and 31.9 percent of placebo patients. Hypericum did not differ from placebo on any of the secondary outcome measures. At week 8, sertraline was significantly better than placebo on the CGI-I score ($p = 0.02$). In a later analysis it was also found to be superior to hypericum ($p = 0.01$).

Side effects
No serious adverse effects occurred. Rates of nausea, diarrhea, and sweating (sertraline); anorgasmia (sertraline and hypericum); and frequent urination and swelling (hypericum) were all higher than those of placebo.

Author's comments
According to the available data, hypericum should not be substituted for standard clinical care of proven efficacy, including antidepressant dedications and specific psychotherapies, for the treatment of major depression of moderate severity.

Reviewers' comments
The overall response to sertraline on primary measures was not better than placebo, an outcome that is not uncommon in trials of approved antidepressants. According to the author, this occurs in up to 35 percent of trials on antidepressants. (5, 6)

Clinical Study: LI 160

Extract name	LI 160
Manufacturer	Lichtwer Pharma AG, Germany
Indication	**Electrophysiological effects** in healthy volunteers
Level of evidence	**II**
Therapeutic benefit	**MOA**

Bibliographic reference
Johnson D, Ksciuk H, Woelk H, Sauerwein-Giese E, Frauendorf A (1994).

Effects of *Hypericum* extract LI 160 compared with maprotiline on resting EEG and evoked potentials in 24 volunteers. *Journal of Geriatric Psychiatry and Neurology* 7 (Suppl. 1): S44-S46. (Also published in Johnson D, Ksciuk H, Woelk H, Sauerwein-Giese E, Frauendorf A [1993]. Wirkungen von Johanniskraut-extrakt LI 160 im vergleich Maprolitin auf Ruhe-EEG und evozierte potentiale bei 24 probunden. *Nervenheilkunde* 12: 328-330.)

Trial design
Parallel. Pretrial washout phase of one week. Subjects were either given LI 160 or maprotiline (3 × 10 mg daily).

Study duration	1 month
Dose	3 (300 mg) tablets daily
Route of administration	Oral
Randomized	Yes
Randomization adequate	No
Blinding	Double-blind
Blinding adequate	Yes
Placebo	No
Drug comparison	Yes
Drug name	Maprotiline
Site description	Not described
No. of subjects enrolled	24
No. of subjects completed	Not given
Sex	Male and female
Age	18-45 years (mean: 28)

Inclusion criteria
Healthy volunteers.

Exclusion criteria
All concomitant medications, apart from contraceptives, were not allowed.

End points
Subjects were assessed at baseline and after two, four, and five weeks. Resting EEG was recorded for five minutes over the frequency range of 0.1 to 200 Hz using the Cz-Fz and Oz-T6 leads. Subjects also rated their well-being using the von Zerssen scale (Bf-S).

Results
Changes at various frequencies in the resting EEGs were associated with both treatments. Changes in the theta region were in opposite directions; all of the other changes were in the same direction. For auditory evoked poten-

tials in the theta region, no relevant changes in amplitude P320 occurred with either drug, but the *Hypericum* group showed a clear reduction in latent times for amplitudes N80, P150, and N240. Clear reductions in latent times for visually evoked potentials were seen in all amplitudes for both groups.

Side effects
None mentioned.

Authors' comments
After four weeks of treatment with *Hypericum,* enhanced activation was seen in the theta and beta-2 regions, which can be interpreted as a relaxing but not sedative effect. In general the evoked potentials showed shortened latency, suggesting more rapid general information processing by the brain. It is clear from the results of measurements of visually evoked potentials in the beta region that similarities exist between the neurophysiologic effect profiles of *Hypericum* extract and maprotiline.

Reviewers' comments
Mode-of-action study exploring changes in EEG following treatment. (2, 4)

Clinical Study: Jarsin® 300

Extract name	LI 160
Manufacturer	Lichtwer Pharma AG, Germany
Indication	**Neuroendocrine effects** in healthy volunteers
Level of evidence	**II**
Therapeutic benefit	**MOA**

Bibliographic reference
Franklin M, Chi J, McGavin C, Hockney R, Reed A, Campling G, Whale RWR, Cowen PJ (1999). Neuroendocrine evidence for dopaminergic actions of *Hypericum* extract (LI 160) in healthy volunteers. *Biological Psychiatry* 46 (4): 581-584.

Trial design
Crossover design. Treatment periods were separated by at least one week.

Study duration	1 day
Dose	9 (300 mg) tablets LI 160
Route of administration	Oral
Randomized	No

Randomization adequate	No
Blinding	Double-blind
Blinding adequate	Yes
Placebo	Yes
Drug comparison	No
Site description	Single center
No. of subjects enrolled	12
No. of subjects completed	8
Sex	Male
Age	22-49 years (mean: 32.5)

Inclusion criteria
Healthy male volunteers not taking any psychotropic medication.

Exclusion criteria
Patients with elevated baseline growth hormone values were eliminated from the analysis.

End points
Subjects fasted after a light breakfast and came to the research unit at 12:30 p.m., when an indwelling venous cannula was inserted and maintained with heparinized saline. Two baseline blood samples were taken during the next half hour, following which either hypericin or placebo was administered. Blood samples were removed at 30-minute intervals for the following 240 minutes for assay. Plasma concentrations of growth hormone (GH), prolactin (PRL), cortisol, as well as hypericin and hyperforin were measured.

Results
Following hypericum administration, plasma GH levels increased, peaking at about 120 min. Plasma PRL was significantly lowered following hypericum treatment relative to placebo, with the lowest point occurring at 180 minutes. Plasma cortisol profiles were similar in both treatments. Plasma hypericin concentrations increased initially from 150 minutes after administration of LI 160, and were still rising at the end of the test period. Plasma mean hyperforin concentrations rose from 60 minutes after LI 160 treatment and peaked at 210 minutes. Neither peak plasma hypericin nor plasma hyperforin concentrations correlated significantly with any of the peak changes in hormone responses (all p values > 0.05)

Side effects
Flatulence in two subjects.

Authors' comments
The most likely explanation for our neuroendocrine findings is that LI 160 en-

hances some aspects of dopamine neurotransmission. This is because dopamine pathways facilitate growth hormone release and suppress prolactin secretion. Plasma concentrations of hypericin, one of the possible active components of LI 160, were not detectable until 150 minutes into the test, and were still rising at the end of the test. The plasma profile suggests that hypericin was not involved either in the increase of growth hormone or in the decrease of prolactin found in this study. In contrast, plasma concentrations of hyperforin rose from 60 minutes after treatment, and peaked at 210 minutes. Although plasma concentrations of hyperforin did not correlate with hormone responses, the time course of hormonal changes are more consistent with an effect of hyperforin than of hypericin.

Reviewers' comments
This study indicates that LI 160 may increase some aspects of dopamine function. The dose used is two times greater than the usual therapeutic dose. (3, 5)

Product Profile: Perika™

Manufacturer	**Dr. Willmar Schwabe GmbH & Co., Germany**
U.S. distributor	**Nature's Way Products, Inc.**
Botanical ingredient	**St. John's wort aerial parts extract**
Extract name	**WS 5572**
Quantity	300 mg
Processing	Plant to extract ratio 2.5-5:1, 60% ethanol (w/w)
Standardization	A minimum of 3% hyperforin
Formulation	Tablet

Recommended dose: Take 1 tablet three times daily with water at mealtimes. Benefits are best realized after two to four weeks of regular usage.

DSHEA structure/function: Scientifically advanced to maintain a healthy emotional outlook.

Cautions: Do not use this product while taking any prescription drug without the advice of your prescribing physician. Avoid excessive exposure to UV radiation (e.g., sunlight; tanning) when using this product. Not recommended for use by pregnant or lactating women.

Other ingredients: Vitamin C (ascorbic acid, 4 mg), cellulose, modified cellulose, starch, silica, magnesium stearate, titanium dioxide.

Comments: WS 5572 is sold in Europe as Neuroplant, Neuroplant 300, and Neuroplant forte.

Source(s) of information: Product label (© Nature's Way Products, Inc., 2000); information provided by distributor.

Product Profile: Movana™

Manufacturer	**Dr. Willmar Schwabe GmbH & Co., Germany**
U.S. distributor	**Pharmaton Natural Health Products**
Botanical ingredient	**St. John's wort flower and leaves extract**
Extract name	**WS 5572**
Quantity	300 mg
Processing	Plant to extract ratio 2.5-5:1, 60% ethanol (w/w)
Standardization	A minimum of 3% hyperforin
Formulation	Tablet

Recommended dose: Take one tablet three times per day. Optimal effectiveness has been shown in as little as two weeks with continued use. Doses above 900 mg per day have not shown any greater effectiveness.

DSHEA structure/function: Mood support dietary supplement. Balances emotions and promotes a feeling of well-being. Maintains healthy motivation and self-esteem. Acts safely and naturally to promote normal levels of neurotransmitters responsible for maintaining positive emotions.

Cautions: St. John's Wort may reduce the effect of many prescription drugs, including drugs used to treat conditions such as heart disease, depression, seizures, certain cancers or to prevent conditions such as transplant rejection or pregnancy (oral contraceptives). Ask a healthcare professional before using this product if you are taking a prescription medication, are pregnant, or are nursing a baby. If you have fair skin, avoid prolonged direct sunlight, as photosensitivities may occur. There have been rare reports (< 1 percent) of gastrointestinal disturbances, allergic reactions, unrest or fatigue. In case of accidental ingestion/overdose, seek the advice of a healthcare professional immediately.

Other ingredients: Microcrystalline cellulose, corn starch, croscarmellose sodium, hydroxypropyl methylcellulose, PEG-4000, magnesium stearate, silicon dioxide, ascorbic acid, synthetic iron oxides, titanium dioxide, talc, vanillin.

Comments: WS 5572 is sold in Europe as Neuroplant, Neuroplant 300, and Neuroplant forte.

Source(s) of information: Product package (© Boehringer Ingelheim Pharmaceuticals, Inc., 2000); information about Perika™ from Nature's Way Products, Inc.

Clinical Study: WS 5572

Extract name	WS 5572
Manufacturer	Dr. Willmar Schwabe GmbH & Co., Germany
Indication	**Depression**
Level of evidence	**I**
Therapeutic benefit	**Yes**

Bibliographic reference
Laakmann G, Schüle C, Baghai T, Kieser M (1998). St. John's wort in mild to moderate depression: The relevance of hyperforin for the clinical efficacy. *Pharmacopsychiatry* 31 (Suppl. 1): 54-59. (Also published in Laakmann G, Dienel A, Kieser M [1998]. Clinical significance of hyperforin for the efficacy of *Hyperium* extracts on depressive disorders of different severities. *Phytomedicine* 5 [6]: 435-442.)

Trial design
Parallel. Pretrial run-in with placebo for three to seven days. WS 5573 (0.5 percent hyperforin) was compared to WS 5572 (5 percent hyperforin) and placebo.

Study duration	6 weeks
Dose	3 × 300 mg WS 5573 or WS 5572 daily
Route of administration	Oral
Randomized	Yes
Randomization adequate	Yes
Blinding	Double-blind
Blinding adequate	Yes
Placebo	Yes

Drug comparison   Yes
Drug name   WS 5573

Site description   11 centers

No. of subjects enrolled   147
No. of subjects completed   138
Sex   Male and female
Age   Mean: 49 ± 12.1 years

Inclusion criteria

Outpatients with mild or moderate depression according to DSM-IV criteria (either single or recurrent episode). Patients had to be between 18 and 65 years of age, and were required to have an initial score of at least 17 on the Hamilton Rating Scale for Depression (HAM-D).

Exclusion criteria

Risk of suicide or a score of at least 2 on the HAM-D item 3 (suicidality), organic brain syndrome, compulsive, schizophrenic or other delusive disorders, serious organic or metabolic disorders, pregnancy or lactation, and known hypersensitivity to hypericum preparations. The use of other antidepressants, benzodiazepines, and neuroleptics was prohibited.

End points

Patients were assessed at baseline and on days 7, 14, 28, and 42 using the HAM-D and the Depression Self-Rating Scale (D-S) according to von Zerssen. The primary efficacy variable was the change in the HAM-D total score between day 0 and the end of the study. At prestudy, as well as on days 0 and 42, the investigators also rated the patients' severity of illness and changes from the last visit with the Clinical Global Impressions scale (CGI). A global assessment of the patients' overall condition (similar to the CGI, but self-rated by the patients) was obtained on days 0 and 42. Adverse events were documented at all visits.

Results

Patients receiving WS 5572 showed the largest HAM-D reduction between day 0 and treatment end (10.3 points), followed by the WS 5573 group (8.5 points) and placebo group (7.9 points). In pairwise comparison, WS 5572 was significantly superior to placebo ($p = 0.004$). No statistically significant differences were found between WS 5573 (0.5 percent hyperforin) and placebo. 49 percent of the individuals treated with WS 5572 had treatment end scores that were at least 50 percent lower than at baseline, compared to 32.7 percent and 38.8 percent for WS 5573 and placebo, respectively. The results from D-S and CGI support the HAM-D findings.

Side effects
One-third of patients in each treatment group experienced adverse events during the trial.

Authors' comments
This study demonstrated a clear-cut relationship between hyperforin dose and antidepressant efficacy. WS 5572 (5 percent hyperforin extract) is an effective antidepressant in the treatment of mild to moderate depression. The improvements from baseline achieved using WS 5573 were too narrow to conclude systematic superiority of the 0.5 percent hyperforin extract over placebo. To arrive at extracts with comparable antidepressant potency, the hyperforin rather than the hypericin content of St. John's wort preparations should be standardized.

Reviewers' comments
This study indicates that hyperforin may be an important active ingredient in St. John's wort preparations used for depression. A trend analysis indicates that the number of individuals improving is greater for the higher concentration of hyperforin. Side effects were not an issue. (5, 6)

Clinical Study: WS 5570

Extract name	WS 5570
Manufacturer	Dr. Willmar Schwabe GmbH & Co., Germany
Indication	**Depression**
Level of evidence	**II**
Therapeutic benefit	**Yes**

Bibliographic reference
Lecrubier Y, Clerc G, Didi R, Kieser M (2002). Efficacy of St. John's wort extract WS 5570 in major depression: A double-blind, placebo-controlled trial. *The American Journal of Psychiatry* 159 (8): 1361-1366.

Trial design
Parallel. Single-blind placebo run-in phase of three to seven days.

Study duration	6 weeks
Dose	1 (300 mg) tablet 3 times daily
Route of administration	Oral
Randomized	Yes
Randomization adequate	No

Blinding	Double-blind
Blinding adequate	Yes
Placebo	Yes
Drug comparison	No
Site description	Multicenter
No. of subjects enrolled	375
No. of subjects completed	332
Sex	Male and female
Age	18-66 years (mean: 40)

Inclusion criteria
Outpatients ages 18 to 65 years giving written informed consent with a current major depressive episode of at least two weeks duration (meeting the DSM-IV code 296.21, 296.22, 296.31, or 296.32 criteria), and a total score of between 18 and 25 on the Hamilton Depression Scale (HAM-D) (including a score of 2 or higher on item 1 ["depressed mood"] at screening and at baseline).

Exclusion criteria
Depression of any other type, any serious psychiatric disease other than depression, serious suicidal risk (score of 3 or higher on item 3 of the HAM-D), or response to placebo in the run-in phase (25 percent or greater reduction of the HAM-D score).

End points
Efficacy was evaluated after one, two, four, and six weeks of treatment. The primary end point was the change from baseline in the total score on the 17-item HAM-D. Secondary end points included the total score on the Montgomery-Åsberg Depression Rating Scale (MADRS), the Clinical Global Impression (CGI), and the 58-item version of the Symptom Check List (SCL-58). Physical examinations and laboratory tests were also carried out before and after the treatment.

Results
Initial mean value for the HAM-D for all subjects was 21.9. Treatment with WS 5570 caused a significantly greater reduction in the HAM-D total score (9.9) compared to placebo (8.1). Also compared to placebo, significantly more patients in the WS 5570 group experienced a treatment response (WS 5570: 52.7 percent, placebo: 42.3 percent, $p < 0.05$) or remission (24.7 percent, 15.9 percent, respectively, $p = 0.03$). The WS 5570 group also saw greater reductions on the MADRS and the depression subscore of the SCL, but these differences were not significant. The score difference on the Bech melancholia subscale of the HAM-D was significantly different (mean decrease WS 5570: 5.5; placebo: 4.4, $p = 0.001$).

Side effects
More patients in the placebo group (37 percent) experienced adverse events, compared to the WS 5570 group (30.6 percent). The adverse events included nausea, headache, dizziness, abdominal pain, and insomnia. However, they did not indicate any treatment-emergent risks associated with WS 5570.

Authors' comments
This study demonstrates the existence of an antidepressant effect of *Hypericum perforatum* in mildly and moderately depressed patients.

Reviewers' comments
This was a phase III trial showing efficacy for mild to moderate depression according to ITT analysis. Interestingly, the decrease from baseline in HAM-D scores for the subset with initial scores equal to or greater than 22 was greater than the placebo group, while the decrease for the subset with initial scores between 10 and 21 was not. (3, 6)

Clinical Study: Neuroplant® 300

Extract name	WS 5572
Manufacturer	Dr. Willmar Schwabe GmbH & Co., Germany

Indication	**Depression**
Level of evidence	I
Therapeutic benefit	**Yes**

Bibliographic reference
Kalb R, Trautmann-Sponsel RD, Kieser M (2001). Efficacy and tolerability of hypericum extract WS 5572 versus placebo in mildly to moderately depressed patients. A randomized, double-blind, multicenter clinical trial. *Pharmacopsychiatry* 34 (3): 96-103.

Trial design
Parallel. Study was preceded by a three- to seven-day (three days in patients without premedication, seven days in patients with premedication), single-blind, placebo run-in phase.

Study duration	6 weeks
Dose	3 (300 mg) hypericum tablets daily
Route of administration	Oral
Randomized	Yes

Randomization adequate	Yes
Blinding	Double-blind
Blinding adequate	Yes
Placebo	Yes
Drug comparison	No
Site description	Multicenter
No. of subjects enrolled	72
No. of subjects completed	65
Sex	Male and female
Age	24-70 years (mean: 48.5)

Inclusion criteria

Outpatients between 18 and 65 years of age; total score for the Hamilton Rating Scale for Depression (HAM-D, 17-item version) of at least 16 at study entry and during subsequent baseline investigation (three to seven days later); diagnosis of mild or moderate major depressive disorder with single or recurrent episodes according to DSM-IV criteria (diagnostic codes 296.21, 296.31, 296.22, or 296.32).

Exclusion criteria

Suicidal tendency (known attempted suicide or a score of 2 or greater on item 3 [suicide] of HAM-D); organic brain syndrome; major psychiatric diseases (other than depression); disorders caused by psychotropic substances; pretreatment with fluoxetine during the last six weeks, with paroxetine or doxepin during the last two weeks before baseline; concomitant medication with other antidepressants, psychotropic drugs, or reserpine; severe metabolic, internal, or neoplastic diseases; substance abuse; pregnancy or lactation period. Concomitant medication doses required for the treatment of nonpsychiatric conditions were required to be maintained unchanged during the course of the study (where possible).

End points

HAM-D scores were assessed on days 7, 14, 28, and 42, and the differences in scores were compared to baseline. Additional end points were self-rating by patients using von Zerssen's Depression Scale (D-S), evaluation based on the Clinical Global Impressions (CGI), and the Global Patient Assessment (GPA).

Results

Patients treated with hypericum showed a larger HAM-D total score reduction between day 0 and treatment end, with superiority over placebo reaching statistical significance by days 28 ($p = 0.011$) and 42 ($p = 0.001$). The two study groups showed rates of 50 percent responders of 62.2 percent and 42.9 percent for hypericum and placebo, respectively. More pronounced differences were determined for 60 percent responders (hypericum: 51.4 percent; placebo: 17.1 percent). The total score time course of the D-S showed increasingly large treatment group differences in favor of hypericum, $p = 0.002$ (day 14), $p = 0.001$ (day 28) and $p = 0.0002$ (day 42). In CGI item 2 (global improvement) and in the global patient self-rating, more than twice as many patients were evaluated as very much improved under hypericum extract than in the placebo group.

Side effects
Five adverse reactions were noted, three of which were seen in the hypericum group (bronchitis, sinusitis, influenza). These were not considered to be related to the treatment.

Authors' comments
The data substantiate the superior antidepressant efficacy of *Hypericum* extract WS 5572 versus placebo in the treatment of mild to moderate depression. With an adverse event rate comparable to placebo, the excellent benefit-risk ratio is impressive.

Reviewers' comments
This is a well-conducted trial in which *Hypericum* performed better than placebo. (5, 6)

Clinical Study: Neuroplant®

Extract name	WS 5572
Manufacturer	Spitzner Arzneimittelfabrik/ Pharmaceutical, Germany (Dr. Willmar Schwabe GmbH & Co., Germany)

Indication	**Depression**
Level of evidence	**III**
Therapeutic benefit	**Undetermined**

Bibliographic reference
Reh C, Laux P, Schenk N (1992). *Hypericum* extract in depressions—An effective alternative. *Therapiewoche* 42: 1576-1581.

Trial design
Parallel. Pretrial washout phase of two weeks.

Study duration	2 months
Dose	2 capsules

Route of administration	Oral
Randomized	Yes
Randomization adequate	No
Blinding	Double-blind
Blinding adequate	Yes
Placebo	Yes
Drug comparison	No
Site description	Not described
No. of subjects enrolled	50
No. of subjects completed	50
Sex	Male and female
Age	Mean: 48.3 ± 8.1 years

Inclusion criteria
Mild to medium severe depression according to ICD classifications 300.4 (neurotic depression), 309.0 (short-term depression), and 311.0 (different, non-classifiable depressive symptoms); and Hamilton Depression Scale (HAM-D) scores between 13 and 25 points. Treatment of accompanying pathological conditions was continued unchanged. In cases of preceding treatment with psychotropic drugs, medication was discontinued two weeks prior to trial start.

Exclusion criteria
Patients suffering from severe or chronic depression, disclosing an attempted suicide in their patient history, as well as patients with severe organic damage were not included in the study.

End points
The following tests were used to monitor patients before and after two, four, six, and eight weeks of treatment: HAM-D, Hamilton Anxiety Scale (HAM-A), Depressivity Scale according to von Zerssen (D-S), and the Clinical Global Impressions scale (CGI). Efficacy and tolerance were also recorded by the patients at each monitoring date. Responder criteria for the HAM-D scale was a reduction in score by at least 50 percent or a final score of 10 or less.

Results
After eight weeks of treatment, the total HAM-D score was reduced by 70 percent in the hypericum group and by 45 percent in the placebo group (significant difference $p < 0.05$). In addition, 80 percent of the hypericum group versus 44 percent of the placebo group had achieved a HAM-D score of less than 10 (significant difference $p < 0.02$). The most positively influenced aspects were depressive instability, disturbances falling or remaining asleep, and work or other activities. The HAM-A scale showed similar results, with

the symptom "mental anxiety" showing particular improvement in the hypericum group. The D-S and the CGI scale also yielded results similar to the HAM-D scale.

Side effects
No adverse drug reactions occurred during the trial.

Authors' comments
Therapy with this St. John's wort extract represents an effective and low-risk alternative to synthetic antidepressants for patients who usually complain only of mild to medium severe conditions of emotional instability, particularly in the case of first treatment where ambulant, depressive patients are concerned.

Reviewers' comments
This is a longer trial than other studies, but the inclusion/exclusion criteria were not clear and the statistical methods were not described adequately. Overall, insufficient information exists to replicate the study. (2, 3)

Clinical Study: Neuroplant® forte

Extract name	WS 5572
Manufacturer	Dr. Willmar Schwabe GmbH & Co., Germany
Indication	**Depression/electrophysiological effects**
Level of evidence	**II**
Therapeutic benefit	**Trend**

Bibliographic reference
Woelk H, Johnson D, Frauendorf A, Ksciuk H, Sauerwein-Geisse E (1996). Study to evaluate the effects of Neuroplant forte (extr. *Hypericum perforatum* L., St. John's wort) compared to trimipramine on cerebral activity in depressed patients. Internal report.

Trial design
Parallel. After a one-week run-in phase, patients took hypericum or trimipramine (2 × 12.5 mg daily) for six weeks, followed by one-week postobservation period, after which a final control was performed.

Study duration	6 weeks
Dose	2 (112-138 mg extract, 0.5 mg total hypericin) capsules daily

Route of administration   Oral

Randomized   Yes
Randomization adequate   No
Blinding   Double-blind
Blinding adequate   No

Placebo   No
Drug comparison   Yes
Drug name   Trimipramine

Site description   Single center

No. of subjects enrolled   48
No. of subjects completed 48
Sex   Male and female
Age   Mean: 48 years

Inclusion criteria
Patients were at least 18 years of age and had a history of depression; mild to moderately depressed patients according to DSM-III-R (296.21, 296.22, 296.31, 296.32).

Exclusion criteria
Patients with endogenic or pharmacogenic depressions; patients who received any prescribed systemic or topical medications within two weeks of the study; alcoholic consumption greater than 100 g alcohol/week or 10 g/day; systemic or topical nonprescription medications within 48 hours of the study; participation in a clinical trial within three months; a history of alcohol or chemical/drug abuse; clinically important psychiatric illness other than depression; serious hepatic, biliary, renal, cardiac, or metabolic disorder; another clinically important illness within two weeks of the study; drug allergies, asthma, or a general history of allergic reactions; pregnant or lactating women; women without adequate contraception; acute deliria; heavily disturbed conduction; MAO inhibitor use; patients with a known history of attempted suicide or a value of 4 on the Hamilton Depression Scale (HAM-D) scale, point 3; and patients with narrow-angle glaucoma.

End points
Assessments were made at baseline and after two, four, six, and seven weeks. Efficacy was measured by changes in latency of visually and acoustically evoked potentials (VEP, AEP), changes in EEG spectra, and psychometric tests (HAM-D, Clinical Global Impressions [CGI] scale, Befindlichkeits-skala [Bf-S], State Trait Anxiety Inventory [STAI], and other tests). Safety was evaluated by measurements of blood, circulatory, and urine parameters.

Results
Results from the EEG and cortical evoked potentials indicated an improvement in cortical function with Neuroplant forte, that is, after two weeks a decrease in power in the alpha range (activation) under resting and controlled vigilance. No significant effect on the beta range was measured. Trimipramine showed an increase in the alpha (relaxation) range and a decrease in the delta and gamma ranges. Trimipramine showed a latency increase in AEP on the component P200 after four weeks of treatment (minimal effect) and a latency decrease for one component of the VEP (N270) after six weeks. Neuroplant forte showed no effect on AEPs or VEPs. Under the HAM-D test and the CGI scale, significant improvement was seen in both treatment groups. Initial HAM-D scores of 13.0 (trimipramine) and 11.2 (Neuroplant forte) dropped to 7.9 and 7.7, respectively, with no significant difference between groups before or after treatment. Both groups made fewer mistakes under monotone stress conditions with the MackWorth Clock.

Side effects
No clinically relevant side effects were measured.

Authors' comments
Neuroplant forte appears to show mild central effects corresponding to antidepressant activity at low dose, i.e., central nervous system (CNS) activation under vigilance and resting conditions. These are seen after two to six weeks. The subjective state was stable during the study period or improved. Neuroplant forte even showed superiority to trimipramine in the EEG and some psychometric parameters such as anxiety reduction, sleep, and general mental state.

Reviewers' comments
Neuroplant forte had similar antidepressant effects to the low dose of trimipramine in this small study. (5, 5)

Clinical Study: WS 5572

Extract name	WS 5572
Manufacturer	Dr. Willmar Schwabe GmbH & Co., Germany
Indication	**Electrophysiological effects** in healthy volunteers
Level of evidence	**II**
Therapeutic benefit	**MOA**

Bibliographic reference
Schellenberg R, Sauer S, Dimpfel W (1998). Pharmacodynamic effects of two different hypericum extracts in healthy volunteers measured by quantitative EEG. *Pharmacopsychiatry* 31 (Suppl. 1): 44-53.

Trial design
Parallel. WS 5573 (0.5 percent hyperforin) was compared to WS 5572 (5 percent hyperforin) and placebo.

Study duration	8 days
Dose	900 mg daily of either WS 5573 or WS 5572
Route of administration	Oral
Randomized	Yes
Randomization adequate	No
Blinding	Double-blind
Blinding adequate	Yes
Placebo	Yes
Drug comparison	Yes
Drug name	WS 5573
Site description	Not described
No. of subjects enrolled	55
No. of subjects completed	53
Sex	Male and female
Age	18-35 years

Inclusion criteria
Healthy volunteers free of any concomitant medication, except for oral contraceptives, for two weeks prior to entering the study, and negative drug and alcohol tests.

Exclusion criteria
Volunteers with pathological findings of any kind, clinically relevant diseases, or a history of serious physical illness were excluded from the study.

End points
Quantitative topographic electroencephalography (qEEG) was performed on days 1 and 8, prior to application of the trial medication and two, four, six, eight, and ten hours after administration. Immediately prior to each qEEG recording, blood pressure and heart rate were measured and blood samples were taken.

Results

The qEEG results of both WS 5572 and WS 5573 showed power increases in the delta, theta, and alpha-1 frequency bands compared to placebo. A peak effect was seen between four and eight hours after administration. The extract containing 5 percent hyperforin produced higher increases in qEEG baseline power performances than the one containing 0.5 percent hyperforin. Compared to placebo, there was a significant increase in qEEG power performance in the delta and beta-1 frequency exclusively for the extract containing 5 percent hyperforin. The effect on theta and alpha-1 frequencies was stronger on day 8 than on day 1. Following the first dose of the 5.0 percent extract, the maximum concentration was attained after 2.9 hours (Tmax). Tmax after administration of the 0.5 percent extract was 3.9 hours. On day 8, Tmax for both extracts was three hours. Pharmacokinetic data and EEG power values did not correlate.

Side effects

None that could be attributable to the trial medication.

Authors' comments

It may be concluded that extracts of St. John's Wort induce significant line-dependent changes in the electrical power performance of lower frequencies in the qEEG, and that repetitive, once-daily administration leads to stabilization of their effects, in particular with the extract containing 5 percent hyperforin. However, the relationship between acute EEG effects of antidepressants and clinical effectiveness is far from understood.

Reviewers' comments

This was a mode-of-action study that demonstrated the central effects of an extract standardized to 5 percent hyperforin compared to 0.5 percent hyperforin and placebo. (3, 6)

Clinical Study: WS 5570

Extract name	WS 5570
Manufacturer	Dr. Willmar Schwabe GmbH & Co., Germany
Indication	**Neuroendocrine effects** in healthy volunteers
Level of evidence	III
Therapeutic benefit	**MOA**

Bibliographic reference
Schüle C, Baghai T, Ferrera A, Laakmann G (2001). Neuroendocrine effects of *Hypericum* extract WS 5570 in 12 healthy male volunteers. *Pharmacopsychiatry* 34 (Suppl. 1): S127-S133.

Trial design
Crossover. On three different test days, subjects were given either placebo, 300 mg WS 5570, or 600 mg WS 5570. Subjects were instructed not to consume alcohol in the 24 hours before each test and to abstain from medication beginning four weeks before the study start.

Study duration	1 day
Dose	300 or 600 mg
Route of administration	Oral
Randomized	Yes
Randomization adequate	No
Blinding	Not described
Blinding adequate	No
Placebo	Yes
Drug comparison	No
Site description	Laboratory
No. of subjects enrolled	12
No. of subjects completed	12
Sex	Male
Age	Between 20 and 35 years

Inclusion criteria
Healthy subjects (determined via psychiatric and medical history, physical examination, and laboratory parameters) between 20 and 35 years of age with normal weight.

Exclusion criteria
None mentioned.

End points
After fasting overnight, subjects were fitted with an intravenous catheter kept open with physiological saline solution. Blood was drawn one hour before and at the time of administration of treatment or placebo as well as every 30 minutes thereafter for up to five hours. Primary end points included plasma concentrations of cortisol (COR), growth hormone (GH), and prolactin (PRL). Blood pressure, heart rate, and side effects were also recorded every half hour.

Results

The 300 mg dose of WS 5570 and placebo had no effect on COR levels. However, the 600 mg dose WS 5570 caused a clear-cut stimulation of COR secretion between 30 and 90 minutes after treatment application. A significant difference in comparison to placebo appeared after 30 minutes ($p < 0.05$), and significance increased until 90 minutes ($p < 0.01$). The area under the curve for GH was significantly greater for the 300 mg WS 5570 group compared to placebo ($p < 0.05$). The 600 mg dose produced levels of GH comparable to placebo. WS 5570 did not have any influence on PRL secretion. There was also no influence on blood pressure or heart rate.

Side effects

No side effects occurred during the study.

Authors' comments

The cortisol stimulation caused by 600 mg WS 5570 suggests that the extract is able to influence noradrenalin reuptake and serotonin reuptake, thereby causing the effects on cortisol release. The best explanation for the significant elevation of growth hormone values after 300 mg of WS 5570 compared to placebo is that the elevation was caused by spontaneous episodes of growth hormone hypersecretion in 2 of the 12 volunteers. We could not replicate the findings of Franklin et al. (1999) that Saint John's wort extracts may stimulate GH release and inhibit PRL secretion. The reason for these conflicting results is probably the fact that the dosages given to the male volunteers differed to a considerable extent (300 and 600 mg in our study; 2,700 mg in Franklin et al. [1999]).

Reviewers' comments

This mode-of-action study is similar to Franklin et al. (1999), but with different results. (1, 6)

Product Profile: St. John's Wort Ze 117™

Manufacturer	**Zeller AG, Switzerland**
U.S. distributor	**General Nutrition Corporation**
Botanical ingredient	**St. John's wort flowering tops extract**
Extract name	**Ze 117**
Quantity	500 mg
Processing	Plant to extract ratio 4-7:1, ethanol 50% (w/w)
Standardization	0.2% hypericin, less than or equal to 0.2% hyperforin
Formulation	Tablet

Recommended dose: Take one tablet daily.

Cautions: May cause skin sensitivity. Care should be taken during exposure to sunlight. Avoid excessive UV sources and discontinue use if sensitivity occurs.

Other ingredients: Cellulose, titanium dioxide (natural mineral whitener), ferric oxide (colorant).

Comments: Ze 117 is also sold as Remotiv and Rebalance (Zeller AG, Switzerland); Valverde Hyperval (Novartis, Switzerland); Remotiv (Bayer, Germany/Hungary/South America); Esbericum forte (Schaper and Brümmer, Germany).

Source(s) of information: Woelk, 2000; Schrader, 2000; Brattström, 2002; product label; personal correspondence with manufacturer.

Product Profile: St. John's Wort (Ze 117™)

Manufacturer	**Zeller AG, Switzerland**
U.S. distributor	**Rexall Sundown, Inc.**
Botanical ingredient	**St. John's wort flowering tops extract**
Extract name	**Ze 117**
Quantity	500 mg
Processing	Plant to extract ratio 4-7:1, ethanol 50% (w/w)
Standardization	0.2% hypericin, less than or equal to 0.2% hyperforin
Formulation	Caplet

Recommended dose: One caplet per day.

DSHEA structure/function: Advanced mood enhancement.

Cautions: Do not use this product if you are pregnant or nursing. If you are under a physician's care or taking medication, consult with your health professional before using this product. Do not take with antidepressant medications. May cause skin sensitivity. Care should be taken during exposure to sunlight. Avoid excessive UV sources and discontinue use if sensitivity develops. Discontinue use two weeks prior to surgery.

Other ingredients: Microcrystalline cellulose, croscarmellose sodium, hydroxypropyl methylcellulose, PEG, titanium dioxide (color), madgesium stearate, ferric oxide (color), stearic acid, silica.

Comments: Ze 117 is also sold as: Remotiv® (Zeller AG, Switzerland); Valverde Hyperval (Novartis, Switzerland); Remotiv® (Bayer, Germany/Hungary/South America); Esbericum forte (Schaper and Brümmer, Germany).

Source(s) of information: Woelk, 2000; Schrader, 2000; Brattström, 2002; product label; personal correspondence with manufacturer.

Clinical Study: Ze 117™

Extract name	Ze 117
Manufacturer	Zeller AG, Switzerland
Indication	**Depression**
Level of evidence	**I**
Therapeutic benefit	**Yes**

Bibliographic reference
Schrader E, Meier B, Brattström A (1998). *Hypericum* treatment of mild-moderate depression in a placebo-controlled study: A prospective, double-blind, randomized, placebo-controlled, multicenter study. *Human Psychopharmacology* 13 (3): 163-169.

Trial design
Parallel.

Study duration	6 weeks
Dose	2 (250 mg) tablets daily
Route of administration	Oral
Randomized	Yes
Randomization adequate	Yes
Blinding	Double-blind
Blinding adequate	Yes
Placebo	Yes
Drug comparison	No
Site description	16 centers
No. of subjects enrolled	162
No. of subjects completed	136
Sex	Male and female
Age	30-60 years

Inclusion criteria

Patients over the age of 18 presenting with mild-moderate depression defined according to ICD-10 (F32.0; F32.1) and who had total scores between 16 and 24 on the Hamilton Depression Scale (HAM-D) were admitted to the study. Medication that might interfere with the trial medication was withdrawn one week prior to the start of the study, extended to four weeks for patients taking fluoxetine. Any preexisting therapy that could not be discontinued was maintained at the same dosage.

Exclusion criteria

Patients who had taken part in other clinical trials in the previous four weeks or during the study itself, psychiatric disorders that might impair accurate history, those unable to give consent, the presence of neoplasia, Parkinson's or Alzheimer's disease, pregnancy or inadequate contraception, risk of suicide (score of at least 2 on the suicidality item of HAM-D), known hypersensitivity to St. John's wort, severe concomitant systemic diseases, chronic alcohol or drug abuse, and concomitant psychotherapy or drug therapy that could influence the assessment of efficacy variables.

End points

Patients were assessed after one, two, three, four, and six weeks with the 21-item HAM-D, the Clinical Global Impressions (CGI) scale, and patient self-assessment on a visual analogue scale (VAS). Criteria for clinically relevant response were a reduction of at least 50 percent in HAM-D score from baseline and/or a score of 10 or less on the final HAM-D.

Results

Both intention-to-treat and protocol-compliant analysis showed that treatment with Ze 117 was associated with significantly superior efficacy than placebo ($p < 0.001$). The responder rate on the HAM-D test was 56 percent with Ze 117 and 15 percent with placebo. A significant difference between the two treatment arms in the CGI and patient self-rated VAS ($p < 0.001$) was also observed.

Side effects

Adverse events occurred in five placebo patients and six hypericum patients. The most common were nonspecific gastrointestinal problems.

Authors' comments

This clinical study, involving a sufficiently large sample size to allow robust statistical evaluation, demonstrated that the hypericum extract (Ze 117) is a safe and effective treatment for mild to moderate depressive episodes. Further clinical trials will be required to evaluate conclusively the efficacy of hypericum in more severe depression.

Reviewers' comments
This was a good intent-to-treat study with protocol-compliant analysis and adequate washout. The treatment was better than placebo, with few side effects for treatment of mild to moderate major depression. (5, 6)

Clinical Study: Remotiv®

Extract name	Ze 117
Manufacturer	Zeller AG, Switzerland
Indication	**Depression**
Level of evidence	I
Therapeutic benefit	**Yes**

Bibliographic reference
Woelk H (2000). Comparison of St. John's wort and imipramine for treating depression: Randomised controlled trial. *British Medical Journal* 321 (7260): 536-539.

Trial design
Parallel. To ensure that participants could tolerate imipramine, the dose was increased from 25 mg twice daily (three days) to 50 mg twice daily (four days), and then to the final dose of 75 mg twice daily on the eighth day.

Study duration	6 weeks
Dose	2 × 250 mg hypericum
Route of administration	Oral
Randomized	Yes
Randomization adequate	Yes
Blinding	Double-blind
Blinding adequate	Yes
Placebo	No
Drug comparison	Yes
Drug name	Imipramine
Site description	40 outpatient clinics
No. of subjects enrolled	324
No. of subjects completed	277
Sex	Male and female
Age	Mean: 46 ± 12.8 years

Inclusion criteria

Participants ages 18 or older, with mild to moderate depression, without increased suicidal ideation, who fulfilled ICD-10 criteria for a depressive episode or recurrent depressive disorder (ICD-10 codes F32.0 or F33.0 and F32.1 or F33.1), and had a score of at least 18 on the 17-item Hamilton Depression Scale (HAM-D) on two consecutive visits.

Exclusion criteria

Pregnant or breast feeding, not using contraception, known to be allergic to the drugs being studied, serious disease, abnormal thyroid function, other relevant abnormalities, bipolar disorder, previous serious psychiatric disease, or alcohol or drug abuse histories. Participants who had taken any of the following medications within two weeks of the trial start: monoamine oxidase inhibitors, antidepressant drugs, lithium, antipsychotic drugs, neuroleptic drugs, cimetidine, oral corticosteroids, anticonvulsants, theophylline, or thyroid hormones.

End points

HAM-D was completed during the screening visit, when allocated to treatment, at the third visit (week 1), fourth visit (week 3), and fifth visit (week 6). The Clinical Global Impressions (CGI) scale was completed by the clinicians during the third, fourth, and fifth visits. Participants completed a global impressions scale the first time they were seen, during treatment (third visit), and at the end of the trial (fifth visit). Benzodiazapines were allowed at a maximum daily dose of 10 mg diazepam for no longer than three consecutive days on not more than three occasions over the six-week study.

Results

The two treatments were therapeutically equivalent with regard to overall effect on depression. Among the 157 subjects taking hypericum, mean HAM-D scores decreased from 22.4 at baseline to 12.00 at end point. Among the 167 subjects taking imipramine, mean HAM-D scores fell from 22.1 to 12.75. All secondary analyses of efficacy supported the conclusions of the primary analysis, although in one exploratory parameter (the anxiety-somatization subscale of the HAM-D scale) hypericum had a significant advantage. Rates of response to treatment were essentially similar.

Side effects

Participants tolerated hypericum better than imipramine ($p < 0.01$). The most common side effect in the hypericum group (8 percent) was dry mouth.

Author's comments

Hypericum is therapeutically equivalent to imipramine, but is better tolerated by patients. In view of the mounting evidence of hypericum's comparable efficacy to other antidepressants and its safety record, hypericum should be considered for first-line treatment in mild to moderate depression, especially in the primary care setting.

Reviewers' comments
This study had a large number of participants at many sites, and the coordinators made an effort to train on HAM-D. The dose of imipramine was still on the lower end of therapeutic dose (normal therapeutic range is between 150 to 250 mg). It is also unfortunate that the report gives the HAM-D scores at baseline and week six only (not in times between). (5, 6)

Clinical Study: Ze 117™

Extract name	Ze 117
Manufacturer	Zeller AG, Switzerland
Indication	**Depression**
Level of evidence	**II**
Therapeutic benefit	**Yes**

Bibliographic reference
Schrader E (2000). Equivalence of St. John's wort extract (Ze 117) and fluoxetine: A randomized, controlled study in mild-moderate depression. *International Clinical Psychopharmacology* 15 (2): 61-68.

Trial design
Parallel. Patients received either hypericum or fluoxetine (20 mg daily). Patients treated with monoamine oxidase (MAO) inhibitors underwent a two-week washout period, which was extended to five weeks for SSRIs (selective seratonin reuptake inhibitors).

Study duration	6 weeks
Dose	1 (250 mg) hypericum tablet twice daily
Route of administration	Oral
Randomized	Yes
Randomization adequate	No
Blinding	Double-blind
Blinding adequate	Yes
Placebo	No
Drug comparison	Yes
Drug name	Fluoxetine
Site description	7 internal medicine practices

No. of subjects enrolled   240
No. of subjects completed 238
Sex   Male and female
Age   Mean: 46.5 ± 18 years

Inclusion criteria

Patients with mild to moderate depression (ICD-10; depressive episode/ recurrent depressive disorder; F32.0 mild; F32.1 moderate) with entry Hamilton Depressive Scale (HAM-D) 21-item scores in the range of 16 to 24.

Exclusion criteria

Excluded from the study were patients with a history of alcohol/substance abuse or dependence; dementia or other severe intellectual impairment; history of seizures; glaucoma; pituitary deficiency; suicidal ideation (score 2 to 4 on HAM-D item 3); thyroid or parathyroid pathology; Parkinson's disease; pregnant or breast-feeding women; any serious concomitant medical condition; or patients taking quinidine, anticholinergic drugs, cimetidine, cardiac glycosides, neuroleptics, sympathomimetic drugs, MAO inhibitors, tryptophan, and any other antidepressant.

End points

The 21-item HAM-D and Clinical Global Impression (CGI) (item 1) tests, as well as the patient self-evaluation test, were conducted at baseline and at the end of the study. CGI items 2 and 3 were evaluated at end point. Other assessments were patients' self-assessment by a validated visual analogue scale, withdrawal rates, and incidence of adverse events. Responders were those with at least a 50 percent decrease from baseline or final score of 10 or less on the HAM-D. The protocol hypothesis was that hypericum would be considered equivalent to fluoxetine if an improvement in mean HAM-D score for the hypericum group was within 3 points of the improvement observed on the fluoxetine group at end point (alpha = 0.05, one-sided).

Results

Analysis of the main efficacy variable rejected the hypothesis of hypericum being inferior to fluoxetine. In the analysis of secondary variables, a trend was observed in favor of hypericum relative to fluoxetine in improving overall HAM-D ($p = 0.09$), and CGI item I ($p = 0.03$) Similarity of effects of the two treatments was observed in most other parameters. The responder rate for hypericum was significantly greater ($p = 0.005$) than for fluoxetine (60 percent versus 40 percent, respectively).

Side effects

Thirty-four adverse events possibly related to fluoxetine and 13 to hypericum occurred. The most common for hypericum was gastrointestinal disturbance.

Author's comments

Hypericum and fluoxetine are equipotent with respect to all main parameters used to investigate antidepressants in this population. The main difference between the two treatments is safety. *Hypericum* was superior to fluoxetine in overall incidence of side effects, number of side effects, and the type of side effect reported.

Reviewers' comments

This was a strong study using a therapeutic dose of SSRI with a good washout period from other medications. Overall a good study with *Hypericum* equivalent to fluoxetine (Prozac), but with fewer side effects. The randomization process was not described. (3, 6)

Product Profile: Hyperiforce

Manufacturer	**Bioforce AG, Switzerland**
U.S. distributor	None
Botanical ingredient	**St. John's wort aerial parts (shoots and tips) extract**
Extract name	None given
Quantity	40-73 mg
Processing	Extract of the fresh plant, ratio 3.9-5.0:1, 60% alcohol
Standardization	0.33 mg dianthrones (total hypericin)
Formulation	Tablet

Recommended dose: Take one tablet three times daily.

Other ingredients: Microcrystalline cellulose, corn starch, polysaccharide of soy, oil (1.3 mg).

Source(s) of information: Information provided by Bioforce USA.

Clinical Study: Hyperiforce

Extract name	None given
Manufacturer	Bioforce AG, Switzerland
Indication	**Depression**
Level of evidence	**II**
Therapeutic benefit	**Undetermined**

Bibliographic reference
Lenoir S, Degenring FH, Saller R (1997). Hyperiforce tablets for the treatment of mild to moderate depression. *Schweizerische Zeitschrift für Ganzheits Medizin* 9 (5): 226-232.

Trial design
Parallel. Dose comparison study with tablets containing one-sixth, one-third, or the usual amount of the same crude extract.

Study duration	6 weeks
Dose	3 tablets providing either 1.0, 0.33, or 0.16 mg hypericin per day in either 180, 60, or 30 mg extract
Route of administration	Oral
Randomized	Yes
Randomization adequate	No
Blinding	Double-blind
Blinding adequate	Yes
Placebo	No
Drug comparison	No
Site description	38 centers
No. of subjects enrolled	348
No. of subjects completed	260
Sex	Male and female
Age	19-94 years

Inclusion criteria
Patients with mild to moderate depression (HAM-D score ≥ 10) of at least 20 years of age, with an initial diagnosis in accordance with ICD-10 criteria of: depressive episodes, recurrent depressive disorder, persistent affective disorder, anxiety disorder, stress and adjustment disorder, and other conditions with accompanying affective mood disorders.

Exclusion criteria
Allergy to St. John's wort; treatment with antidepressants, tranquilizers, hypnotics, or neuroleptics within the last two weeks prior to the study; or acute risk of suicide.

End points
Assessments were made at baseline and after one and six weeks of treatment with the Hamilton Depression Scale (HAM-D)-17 and -21 scores, by the physician with the Clinical Global Impressions (CGI) scale, and with a self-

assessment by the patient using the HAD (Hospital Anxiety and Depression) scale.

Results

During the course of the six weeks of treatment, the HAM-D-17 score decreased appreciably in all three groups ($p < 0.001$). Related efficacy was about 4 percent better in the highest dose group than in the group receiving the lowest dose (no significant difference). The response rate established on the basis of the HAM-D score was about 39 percent after 14 days, and 62 to 68 percent by the end of the treatment period. In the assessment of the physicians, severity of the disease (CGI scale) decreased on average from moderate to marked before treatment to mild at the end of treatment. Self-assessment scores of the patients for anxiety and depression (HAD) decreased appreciably in all three treatment groups.

Side effects

In the assessment of the physicians, tolerability was good, namely 84 percent (high dose), 95 percent (medium dose), and 90 percent (low dose), with no clear differences between the doses. Eighty-two events were observed in 74 patients affecting the nervous system, gastrointestinal tract, and general well-being. An increase in events of "questionable" causality was seen in the high dose group, but no difference in effects of "possible" or "probable" causality was observed.

Authors' comments

The response rates of between 62 and 68 percent, including that of the lowest daily dose of 0.17 mg hypericin, were better than the 55 percent reported by other hypericum studies employing 0.5 to 2.7 mg hypericin/day. It is possible that this reflects the advantage of using only the fresh shoot tips of St. John's wort. On the basis of these results, it may be recommended that treatment with Hyperiforce tablets could be started at a dose of one tablet three times a day, and then continued over the long term with one to two tablets per day.

Reviewers' comments

The study was flawed by the lack of a placebo group. The placebo comparison, which is important when comparing different doses of the same preparation, was especially important because of the authors' unusual findings that no statistical differences existed between the doses. In addition, no description was provided of how patients were randomized. (3, 6)

Product Profile: STEI 300

Manufacturer	**Steiner Arzneimittel, Germany**
U.S. distributor	None
Botanical ingredient	**St. John's wort extract**
Extract name	**STEI 300**
Quantity	350 mg
Processing	Extracted with 60% ethanol (w/w)
Standardization	0.2%-0.3% hypericin and pseudohypericin and 2%-3% hyperforin
Formulation	Capsule

Source(s) of information: Philipp, Kohnen, and Hiller, 1999.

Clinical Study: STEI 300

Extract name	STEI 300
Manufacturer	Steiner Arzneimittel, Germany
Indication	**Depression**
Level of evidence	**II**
Therapeutic benefit	**Yes**

Bibliographic reference
Philipp M, Kohnen R, Hiller KO (1999). *Hypericum* extract versus imipramine or placebo in patients with moderate depression: Randomised multicenter study of treatment for eight weeks. *British Medical Journal* 319 (7224): 1534-1538.

Trial design
Parallel. Trial was preceded by a one-week washout period. *Hypericum* was given in a constant dose of 1,050 mg/day throughout the study. Imipramine doses were increased from 50 mg on day 1, to 75 mg (days 2 through 4), and to 100 mg thereafter.

Study duration	8 weeks
Dose	1,050 mg daily
Route of administration	Oral
Randomized	Yes
Randomization adequate	Yes

Blinding	Double-blind
Blinding adequate	Yes
Placebo	Yes
Drug comparison	Yes
Drug name	Imipramine
Site description	18 general practices
No. of subjects enrolled	263
No. of subjects completed	251
Sex	Male and female
Age	Mean: 47 ± 12 years

Inclusion criteria
Patients ages 18 to 65 with a diagnosis of moderate depressive according to ICD-10 codes F32.1 and F33.1; minimum score of 18 on the Hamilton Depression scale (HAM-D), Clinical Global Impressions (CGI) rating of severity of moderately, markedly, or severely ill; minimum depression duration of four weeks and maximum of two years.

Exclusion criteria
Mild and severe depressive disorders; bipolar disorders; comorbidity from alcohol or drug dependence; suicidal risk; long-term prophylaxis with lithium or carbamazepine; nonsufficient washout phase of previous psychotropic drug; any interfering psychotropic drug taken concurrently; any previous long-term (> 3 months) treatment with benzodiazapines; and patients at general and specific risk (imipramine contraindications).

End points
Efficacy and safety were evaluated after one, two, four, six, and eight weeks with the 17-item HAM-D, the Hamilton Anxiety scale (HAM-A), the CGI scale, Zung self-rating depression scale (ZSDS), and quality of life was determined using the 36-item short form health survey (SF-36). The hypericum group was compared to placebo after six weeks and to imipramine after eight weeks. Data for evaluation of safety comprised of adverse events, clinically relevant changes in electrocardiogram, measurements of vital signs, and physical examination.

Results
Hypericum extract was more effective at reducing HAM-D scores than placebo, and as effective as imipramine (mean −15.4, −12.1 and −14.2, respectively). The HAM-A, ZSDS, and SF-36 had similar results to those obtained with the HAM-D. Compared with placebo (50 percent), the number of patients who improved in the CGI was noticeably higher under active treatments: 74 percent in the hypericum group and 71 percent in the imipramine group.

Side effects

Adverse events were reported for 22 percent of the hypericum group, compared with 19 percent for placebo and 46 percent for the imipramine group. The most frequent (8 percent) side effect in the hypericum group was nausea.

Authors' comments

Hypericum extract, 350 mg three times daily, was more effective than placebo, and at least equally effective to 100 mg imipramine daily, in the treatment of moderate depression. Treatment with hypericum extract is safe and improves the quality of life.

Reviewers' comments

This is a good study, but unfortunately a low dose (subtherapeutic) of imipramine was used. Also the report did not specify the number of dropouts/withdrawals. (4, 6)

Product Profile: Dysto-lux®

Manufacturer	**Dr. Loges & Co. GmbH, Germany**
U.S. distributor	None
Botanical ingredient	**St. John's wort extract**
Extract name	**LoHyp-57**
Quantity	200 mg
Processing	Plant to extract ratio 5-7:1, ethanol 60% (w/w)
Standardization	No information
Formulation	Tablet

Source(s) of information: Harrer et al., 1999.

Clinical Study: Dysto-lux®

Extract name	LoHyp-57
Manufacturer	Dr. Loges & Co. GmbH, Germany
Indication	**Depression in elderly patients**
Level of evidence	**II**
Therapeutic benefit	**Yes**

Bibliographic reference

Harrer G, Schmidt U, Kuhn U, Biller A (1999). Comparison of equivalence between the St. John's wort extract LoHyp-57 and fluoxetine. *Arzneimittel-Forschung/Drug Research* 49 (4): 289-296.

Trial design

Parallel. Patients received either hypericum or fluoxetine (20 mg daily).

Study duration	6 weeks
Dose	2 (200 mg) tablets twice daily
Route of administration	Oral
Randomized	Yes
Randomization adequate	Yes
Blinding	Double-blind
Blinding adequate	Yes
Placebo	No
Drug comparison	Yes
Drug name	Fluoxetine
Site description	17 centers
No. of subjects enrolled	161
No. of subjects completed	137
Sex	Male and female
Age	Mean: 69 years

Inclusion criteria

Patients ages 60 to 80, suffering from their first psychiatric illness, with symptoms diagnosed as F32.0 and F32.1 according to the ICD-10.

Exclusion criteria

Patients with a dementia disorder according to the Mini Mental Status Test.

End points

Hamilton Global 17-item (HAM-D-17) scores were determined on entry to the study and at the end of one, two, four, and six weeks of treatment. Responders were defined as patients who decreased their HAM-D score by at least 50 percent or to below 10. Secondary target parameters were the Self-rating Depression Scale (SDS), the Everyday Life questionnaire (AL), and the Clinical Global Impressions scale (CGI). At all visits, doctors and patients were asked to provide assessment of efficacy and tolerability, patient satisfaction with the medication, and adverse events.

Results

During the six-week treatment, HAM-D scores fell in both groups, from

16.60 to 7.91 in the hypericum group, and from 17.18 to 8.11 in the fluoxetine group. In patients with mild depression, scores showed a mean fall from 14.21 to 6.21 on LoHyp-57, and from 15.21 to 7.46 on fluoxetine. In patients with moderate depression, mean scores fell from 18.73 to 9.43 on LoHyp-57, and from 19.10 to 8.75 on fluoxetine. Equivalence of the two treatments was confirmed for both the total sample and for the two subgroups. At the end of week 6, the response rate in the LoHyp-57 group was 71.4 percent, whereas it was 72.2 percent in the fluoxetine group. CGI and SDS data support the HAM-D findings.

Side effects
Twelve patients in the hypericum group and 17 patients in the fluoxetine group reported adverse events.

Authors' comments
The St. John's wort extract LoHyp-57 was found to be both statistically and clinically equivalent to fluoxetine in its efficacy in the sample of elderly patients investigated here. For elderly patients who often have multiple pathologies and are consequently subjected to multiple drug treatments, hypericum has the advantage over the tricyclics and SSRIs in that it does not cause drug interactions.

Reviewers' comments
This good trial included severity in relation to side effects and used well-trained examiners at all sites. However, the authors did not give actual HAM-D scores as allowance for comparison, and thus readers can only compare response rate (which does not allow enough information). In addition, it is unclear whether patients with any coexisting psychiatric medical treatment were excluded. (5, 5)

Valerian

Other common names: **Garden heliotrope, garden valerian**
Latin name: *Valeriana officinalis* **L.** [Valerianaceae]
Latin synonyms: *Valeriana exaltata* **J.C. Mikan**
Plant part: **Root**

PREPARATIONS USED
IN REVIEWED CLINICAL STUDIES

Valerian species grow worldwide. The root (or more precisely the underground parts including the rhizome, roots, and stolons) of European valerian, *Valeriana officinalis* L., is used as an official drug in many European countries. There is no scientific agreement regarding valerian's active constituents, but sesquiterpenes, valerenic acid, and acetoxyvalerenic acid have been used as quality control markers, usually described simply as valerenic acid. Pharmaceutical products are produced mainly from aqueous extracts or aqueous alcoholic extracts. The two extract types are not equivalent. The aqueous extracts are based on traditional teas with an herb to extract ratio of 5:1 (2 g herb resulting in 400 mg extract). Aqueous alcoholic extracts are often made with 70 percent ethanol, and have an herb to extract ratio of 4 to 7:1 (Schulz, Hänsel, and Tyler, 2001).

Valerian products are commonly formulated with lemon balm, hops, or passionflower. In fact, the German Commission E has approved the use of combinations in fixed proportions of passionflower herb, valerian root, and lemon balm, as well as valerian with hops (see the Information from Pharmacopoeial Monographs section) (Blumenthal et al., 1998).

Sedonium™, manufactured by Lichtwer Pharma GmbH, Germany, and distributed in the United States by Lichtwer Pharma U.S., Inc., contains an aqueous alcoholic valerian extract named LI 156 (ratio 3 to 7:1, 300 mg extract/tablet).

VALERIAN SUMMARY TABLE

Product Name	Manufacturer/ U.S. Distributor	Product Characteristics	Dose in Trials	Indication	No. of Trials	Benefit (Evidence Level-Trial No.)
Single Ingredient Products						
Sedonium™	Lichtwer Pharma AG, Germany/ Lichtwer Pharma US, Inc.	Ethanolic extract (LI 156)	2 (300 mg) tablets an hour before bed	Insomnia	4	Yes (I-2) Trend (III-1) Undetermined (III-1)
				Mental stress	1	Undetermined (III-1)
				Cognitive functioning	1	Yes (III-1)
Valdispert® (EU), Baldrian-Dispert® (EU)	Solvay Arzneimittel GmbH, Germany/ None	Aqueous alkaline dry extract	3 (135 mg extract) tablets 3 times daily	Insomnia	1	Undetermined (III-1)
				Nervous disorders	1	Undetermined (III-1)
Generic, aqueous extract	None/None	Freeze-dried aqueous extract	400 to 900 mg per day	Insomnia	1	Trend (III-1)
				Sleep quality	2	Trend (II-2) Undetermined (III-1)

Combination Products

Valerian Night-time™ (US), Euvegal® forte (EU)	Dr. Willmar Schwabe GmbH & Co., Germany/ Nature's Way Products, Inc.	Aqueous/ ethanolic extracts of valerian root and lemon balm leaf	1 to 4 (valerian: 160 mg/lemon balm: 80 mg) tablets daily	Insomnia	1	Yes (II-1)
				Sleep quality	1	Undetermined (III-1)
Songha Night® (EU)	Pharmaton S.A., Switzerland/None	Extracts of valerian root and lemon balm leaf	3 (valerian 120 mg/lemon balm: 80 mg) tablets daily	Sleep quality	1	Undetermined (II-1)
Alluna™ Sleep (US), IVEL® (EU), ReDormin® (EU)	Zeller AG, Switzerland/ GlaxoSmithKline	Extracts of valerian root and hops (Ze 91019)	1-3 (valerian 500 mg/hops 120 mg) tablets daily	Electrophysiological effects	1	MOA (III-1)

Valdispert®, or Baldrian-Dispert®, is manufactured by Solvay Arzneimittel GmbH in Germany, and is not available in the United States. It is an aqueous alcoholic extract with a ratio of 5 to 6:1. The tablets contain 135 mg extract.

Several trials were conducted with a generic aqueous extract characterized with a plant-to-extract ratio of 2.8 to 3.1:1.

A valerian and lemon balm (*Melissa officinalis* L.) product known as Valerian Nighttime™ in the United States and Euvegal® forte in Europe is manufactured by Dr. Willmar Schwabe GmbH & Co. in Germany and distributed in the United States by Nature's Way Products, Inc. Each tablet contains 160 mg valerian extract (ratio 4.5:1) and 80 mg lemon balm (ratio 5.5:1).

Another valerian (120 mg, ratio 4.5:1) and lemon balm (80 mg, ratio 5:1) product produced by Pharmaton S.A. in Switzerland is sold in Europe with the name of Songha Night®.

A valerian and hops (*Humulus lupulus* L.) combination called Alluna™ Sleep is manufactured in Switzerland by Zeller AG and distributed in the United States by GlaxoSmithKline. Each tablet contains 250 mg valerian (ratio 4 to 6:1) and 60 mg hops (ratio 5 to 7:1) extracts in a combination called Ze 91019. Ze 91019 is sold as IVEL® and ReDormin® in Europe.

SUMMARY OF REVIEWED CLINICAL STUDIES

Traditional uses for valerian products include states of tension, restlessness, irritability, unrest, and insomnia. Insomnia, is one of several sleep disorders, defined as difficulty falling asleep, difficulty sleeping through the night, frequent night awakenings, early awakening, or unrefreshing sleep. It is most commonly a transient problem of less than two weeks, but it can also be chronic. Primary insomnia is a sleeping problem not associated with any other health problem. Secondary insomnia is related to a health condition, such as depression, heartburn, cancer, asthma, pain, or related to administration of a medication or alcohol.

Sleep stages have been defined according to polysomnographic recordings, including electroencephalograms (EEG). Stage 1 sleep is the transition from drowsy wake to sleep, and Stage 2 is light sleep. Stages 3 and 4 are deep sleep, also known as slow wave or delta sleep. REM (rapid eye movement) sleep occurs in Stage 5, in which dreaming occurs. Sleep stages occur in cycles throughout the night (Pagel and Parnes, 2001).

Sedative/hypnotic agents are commonly prescribed to treat insomnia. The benzodiazepines (i.e., flurazepam, oxazepam, trizolam) are very effective at inducing sleep, but they also can suppress REM sleep, may result in dependence, and can cause hangover effects the morning after. Ethanol can assist with sleep, but can cause tolerance, dependency, and diminished sleep efficiency and quality. Antihistamines can help, but may lead to daytime sleepiness. Antidepressants have also been used with some success if the individual also has symptoms of depression (Pagel and Parnes, 2001).

We include 15 controlled clinical trials using valerian to improve sleep or reduce stress that studied both single-ingredient valerian products and valerian in combination with either lemon balm or hops. Of these studies, six were considered to be of sufficient quality to substantiate findings of subjective reports of improvement in sleep quality and/or improvements in objective measures of sleep structure.

Sedonium (LI 156)

We reviewed five studies conducted on LI 156 related to insomnia and/or stress and one study that examined morning alertness, concentration, or reaction time compared to a benzodiazepine sleep aid. Two good-quality insomnia studies indicated a significant improvement in insomnia following a dose of 600 mg for at least two weeks. A comparative study found that valerian was equal to the benzodiazepine oxazepam in treating insomnia. A pilot study compared the effects of kava and valerian on stress-induced insomnia. Another trial evaluated the effects of valerian and kava on blood pressure and heart rate before and during a mental performance task.

Insomnia

The largest sleep study with Sedonium is a double-blind, placebo-controlled trial with 117 subjects with primary (nonorganic) insomnia (according to the World Health Organization's [1992] *International Classification of Diseases,* Tenth Revision [ICD-10]) given either two tablets Sedonium (600 mg extract) or placebo one hour before bed for 28 days. According to sleep questionnaires, significant improvements were seen in the degree of insomnia, the restored feeling after sleep, and general well-being compared to placebo. Some improvement was described after 14 days, and after 28 days it was more pronounced (Vorbach, Görtelmeyer, and Brüning, 1996).

A pilot crossover trial with 16 patients, with primary insomnia, used objective measures of sleep, as recorded with polysomnographic recordings, as well as questionnaires to measure sleep efficiency. Subjects were rotated through two 14-day treatment periods of two tablets Sedonium or placebo one hour before bed. After a single dose of valerian, no significant effect was observed on sleep structure or subjective sleep assessment. After 14 days, sleep efficiency increased significantly for both groups. However, Sedonium produced a comparative reduction in slow-wave sleep latency and an increase in the percentage of time in slow-wave sleep (Stages 3 and 4) (Donath et al., 2000).

Another study with 65 primary (nonorganic, nonpsychiatric) insomniacs (as defined by ICD-10) compared the effectiveness of two tablets Sedonium to 10 mg oxazepam. According to sleep questionnaires, valerian caused an improvement in sleep quantity after one month that was equivalent to that from oxazepam (Dorn, 2000). Although the addition of a placebo group would have strengthened the evidence, the quality of the study was still considered to be good.

A pilot crossover trial included 19 subjects with stress-induced insomnia (not defined) who were treated with kava (120 mg LI 150), valerian (120 mg per day LI 156), and both kava and valerian together. Each subject received each of the three treatments for a six-week period, in the order given earlier. Each treatment was separated by a two-week washout period. The subjects assessed their degree of stress and insomnia using a subjective visual analogue scale. As a result, a significant decrease in stress was observed during the first six weeks with kava, but no subsequent change during the washout period or treatments with valerian or the combination of the two. A similar pattern was observed with insomnia, with a significant decrease with initial kava treatment and no further decrease with valerian. Here, however, there was another decrease during treatment with both kava and valerian (Wheatley, 2001). This study was neither double-blinded nor placebo-controlled. In addition, all subjects were treated in the same order, and that may have had an influence on the outcome.

Mental Stress

A parallel study with 54 healthy volunteers compared the effects of valerian to kava or no treatment on psychological stress induced under laboratory conditions. The authors of the study suggested that both preparations might be beneficial in reducing physiological reactions to stressful situations. A standardized color/word mental stress task was performed before and after seven days of treatment with valerian extract (600 mg LI 156 per day), kava extract (120 mg LI 150 per day), or nothing. Comparing the resting state of groups before and after treatment, in the valerian group there was a significant reduction in systolic blood pressure and heart rate, but an insignificant reduction in diastolic blood pressure. In the kava group, a significant reduction in diastolic blood pressure was observed. No changes occurred in the control group. Comparing the response to the stress task before and after treatment revealed significant reductions in systolic blood pressure for both the valerian and kava groups with no significant change for the control group. No change was observed in diastolic blood pressure for any group. A significant reduction in heart rate was observed in the valerian group but no change was seen in the kava or control groups. Both the valerian and kava groups reported a reduction in mental pressure following treatment both before and during the task. The control group did not indicate any change in mental pressure (Cropley et al., 2002).

Cognitive Functioning

The effect of valerian extract (LI 156) on morning alertness, concentration, and reaction time was tested in a two-part study using 91 healthy volunteers. In the first part, one dose of 600 mg LI 156 extract was compared with one dose of 1 mg flunitrazepam (a benzodiazepine) taken before bed. The next morning, reaction time and performance were decreased by flunitrazepam, but not by LI 156. In the second part of the study, valerian was compared to placebo following two weeks of treatment. No negative impact on morning alertness, concentration, or reaction time was observed (Kuhlmann et al., 1999).

Valdispert

The effectiveness of Valdispert forte, 405 mg three times daily, was deemed undetermined in two poor-quality trials with elderly persons with insomnia or nervous disorders.

Insomnia

The first was a placebo-controlled pilot study with 14 elderly patients who complained of primary insomnia. Polysomnography was conducted on three nights at one-week intervals: on an adaptation night, after one dose, and after one week of treatment. There was no effect on sleep after one dose. However, after one week, subjects in the valerian group showed an increase in slow-wave sleep (sleep Stages 3 and 4) and a decrease in sleep Stage 1 compared to baseline. There was no effect on REM sleep. There was also no difference from placebo in self-rated sleep quality (Schulz, Stolz, and Muller, 1994).

Nervous Disorders

The second study with Valdispert used 78 elderly subjects with low scores in a questionnaire measuring subjective "well-being," and with behavioral disorders. Valerian increased scores for "well-being," improved behavior, and improved sleep compared with placebo (Kamm-Kohl, Jansen, and Brockmann, 1984). However, efficacy in this trial was rated as undetermined because method details, including randomization, blinding, and inclusion and exclusion criteria, were not well described.

Generic

Insomnia and Sleep Quality

Three trials with crossover designs rated as moderate to poor in methodology were conducted on a generic aqueous extract. The first study was a single-blind, placebo-controlled crossover trial conducted with 128 volunteers. Approximately half described themselves as poor or irregular sleepers, and the other half described themselves as good sleepers. Each person received three different preparations to be taken on three nonconsecutive nights for a total study length of nine days. The treatments were a generic aqueous valerian extract, a commercial preparation of valerian and hops (Hova® tablets [Zyma S.A., Switzerland] containing 60 mg valerian extract and 30 mg hops flower extract), and placebo. Both valerian preparations delivered a dose of 400 mg valerian extract per evening. Sleep was assessed using a subjective questionnaire. Sleep quality increased and time to fall asleep decreased with both valerian preparations compared to placebo. The effect was most notable for those who considered themselves poor sleepers. Little change was seen in those with normal sleep patterns. The participants reported being sleepier than normal the next morning after taking Hova (valerian/hops combination) but not the generic valerian preparation (Leathwood et al., 1982).

Another crossover study included seven volunteers who complained that they usually have problems falling sleep. In three blocks of four nights each, 450 and 900 mg aqueous valerian extract were compared to placebo. Using the criteria of five minutes without movement as monitored by a wrist-worn activity meter to determine sleep start, both doses of valerian significantly decreased the time taken to fall asleep. A sleep questionnaire that subjects filled out also indicated a decrease in time to sleep for valerian. Increasing the dose from 450 mg to 900 mg extract did not increase the effect on sleep, but did cause subjects to feel sleepier the next morning compared to placebo (Leathwood and Chauffard, 1985).

One more crossover trial included ten healthy volunteers who slept at home and eight who slept in the laboratory. The home study monitored the effects of 450 and 900 mg aqueous extract and placebo using questionnaires. One dose of 900 mg extract reduced the time taken to fall asleep and time spent awake after falling asleep by 50 percent. The lower dose had less of an effect. The laboratory study compared one dose of 900 mg extract to placebo, and used objective polysomnographic recordings. In this study, no significant differences from placebo were observed, although some trends toward improvement of sleep were noted (Balderer and Borbely, 1985).

Valerian Nighttime (Euvegal forte)

Valerian Nighttime (valerian/lemon balm combination) was studied for its effect on sleep in both a placebo-controlled trial and in comparison with the benzodiazepine, triazolam.

Insomnia

In a good-quality, placebo-controlled, double-blind study, 66 sub-jects with mild insomnia according to the *Diagnostic and Statistical Manual of Mental Disorders,* Third Edition, Revised (DSM-III-R), (American Psychiatric Association, 1987) or ICD-10 were given ei-ther two tablets Euvegal forte or placebo for two weeks. According to sleep questionnaires, sleep quality increased in both groups, but the extent of improvement was greater with treatment than placebo. No hangover effects or rebound insomnia were reported following treat-ment (Dressing, Kohler, and Muller, 1996).

Sleep Quality

A poorly described, comparison, crossover trial included 20 healthy volunteers monitored in a sleep laboratory. Effects of a single dose of one tablet Euvegal forte or 0.125 mg triazolam were com-pared to placebos in a double dummy design. Triazolam caused sig-nificant increases in sleep efficiency and a decrease in time to fall asleep. However, the latency for REM sleep was significantly length-ened. No significant effect on sleep was reported for Euvegal (va-lerian/lemon balm combination) until the volunteers were divided into groups of "good" and "bad" sleepers according to the median of sleep efficiency for the placebo group. In the subgroup of bad sleep-ers who received Euvegal, there was a significant increase in sleep ef-ficiency compared to placebo and a tendency toward an increase in deep sleep (sleep Stages 3 and 4) (Dressing et al., 1992).

Songha Night

Sleep Quality

Songha Night (valerian/lemon balm combination) was studied in a placebo-controlled trial with 95 healthy volunteers given three tablets before bed for one month. The treatment produced a trend toward im-proving subjective sleep quality, with 33 percent of the treatment group reporting a higher quality of sleep compared to 9 percent of the placebo group (Cerny and Schmid, 1999).

Alluna Sleep

Electrophysiological Effects

Alluna Sleep (valerian/hops combination) was tested in a small trial, with 12 healthy young adults, in which quantitative topographical electroencephalograms (qEEG) were recorded following administration of a low dose (two tablets) and high dose (six tablets). The authors suggested that the slight power reduction in beta2-frequency band after administration of the higher dose might be in agreement with the benefits for relaxation and sleep disorders (Vonderheid-Guth et al., 2000). In the opinion of our reviewers, Drs. Lynn Shinto and Barry Oken, the high dose led to some EEG changes, although the report included limited methodological detail, and the results were confounded by a large number of variables with no statistical adjustment of p values.

ADVERSE REACTIONS OR SIDE EFFECTS

In the trials we reviewed, valerian was reported to have good tolerability and a low number of side effects. Eight of the 15 studies reported some adverse reactions or side effects during valerian use. These side effects included dizziness, headache, sweating, tremors, nausea, nighttime itching, sleep disturbances, and tiredness. However, more side effects were often reported in the placebo group in these studies, and many of the side effects reported from the placebo groups were similar to those reported in the valerian group.

An open, multicenter field study reported that side effects occurred in eight out of 1,448 patients, an incidence rate of 0.55 percent. Patients received three to nine tablets of Baldrian Dispert (Valdispert) for ten days. The side effects that were recorded were headache and gastrointestinal complaints (Siefert, 1988).

A randomized, placebo-controlled, double-blind study with 54 participants concluded that administration of Euvegal forte did not affect concentration or attentiveness required to drive vehicles or operate machinery and that there was no additive effect with alcohol. Healthy volunteers were given four tablets per day of the valerian/lemon balm product or placebo for three weeks. After this time, the participants additionally received sufficient 70 percent ethanol in juice to obtain blood alcohol levels of 0.5 percent. They were then subjected to a battery of psychometric tests (Albrecht et al., 1995).

INFORMATION FROM PHARMACOPOEIAL MONOGRAPHS

Sources of Published Therapeutic Monographs

American Herbal Pharmacopoeia
British Herbal Compendium
European Scientific Cooperative on Phytotherapy
German Commission E
United States Pharmacopeia—Drug Information
World Health Organization

Indications

The German Commission E approves the use of valerian root (fresh underground plant parts, carefully dried below 40°C) for restlessness and sleeping disorders based on nervous conditions (Blumenthal et al., 1998). The World Health Organization (WHO) states that the subterranean parts of valerian, including the rhizomes, roots, and stolons, carefully dried below 40°C, are used as a mild sedative and sleep-promoting agent for nervous excitation and anxiety-induced sleep disturbances (WHO, 1999). The European Scientific Cooperative on Phytotherapy (ESCOP) and the *British Herbal Compendium (BHC)* also add that valerian can be used for tenseness and restlessness (ESCOP, 1997; Bradley, 1992). Based on pharmacologic literature, the *American Herbal Pharmacopoeia (AHP)* states that valerian fragments or whole, fresh or dried, rhizomes, roots, and stolons are indicated for the symptomatic relief of insomnia, spasms due to nervous tension, and restlessness (Upton et al., 1999). *The United States Pharmacopeia—Drug Information (USP-DI)* botanical monograph series also states that preparations of the rhizome, roots, and/or stolons of valerian are reportedly used for the short-term treatment of insomnia (poor sleep quality and difficulty falling asleep) (*USP-DI*, 1998).

Doses

Infusion: 2 to 3 g of valerian per cup, once to several times per
day (Blumenthal et al., 1998; ESCOP, 1997; WHO, 1999); 1
to 3 g by infusion or dried (Bradley, 1992)

Tincture: ½ to 1 teaspoon (1 to 3 ml), once to several times per
day (Blumenthal et al., 1998); 1:5, ethanol 70 percent v/v
(ESCOP, 1997; WHO, 1999); 3 to 5 ml up to three times daily
(Bradley, 1992)

Essential oil: 0.05 to 0.25 ml (2 to 6 drops) up to two times daily
(Upton et al., 1999)

Extracts: amount equivalent to 2 to 3 g of drug, once to several
times per day (Blumenthal et al., 1998)

External use: 100 g for one full bath (Blumenthal et al., 1998;
WHO, 1999)

Treatment Period

ESCOP lists no restriction for the treatment period, since neither
dependence nor withdrawal symptoms have been reported (ESCOP,
1997).

Contraindications

The Commission E and the *BHC* list no known contraindications
(Blumenthal et al., 1998; Bradley, 1992). However, ESCOP lists va-
lerian as contraindicated for children under three years of age
(ESCOP, 1997), and the WHO states that it should not be used during
pregnancy or lactation (WHO, 1999). The *USP-DI* agrees with both
ESCOP and the WHO (*USP-DI,* 1998).

Adverse Reactions

The Commission E and ESCOP list no known adverse reactions
(Blumenthal et al., 1998; ESCOP, 1997). However, the WHO states
that headaches, excitability, uneasiness, and insomnia have been associated with chronic use of valerian (WHO, 1999). The *AHP* also
cautions that valerian can cause nervousness and heart palpitations in
sensitive individuals and occasional headache and gastrointestinal

distress (Upton et al., 1999). According to the *USP-DI,* no side effects have been reported with the recommended dose, but acute overdose or chronic use of valerian has been associated with restlessness, excitability, headaches, nausea, blurred vision, uneasiness, and cardiac disturbances (*USP-DI,* 1998).

Precautions

ESCOP lists no precautions (ESCOP, 1997), but the WHO and *AHP* warn that valerian may cause drowsiness (WHO, 1999; Upton et al., 1999). The WHO also advises that patients should avoid consuming alcoholic beverages or other sedatives in conjunction with valerian (WHO, 1999). According to the *AHP,* abrupt discontinuation after long-term use may result in withdrawal symptoms (valerian may work like benzodiazepines) (Upton et al., 1999). The *USP-DI* warns that patients that have impaired liver function should use valerian with care (*USP-DI,* 1998).

Drug Interactions

The Commission E and ESCOP list no known drug interactions (Blumenthal et al., 1998; ESCOP, 1997). However, the *AHP* states that valerian potentiates the effects of barbiturates (Upton et al., 1999). The *USP-DI* also states that data from animal studies suggest that valerian may boost the effects of alcohol and those of other medications that depress the central nervous system (*USP-DI,* 1998).

Official Combination with Other Herbs

The German Commission E approves of fixed combinations of valerian with other herbs. A combination consisting of passionflower herb, valerian root, and lemon balm is approved for conditions of unrest and difficulty falling asleep due to nervousness. The individual components must each be present at 30 to 50 percent of the daily dosage given in the monographs for the individual herbs. A combination of valerian and hops is approved for nervous sleeping disorders and conditions of unrest. The individual components must each be present at 50 to 75 percent of the daily dosage given in the monographs for the individual herbs (Blumenthal et al., 1998).

REFERENCES

Albrecht M, Berger W, Laux P, Schmidt U, Martin C (1995). Psychopharmaceuticals and safety in traffic: The influence of a plant-based sedative on vehicle operation ability with or without alcohol. *Zeitschrift fur Allgemeinmedizin* 71: 1215-1221.

American Psychiatric Association (1987). *Diagnostic and Statistical Manual of Mental Disorders,* Third Edition, Revised. Washington, DC: American Psychiatric Association.

Balderer G, Borbely AA (1985). Effect of valerian on human sleep. *Psychopharmacology* 87 (4): 406-409.

Blumenthal M, Busse W, Hall T, Goldberg A, Grünwald J, Riggins C, Rister S, eds. (1998). *The Complete German Commission E Monographs: Therapeutic Guide to Herbal Medicines.* Trans. S Klein. Austin: American Botanical Council.

Bradley PR, ed. (1992). *British Herbal Compendium: A Handbook of Scientific Information on Widely Used Plant Drugs,* Volume 1. Dorset: British Herbal Medicine Association.

Cerny A, Schmid K (1999). Tolerability and efficacy of valerian/lemon balm in healthy volunteers: A double-blind, placebo-controlled, multicenter study. *Fitoterapia* 70 (3): 221-228.

Cropley M, Cave Z, Ellis J, Middleton RW (2002). Effect of kava and valerian on human physiological and psychological responses to mental stress assessed under laboratory conditions. *Phytotherapy Research* 16 (1): 23-27.

Donath F, Quispe S, Diefenbach K, Maurer A, Fietze I, Roots I (2000). Critical evaluation of the effect on valerian extract on sleep structure and sleep quality. *Pharmacopsychiatry* 33 (2): 47-53.

Dorn M (2000). Baldrian versus oxazepam: Efficacy and tolerability in non-organic and non-psychiatric insomniacs: A randomized, double-blind, clinical, comparative study. *Forschende Komplementarmedizin und Klassische Naturheilkunde* 7 (2): 79-84.

Dressing H, Kohler S, Muller WE (1996). Improvement of sleep quality with a high-dose valerian/lemon balm preparation: A placebo-controlled, double-blind study. *Psychopharmakotherapie* 3: 123-130.

Dressing H, Riemann D, Low H, Schredl M, Reh C, Laux P, Muller WE (1992). Insomnia: Are valerian/balm combinations of equal value to benzodiazepine? *Therapiewoche* 42 (12): 726-736.

European Scientific Cooperative on Phytotherapy (ESCOP) (1997). *Valerianae radix:* Valerian root. In *Monographs on the Medicinal Uses of Plant Drugs* (Fascicle 4: p. 10). Exeter, UK: European Scientific Cooperative on Phytotherapy.

Kamm-Kohl AV, Jansen W, Brockmann P (1984). Modern valerian therapy of nervous disorders in elderly patients. *Medwelt* 35: 1450-1454.

Kuhlmann J, Berger W, Podzuweit H, Schmidt U (1999). The influence of valerian treatment on "reaction time, alertness, and concentration" in volunteers. *Pharmacopsychiatry* 32 (6): 235-241.

Leathwood PD, Chauffard F (1985). Aqueous extract of valerian reduces latency to fall asleep in man. *Planta Medica* 51 (2): 144-148.

Leathwood PD, Chauffard F, Heck E, Munoz-Box R (1982). Aqueous extract of valerian root (*Valeriana officinalis* L.) improves sleep quality in man. *Pharmacology, Biochemistry & Behavior* 17 (1): 65-71. (Also published in Leathwood PD, Chauffard F, Munoz-Box [1982]. Effect of *Valeriana officianalis* L. on subjective and objective sleep parameters. Sleep 1982. Sixth European Congress on Sleep Research, Zurich, pp. 402-405.)

Pagel JF, Parnes BL (2001). Medications for the treatment of sleep disorders: An overview. *Primary Care Companion Journal of Clinical Psychiatry* 3 (3): 118-125.

Schulz H, Stolz C, Muller J (1994). The effect of valerian extract on sleep polygraphy in poor sleepers: A pilot study. *Pharmacopsychiatry* 27 (4): 147-151.

Schulz V, Hänsel R, Tyler VE (2001). *Rational Phytotherapy: A Physicians' Guide to Herbal Medicine,* Fourth Edition. Trans. TC Telgar. Berlin: Springer-Verlag.

Siefert T (1988). Therapeutic effects of valerian in nervous disorders: A field study. *Therapeutikon* 2: 94-98.

United States Pharmacopeia—Drug Information (USP-DI) (1998). Botanical Monograph Series: Valerian. Rockville, MD: The United States Pharmacopeial Convention, Inc.

Upton R, Graff A, Williamson E, Bevill A, Ertl F, Reich E, Martinez M, Lange M, Wang W, Barrett M (1999). *Valerian Root,* Valeriana officinalis, *Analytical, Quality Control, and Therapeutic Monograph. American Herbal Pharmacopoeia and Therapeutic Compendium.* Eds. R Upton, C Petrone. Santa Cruz: American Herbal Pharmacopoeia.

Vonderheid-Guth B, Todorova A, Brattstrom A, Dimpfel W (2000). Pharmacodynamic effects of valerian and hops extract combination (Ze

91019) on the quantitative-topographical EEG in healthy volunteers. *European Journal of Medical Research* 5 (4): 139-144.

Vorbach EU, Görtelmeyer R, Brüning J (1996). Treatment of insomnia: Effectiveness and tolerance of a valerian extract. *Psychopharmakotherapie* 3 (3): 109-115.

Wheatley D (2001). Stress-induced insomnia treated with kava and valerian: Singly and in combination. *Human Psychopharmacology and Clinical Experiments* 16 (4): 353-356.

World Health Organization (WHO) (1992). *International Statistical Classification of Diseases and Related Health Problems,* Tenth Revision. Geneva: World Health Organization.

World Health Organization (WHO) (1999). *WHO Monographs on Selected Medicinal Plants,* Volume 1. Geneva: World Health Organization.

DETAILS ON VALERIAN PRODUCTS
AND CLINICAL STUDIES

Product and clinical study information is grouped in the same order as in the Summary Table. A profile on an individual product is followed by details of the clinical studies associated with that product. In some instances, a clinical study, or studies, supports several products that contain the same principal ingredient(s). In these instances, those products are grouped together.

Clinical studies that follow each product, or group of products, are grouped by therapeutic indication, in accordance with the order in the Summary Table.

Index to Valerian Products

Product Profile: Sedonium™

Manufacturer	**Lichtwer Pharma AG, Germany**
U.S. distributor	**Lichtwer Pharma U.S., Inc.**
Botanical ingredient	**Valerian root extract**
Extract name	**LI 156**
Quantity	300 mg
Processing	Plant to extract ratio 3-7:1, 70% (v/v) ethanol
Standardization	Valerenic acid, acetoxyvalerenic acid, and hydroxyvalerenic acid, tested using high-performance liquid chromatography (HPLC)
Formulation	Tablet

Recommended dose: Two tablets one to two hours before retiring. Swallow whole with cool liquid. Sedonium is non-habit forming and can be taken on a regular basis.

DSHEA structure/function: Clinically proven to help promote restful sleep. Awake refreshed and alert. LI 156 formula has been clinically proven to help support normal gamma aminobutyric acid (GABA) production, a neurotransmitter known for its beneficial effect on sleep.

Cautions: If one is taking prescription medicine, pregnant, nursing a baby, or administering to children under the age of 12, a health professional should be consulted before using this product.

Other ingredients: Sucrose, glucose, lactose, talc, powdered cellulose, silicon dioxide, hydroxypropyl methylcellulose, castor oil, polyvinylpyrrolidone, magnesium stearate, polyethylene glycol, gelatin, titanium dioxide, carnauba wax.

Source(s) of information: Product package; Sedonium™: Product information (Lichtwer Pharma, 1996).

Clinical study: Sedonium™

Extract name	LI 156
Manufacturer	Lichtwer Pharma AG, Germany
Indication	**Insomnia**
Level of evidence	**I**
Therapeutic benefit	**Yes**

Bibliographic reference
Vorbach EU, Görtelmeyer R, Brüning J (1996). Treatment of insomnia: Effectiveness and tolerance of a valerian extract. *Psychopharmakotherapie* 3 (3): 109-115.

Trial design
Parallel.

Study duration	1 month
Dose	2 (300 mg extract) tablets 1 hour before bed
Route of administration	Oral
Randomized	Yes
Randomization adequate	Yes

Blinding	Double-blind
Blinding adequate	Yes
Placebo	Yes
Drug comparison	No
Site description	23 practices (general, internal, psychiatric)
No. of subjects enrolled	121
No. of subjects completed	117
Sex	Male and female
Age	24-68 years (mean: 47)

Inclusion criteria
Nonorganic insomnia according to the ICD-10 (F51.0)

Exclusion criteria
Severe organic and mental concomitant illnesses; administration of a synthetic hypnotic more than three times a week 14 days before the trial; taking an herbal remedy to treat sleep disorder; medication with drugs that affect sleeping patterns or waking state; pregnancy, breast feeding, or women wishing to become pregnant; unwillingness to cooperate; and participation in a clinical trial within the previous three months.

End points
Examinations were conducted on day 0 (recruitment) and on days 14 and 28 of treatment. The following methods were used to assess efficacy and tolerance: Gortelmeyer's sleep questionnaire B, form B3 (SF-B); von Zerssen's well-being scale (Bf-S); Clinical Global Impressions (CGI); overall assessment of effectiveness and tolerance by doctor and patient; blood pressure and pulse rate; and documentation of adverse events and compliance.

Results
Significant differences after 28 days of treatment were seen in the following measures: quality of sleep according to the type B (SF-B) sleep questionnaire ($p = 0.035$); restored feeling after sleep ($p = 0.032$); patients' assessment of well-being (Bf-S) ($p = 0.002$); change of condition based upon the CGI scale ($p < 0.001$); degree of severity of insomnia ($p = 0.002$); and assessment of therapeutic effect ($p = 0.001$). The effect of valerian was rated as good or very good by doctors in 61 percent of cases and by patients in 66 percent of cases. In contrast, placebo was rated good or very good in 26 percent of cases by doctors and patients alike.

Side effects
Tolerability was rated very good by doctors among 91.5 percent of patients taking valerian and 72.4 percent of those taking placebo. Five subjects re-

ported "undesirable" effects: three in valerian group (two reports of headache, one report of dizziness in the morning), and two in the placebo group (tiredness, nausea, and vomiting with gastric ulcer).

Authors' comments
The results of the trial show that treatment with the valerian extract LI 156 has significant effects on nonorganic insomnia (ICD-10: F51.0). The absence of potential for dependency, the lack of any hangover effect, and the possibility of long-term treatment are arguments for using herbal sedatives as an initial treatment for insomnia.

Reviewers' comments
This well-designed and well-reported study used subjective measures of sleep (no objective measures). Effects were observed after 14 days, and were more pronounced at 28 days. (Translation reviewed) (5, 6)

Clinical Study: Sedonium™

Extract name	LI 156
Manufacturer	Lichtwer Pharma AG, Germany
Indication	**Insomnia**
Level of evidence	**III**
Therapeutic benefit	**Trend**

Bibliographic reference
Donath F, Quispe S, Diefenbach K, Maurer A, Fietze I, Roots I (2000). Critical evaluation of the effect on valerian extract on sleep structure and sleep quality. *Pharmacopsychiatry* 33 (2): 47-53.

Trial design
Crossover. Two 15-day treatment periods. Patients did not receive any treatment on day one, and received either placebo or valerian from day 2 through day 15. Treatment periods were separated by a 13-day washout period.

Study duration	15 days
Dose	2 (300 mg extract) pills 1 hour before bed
Route of administration	Oral
Randomized	Yes
Randomization adequate	No
Blinding	Double-blind
Blinding adequate	No

Placebo	Yes
Drug comparison	No
Site description	Not described
No. of subjects enrolled	16
No. of subjects completed	16
Sex	Male and female
Age	22-55 years (median: 49)

Inclusion criteria
Primary insomnia (International Classification of Sleep Disorders [ICSD] code 1.A.1.) confirmed by polysomnographic recording throughout one night and subjective sleep disturbances from three months to several years.

Exclusion criteria
Patients suffering from organic or psychiatric diseases that could cause sleep disturbances; sleep apnea syndrome; periodic limb movements or restless-legs syndrome; taking psychotropic drugs, including alcohol, cocaine, benzodiazepines, barbiturates, etc. Patients were not allowed to take any drugs influencing sleep structure and daytime vigilance 14 days before the trial start and until the end of the trial.

End points
Patients underwent eight study nights of polysomnographic recordings, four nights during each treatment phase: day 1 (baseline recording), day 2 (after one day treatment), day 14 (treatment baseline), and day 15 (treatment recording). The target variable of the study was sleep efficiency. Other parameters describing sleep structure were sleep-stage analysis, based on the rules of *Rechtschaffen* and *Kales,* and the arousal index (ASDA criteria). Subjective parameters were assessed by questionnaires.

Results
After a single dose of valerian, no significant effect on sleep structure and subjective sleep assessment was observed. After 14 days of treatment, sleep efficiency increased significantly for both placebo and valerian groups compared to baseline. In both groups, sleep period time and REM sleep percentage increased, whereas NREM 1 percentage decreased. The arousal index did not change with either group. Slow-wave sleep latency was reduced by valerian compared to placebo, $p < 0.05$. The percentage of time in slow-wave sleep was increased by valerian compared to baseline, $p < 0.05$.

Side effects
Three with valerian (migraine, headache, pruritis); 18 with placebo (headache, migraine, gastrointestinal complaints, flu and common cold, left thoracic pain).

Authors' comments
Treatment with an herbal extract of *radix valerianae* at relatively high dose levels demonstrated a number of positive effects on the sleep structure and sleep perception of insomnia patients, and can therefore be recommended for the treatment of patients with mild psychophysiological insomnia.

Reviewers' comments
This was a small pilot trial. Positive effects were reported in the objective measures of sleep structure and slow-wave sleep latency. No difference was seen, however, between the placebo and valerian groups on the primary outcome measure: sleep efficiency. The study had well-defined inclusion and exclusion criteria, but the randomization and blinding were not well described. (1, 5)

Clinical Study: Sedonium™

Extract name	LI 156
Manufacturer	Lichtwer Pharma AG, Germany
Indication	**Insomnia**
Level of evidence	I
Therapeutic benefit	**Yes**

Bibliographic reference
Dorn M (2000). Baldrian versus oxazepam: Efficacy and tolerability in non-organic and non-psychiatric insomniacs: A randomized, double-blind, clinical, comparative study. *Forschende Komplementarmedizin und Klassische Naturheilkunde* 7 (2): 79-84.

Trial design
Parallel. Patients received either valerian or oxazepam (2 x 5 mg) 30 minutes before bed.

Study duration	1 month
Dose	2 (300 mg) valerian capsules
Route of administration	Oral
Randomized	Yes
Randomization adequate	Yes
Blinding	Double-blind
Blinding adequate	Yes
Placebo	No
Drug comparison	Yes

Drug name	Oxazepam
Site description	8 general practices
No. of subjects enrolled	75
No. of subjects completed	65
Sex	Male and female
Age	18-70 years (mean: 52)

Inclusion criteria
Nonorganic, nonpsychiatric insomniacs as defined in ICD-10 (F51.0); ages 18-70.

Exclusion criteria
Persons with known hypersensitivity to valerian and/or oxazepam; participation in a different study within 30 days of the trial start; lack of contraception in premenopausal women; pregnant or breastfeeding; taking other psychotropically active drugs during the study and within four weeks of its start; known medicine/drug/alcohol dependency; poor overall condition; with severe renal or hepatic dysfunctions or illnesses; leukocyto-, granulocyto-, or thrombocytophenia; noncompensated cardiac insufficiency; neurological/psychiatric illnesses (morbus Parkinson, spinal or cerebral ataxia, myasthenia gravis, cerebral organical psychosyndrome, or psychosis); malign diseases; hypotonia; glaucoma; or sleep apnea.

End points
Primary outcome was sleep quality according to Gortelmeyer's sleep questionnaire B (SF-B). Secondary outcomes were other sleep characteristics of the SF-B, Von Zerssen's well-being scale (Bf-S), the Hamilton Anxiety scale (HAM-A), as well as sleep-rating by the doctor. Testing was performed before treatment and after one, two, and four weeks.

Results
In both groups, sleep quality improved significantly ($p < 0.001$), but no statistically significant differences could be found between groups ($p = 0.70$). At the end of the study 55 percent of patients on valerian and 70 percent on oxazepam assessed the treatment as good or very good ($p = 0.6$)

Side effects
Two subjects terminated the trial from the valerian group (sweating, tremors, nausea, night-time pruritis). Three terminated the trial from the oxazepam group (tiredness, hangover, angina pectoris).

Author's comments
The study showed no differences in the efficacy for valerian and oxazepam. Because of the more favorable adverse effect profile of valerian compared to oxazepam, this hypothesis should be confirmed.

Reviewers' comments
This well-designed and well-described study compared valerian with oxazepam. Statistically significant outcomes were seen in both groups on subjective measures for sleep quality. The inclusion of a placebo group would have strengthened the validity of positive outcome findings. The addition of a "withdrawal" effect comparison would have also increased the quality of the study. (Translation reviewed) (5, 6)

Clinical Study: LI 156

Extract name	LI 156
Manufacturer	Lichtwer Pharma AG, Germany
Indication	**Insomnia, stress-induced**
Level of evidence	**III**
Therapeutic benefit	**Undetermined**

Bibliographic reference
Wheatley D (2001). Stress-induced insomnia treated with kava and valerian: Singly and in combination. *Human Psychopharmacology and Clinical Experiments* 16 (4): 353-356.

Trial design
Crossover. Patients received treatments for three six-week periods with two-week washout periods in between. Patients first received kava (LI 150, 120 mg daily), then received valerian (LI 156, 600 mg daily), then received kava and valerian in combination.

Study duration	6 weeks
Dose	120 mg daily
Route of administration	Oral
Randomized	No
Randomization adequate	No
Blinding	Open
Blinding adequate	No
Placebo	No
Drug comparison	Yes
Drug name	Kava extract (LI 150)
Site description	Not described
No. of subjects enrolled	24
No. of subjects completed	19

| Sex | Male and female |
| Age | 23-65 years (mean: 44) |

Inclusion criteria
Outpatients with stress-induced insomnia of varying intensity and duration.

Exclusion criteria
Subjects taking other psychotropic drugs, with symptoms of depressed mood that were severe and/or included suicidal ideation, or women of child-bearing potential not using adequate contraception methods.

End points
To determine the severity of stress, three parameters were studied: social, personal, and life events. An additional three parameters were studied to determine sleep disturbance: time to fall asleep, hours slept, and mood on final waking. The different parameters of stress severity and sleep disturbance were measured by subjects with visual analogue scales (VAS). Subjects made assessments at the beginning, middle, and end of each six-week treatment.

Results
After the first six-week treatment period with kava alone, the mean total stress score was significantly reduced ($p < 0.01$). This reduction was virtually unchanged during subsequent treatment periods with valerian alone and the kava plus valerian, as well as the washout periods in between. The difference between the baseline and final stress score was highly significant ($p < 0.001$). The severity of insomnia was similarly reduced by kava ($p < 0.05$ compared to baseline), with no further decrease with the subsequent treatment with valerian. However, treatment with valerian plus kava produced an additional decrease ($p < 0.05$). The overall decrease from baseline was highly significant ($p < 0.001$).

Side effects
Slightly more subjects experienced side effects with valerian (47 percent) and kava plus valerian (47 percent) than with kava alone (33 percent). The most common side effects for the three groups were vivid dreams for both valerian and kava plus valerian (16 and 21 percent, respectively), dizziness and gastric discomfort with kava (12 percent for each), and dry mouth for kava and kava plus valerian (8 and 11 percent, respectively).

Author's comments
Kava was undoubtedly effective in this study, and would seem to have a number of desirable properties for use as a general hypnotic and anxiolytic. The role of valerian is less clear: it does not appear to be as effective in inducing sleep, but has beneficial effects on the sleep EEG, indicating that it may well improve the quality of sleep. Thus it might be useful in chronic in-

somnia and in the elderly, and to give an additive effect in improving sleep in patients who may be particularly refractory to treatment with kava alone.

Reviewers' comments

The goal of this pilot study was to collect preliminary data to support future research in determining whether kava, valerian, or the combination are safe and effective treatments for stress-induced insomnia. This was an open label study that included no objective outcome measures. The mean stress and insomnia scores reflect no change during the washout phases between treatments, which may indicate that these self-reported measures may be significantly influenced by subjects' knowledge of treatment. Including a laboratory measurement for adverse events, especially liver function tests, would have improved the study design for safety issues. Given that the primary goal of this study was exploratory in nature, the results do provide some evidence for future studies to determine whether the combination of kava and valerian is effective for stress-induced insomnia. (1, 4)

Clinical Study: LI 156

Extract name	LI 156
Manufacturer	Lichtwer Pharma AG, Germany
Indication	**Mental stress**
Level of evidence	**III**
Therapeutic benefit	**Undetermined**

Bibliographic reference

Cropley M, Cave Z, Ellis J, Middleton RW (2002). Effect of kava and valerian on human physiological and psychological responses to mental stress assessed under laboratory conditions. *Phytotherapy Research* 16 (1): 23-27.

Trial design

Parallel. Subjects were randomized to receive either valerian extract (LI 156: 600 mg/day), kava extract (LI 150: 120 mg/day), or nothing (nonplacebo controls). Subjects were asked to refrain from eating and drinking caffeinated or alcoholic drinks, or smoking 1.5 hours before test periods.

Study duration	1 week
Dose	2 (300 mg) tablets daily
Route of administration	Oral
Randomized	Yes
Randomization adequate	No
Blinding	Open

Blinding adequate	No
Placebo	No
Drug comparison	Yes
Drug name	Kava extract (LI 150)
Site description	University psychology lab
No. of subjects enrolled	54
No. of subjects completed	Not given
Sex	Male and female
Age	18-30 years (mean: 24)

Inclusion criteria
Healthy volunteers.

Exclusion criteria
None mentioned.

End points
A standardized color/word mental stress task was performed before (T1) and after seven days of treatment (T2). At each test session heart rate (HR) and blood pressure (BP) were recorded after resting for five minutes, and patients rated their perceived feeling of pressure at that moment. Then the subjects completed the color/word interference task, lasting six minutes. During this task, BP and HR were recorded at 0.5, 2.5, and 4.5 minutes. After completing the task, participants rated the feeling of pressure experienced during the task. After resting five minutes, final HR and BP measurements were taken.

Results
In the resting state at the second testing period (T2), a significant reduction in systolic BP and HR was observed in the group that received valerian compared to T1. Diastolic BP decreased in this group, but not significantly. The kava group experienced a significant decrease in resting diastolic BP at T2 compared to T1. While undergoing the stress task at T2, systolic BP was significantly lower than at T1 (under the same stress conditions) for both kava and valerian (both $p < 0.001$). No differences in diastolic BP were observed for either group, however. Heart rate was significantly reduced at T2 compared to T1 for the valerian group ($p < 0.001$), but was not changed for the kava group. Both the kava and valerian groups reported less pretask pressure at T2 compared to T1 ($p < 0.001$), and a significant reduction in pressure was experienced during the mental stress task for both groups ($p < 0.001$). The control group experienced no changes in BP, HR, or perceived pressure.

Side effects
None mentioned.

Authors' comments
Consistent with expectations, kava and valerian appeared to moderate the subjective effects of stress. Some caution is warranted in the interpretation of the results, since the study incorporated a nonplacebo design.

Reviewers' comments
The primary goal of this study was to investigate whether kava or valerian would moderate physiological and psychological reactivity to laboratory induced stress. Given the goal of this study, a placebo control group should have been included. The physiological outcome measures of HR and BP are known to be influenced strongly by placebo. Therefore, it cannot be determined whether the outcomes of this study reflect treatment or placebo effect. Self-report of stress, one week after completing a stressful mental task, may also be bias-related to the subject's knowledge of treatment. In general, subject demographics by group assignment at baseline, inclusion and exclusion criteria, study medication, dropouts, and adverse events are not well described. (0, 3)

Clinical Study: LI 156

Extract name	LI 156
Manufacturer	Lichtwer Pharma AG, Germany
Indication	**Cognitive functioning** in healthy volunteers
Level of evidence	**III**
Therapeutic benefit	**Yes**

Bibliographic reference
Kuhlmann J, Berger W, Podzuweit H, Schmidt U (1999). The influence of valerian treatment on "reaction time, alertness, and concentration" in volunteers. *Pharmacopsychiatry* 32 (6): 235-241.

Trial design
Study in two sections: (1) three-armed study with a single dose of valerian, flunitrazepam (1 mg), or placebo, and psychometric testing the morning after, followed by a seven-day washout phase; (2) two weeks of valerian or placebo.

Study duration	1 day, 2 weeks
Dose	2 (300 mg valerian extract) capsules or tablets
Route of administration	Oral
Randomized	Yes
Randomization adequate	No
Blinding	Double-blind
Blinding adequate	No
Placebo	Yes
Drug comparison	Yes
Drug name	Flunitrazepam
Site description	Single center
No. of subjects enrolled	102
No. of subjects completed	91
Sex	Male and female
Age	30-60 years (mean: 41)

Inclusion criteria
Healthy volunteers with normal daylight vision, social drinking behavior, low caffeine consumption, and no nicotine consumption.

Exclusion criteria
Usual exclusion criteria, along with any sleep disorder (ICD-10: G47), any disease that was known to lead to secondary sleep disorders, and simultaneous use of psychoactive drugs or other pharmaceuticals that could influence sleep patterns.

End points
The primary evaluation was the median of reaction time measured with the Vienna Determination Unit (VDU). Secondary criteria were the alertness test, tracking test (two-handed coordination), sleep quality (via questionnaires Visuelle Analogskalen abends [VIS-A] and Visuelle Analogskalen morgens [VIS-M], and further VDU paremeters.

Results
Single administration of LI 156 did not impair reaction abilities, concentration, or coordination. In contrast, reaction time and performance were decreased by flunitrazepam. After 14 days, improvement in median reaction time of the valerian group did not differ from the placebo group ($p = 0.4481$). Evaluations of secondary criteria were consistent with the results of the primary criteria. After 14 days of treatment, sleep quality showed a trend toward improvement in the valerian group compared to placebo.

Side effects
Eleven cases of dizziness were reported in the valerian group; 12 adverse events were reported in the placebo group; 19 events were reported in the flunitrazepam group (dizziness, tiredness, hypokinesis, lack of concentration).

Authors' comments
Neither single nor repeated evening administrations of 600 mg LI 156 have a relevant negative impact on reaction time, alertness, and concentration the morning after intake.

Reviewers' comments
This is a good study with well-defined inclusion/exclusion criteria and a good description of ingredients of placebo and active treatment capsules. There is a limited description of blinding and no description of the randomization method (minor flaw). The flaws mentioned do not negate observations that single or repeated evening administration of 600 mg LI 156 have a low negative impact on alertness, concentration, and reaction time. (1, 6)

Product Profile: Valdispert®

Manufacturer	**Solvay Arzneimittel GmbH, Germany**
U.S. distributor	None
Botanical ingredient	**Valerian root extract**
Extract name	None given
Quantity	135 mg
Processing	Plant to extract ratio 5-6:1, aqueous alkaline dry extract
Standardization	Valerenic acid
Formulation	Tablet

Comments: Also sold as Baldrian-Dispert®.

Source(s) of information: Schulz, Stolz, and Muller, 1994; Kamm-Kohl, Jansen, and Brockmann, 1984.

Clinical Study: Valdispert®

Extract name	None given
Manufacturer	Solvay Arzneimittel GmbH, Germany

Indication	**Insomnia** in elderly females
Level of evidence	**III**
Therapeutic benefit	**Undetermined**

Bibliographic reference

Schulz H, Stolz C, Muller J (1994). The effect of valerian extract on sleep polygraphy in poor sleepers: A pilot study. *Pharmacopsychiatry* 27 (4): 147-151.

Trial design

Parallel. Subjects spent three nights in a sleep lab. The first (N_0) was an adaptation night, followed by a week of subjective monitoring of sleep patterns. The second night (N_1) followed the first treatment dose (of either valerian or placebo), and the third night (N_2) followed a week of treatment.

Study duration	3 nights with 1-week intervals
Dose	3 (135 mg extract) tablets 3 times daily
Route of administration	Oral
Randomized	Yes
Randomization adequate	No
Blinding	Double-blind
Blinding adequate	No
Placebo	Yes
Drug comparison	No
Site description	Sleep lab
No. of subjects enrolled	14
No. of subjects completed	14
Sex	Female
Age	Mean: 61.6 years

Inclusion criteria

Elderly females who were poor sleepers and fulfilled at least two of the following subjective inclusion criteria: (1) sleep latency > 30 minutes; (2) more than three awakenings per night and inability to go back to sleep within five minutes; (3) total sleep time < 5 hours. Subjects also had to have a normal, age-related health status, normal clinico-chemical values, and an uneventful anamnesis.

Exclusion criteria

Indications of organic or psychiatric causes of the sleep disturbances; abnormal body weight; or hypnotics, sedatives, or other central nervous system (CNS) active drugs two weeks prior to the study.

End points

Polysomnography was conducted on three nights at one-week intervals (N_0, N_1, N_2). The following parameters were recorded: time in bed, total sleep time (TST), sleep period time, sleep efficiency index, sleep latencies, and sleep stages in minutes and percentages of TST. The density of sleep spindles and K-complexes were also visually evaluated. Sleep was also measured subjectively with sleep questionnaires (Visuelle Analogskalen abends [VIS-A] at night and Schlaf-fragebogen A [SF-A] in the morning), and with a sleep diary, starting after N_0 and until the end of the trial.

Results

At baseline, the two groups differed significantly in sleep period time, sleep efficiency, and in sleep latency. During the second night of polysomnographic measurement (N_1), the two treatment groups differed in none of the sleep parameters. After repeated administration of treatment, slow-wave sleep (SWS) increased in the valerian group ($p = 0.027$), but not in the placebo group. There was a significant decrease in Stage 1 sleep ($p = 0.027$). In the placebo group, a slight reduction of movement time indicates a decrease of large body movements ($p = 0.031$). No effect on REM sleep was observed in either group. The two groups were not significantly different with respect to spindle or K-complex density on any of the three nights. No changes were seen in any of the subjective sleep parameters measured by questionnaires and sleep logs.

Side effects

None mentioned in this paper.

Authors' comments

Various shortcomings in the design of this study restrict interpretation of the results. Even allowing for these limitations, the results suggest that valerian has selective effects on non-REM sleep. We conclude from the present results and those in the literature that valerian has a mild tranquilizing quality.

Reviewers' comments

In this pilot study, the authors list several shortcomings: a small sample size with some resultant baseline differences in two groups, and a lack of good baselines, since only a limited number of polysomnography studies were conducted on each subject. Both groups had no true baseline, so changes in treatment or placebo within groups were compared against the sleep adaptation night. The study had well-defined inclusion and exclusion criteria, but did not describe the randomization process (minor flaw) or blinding techniques. Comparing active and placebo groups, no significant differences in polysomnographic measures were observed, although there were some differences when compared to baseline measures in non-REM sleep, favoring valerian. (1, 5)

Clinical Study: Valdispert® (Baldrian-Dispert®)

Extract name	None given
Manufacturer	Solvay Arzneimittel GmbH, Germany

Indication	**Nervous disorders in elderly patients**
Level of evidence	**III**
Therapeutic benefit	**Undetermined**

Bibliographic reference
Kamm-Kohl AV, Jansen W, Brockmann P (1984). Modern valerian therapy of nervous disorders in elderly patients. *Medwelt* 35: 1450-1454.

Trial design
Parallel.

Study duration	2 weeks
Dose	2 tablets 3 times daily
Route of administration	Oral
Randomized	Yes
Randomization adequate	No
Blinding	Double-blind
Blinding adequate	No
Placebo	Yes
Drug comparison	No
Site description	Senior care facility and geriatric hospital
No. of subjects enrolled	80
No. of subjects completed	78
Sex	Male and female
Age	59-79 years (mean: 70)

Inclusion criteria
Elderly patients suffering from disturbances of subjective well-being and behavioral disorders of nervous origin.

Exclusion criteria
None mentioned.

End points
Patients were evaluated at baseline and on days 7 and 14 of treatment. Psychometric evaluation was based on von Zerssen's scales of subjective well-being (Bf-S) and on the Nurses' Observation Scale for Inpatient Evaluation (NOSIE), an objective rating scale.

Results
Scales for rating subjective well-being indicated improvement in the valerian group compared to the placebo group ($p < 0.01$). Evaluation on the basis of the NOSIE also revealed that patients in the valerian group exhibited a marked improvement in behavior compared to placebo ($p < 0.01$). The ability to fall asleep and sleep through the night improved in the valerian group compared to placebo ($p < 0.001$). Valerian also helped with fatigue ($p < 0.02$).

Side effects
Four patients (two in each group) complained of mild dizziness.

Authors' comments
The study succeeded in confirming the efficacy of Valdispert therapy.

Reviewers' comments
The study is not well described. It has no description of randomization or blinding, and no well-defined inclusion and exclusion criteria. The sample size is appropriate, however, and the outcome measures are clearly defined. (Translation reviewed) (1, 2)

Product Profile: Valerian (Generic)

Manufacturer	None
U.S. distributor	None
Botanical ingredient	**Valerian rhizome extract**
Extract name	None given
Quantity	200-225 mg
Processing	Plant to extract ratio 2.8-3.2:1, freeze-dried aqueous extract
Standardization	No information
Formulation	Capsule

Source(s) of information: Leathwood et al., 1982; Balderer and Borbely, 1985.

Clinical Study: Valerian (Generic)

Extract name	None given
Manufacturer	None

Indication	**Insomnia**
Level of evidence	**III**
Therapeutic benefit	**Trend**

Bibliographic reference

Leathwood PD, Chauffard F (1985). Aqueous extract of valerian reduces latency to fall asleep in man. *Planta Medica* 51 (2): 144-148..

Trial design

Crossover with random treatment order comparing placebo to two doses of valerian extract. Samples were administered in random order four nights a week for three weeks (12 samples total: four samples from each treatment).

Study duration	3 blocks of 4 nights each
Dose	450 mg or 900 mg valerian extract
Route of administration	Oral
Randomized	Yes
Randomization adequate	Yes
Blinding	Double-blind
Blinding adequate	No
Placebo	Yes
Drug comparison	No
Site description	Sleep lab
No. of subjects enrolled	8
No. of subjects completed	7
Sex	Male and female
Age	33-59 years (mean: 45)

Inclusion criteria

Volunteers who complained that they usually have problems falling asleep.

Exclusion criteria

None mentioned.

End points

Subjective sleep ratings were assessed by questionnaire, and movements were recorded throughout the night with wrist-worn activity meters.

Results

Using a criterion of five minutes without movement as the onset of sleep, valerian (450 mg) produced a significant decrease in this measure of time to fall asleep ($p < 0.01$). Increasing the dose to 900 mg led to no further improvement. For the rest of the night, activity levels were similar for all three treatments. There was no evidence of carryover of valerian effects to the next consecutive night. Valerian had no significant effect on total sleep time, nor did it influence the number of minutes with movement or the total number of movements. The subjective ratings of sleep mirrored the results from the objective ratings. Subjects reported feeling more sleepy the next morning with the larger dose of valerian (900 mg) than with placebo ($p < 0.05$).

Side effects
No side effects were reported by patients.

Authors' comments
These results show that an aqueous extract of valerian root decreases sleep latency in people who have problems falling asleep.

Reviewers' comments
This was a small pilot study ($n = 7$) with inadequate inclusion and exclusion criteria. (3, 3)

Clinical Study: Valerian (Generic)

Extract name	None given
Manufacturer	None
Indication	**Sleep quality**
Level of evidence	**II**
Therapeutic benefit	**Trend**

Bibliographic reference
Leathwood PD, Chauffard F, Heck E, Munoz-Box R (1982). Aqueous extract of valerian root (*Valeriana officinalis* L.) improves sleep quality in man. *Pharmacology, Biochemistry & Behavior* 17 (1): 65-71. (Also published in Leathwood PD, Chauffard F, Munoz-Box [1982]. Effect of *Valeriana officianalis* L. on subjective and objective sleep parameters. Sleep 1982. *Sixth European Congress on Sleep Research*, Zurich, pp. 402-405.)

Trial design
Crossover. Each subject received 3 × 3 different samples: (1) aqueous valerian extract; (2) commercial preparation (Hova®, Zyma S.A. Switzerland containing valerian extract and hops extract; patients were given a dose containing 400 mg valerian extract daily); and (3) placebo. Samples were taken in random order on nine nonconsecutive nights. Volunteers were instructed to take one sachet of pills per night, one hour before going to sleep, and to

avoid taking the pills on evenings following abnormal or excessive food intake, drinking, exercise, etc.

Study duration	9 nights
Dose	2 (200 mg) capsules daily
Route of administration	Oral
Randomized	Yes
Randomization adequate	Yes
Blinding	Single-blind
Blinding adequate	No
Placebo	Yes
Drug comparison	Yes
Drug name	Hova
Site description	Not described
No. of subjects enrolled	166
No. of subjects completed	128
Sex	Male and female
Age	59% of subjects were 40 years old or younger, 41% were older

Inclusion criteria
None mentioned.

Exclusion criteria
None mentioned.

End points
Subjects filled out sleep questionnaires the morning after taking each sample.

Results
With valerian, 37 percent of patients had shorter than normal sleep latency, whereas reduced sleep latency was 31 percent with Hova and 23 percent with placebo. The difference between placebo and valerian was statistically significant ($p = 0.01$). Sleep quality was improved with valerian compared with placebo ($p < 0.05$). The effect was most notable among people who consider themselves poor or irregular sleepers, smokers, and people with difficulty falling asleep. With Hova, no significant change was observed in the response pattern. For the whole population, no significant changes were observed either in night awakenings or dream recall. The frequency of "more sleepy than usual" the next morning was significantly greater with Hova than with placebo ($p < 0.01$) or valerian ($p < 0.05$).

Side effects
One patient withdrew from the study due to nausea, but it is unknown which treatment he received. No other side effects were mentioned in study.

Authors' comments
In this study, an aqueous extract of valerian root improved sleep quality of poor or irregular sleepers without producing a detectable hangover effect the next morning.

Reviewers' comments
This is an adequately powered, randomized study with self-rated outcomes in a large group of volunteers, only a subset of which described themselves as poor sleepers. However, no inclusion or exclusion criteria were described. (3, 5)

Clinical Study: Valerian (Generic)

Extract name	None given
Manufacturer	None
Indication	**Sleep quality** in healthy volunteers
Level of evidence	**III**
Therapeutic benefit	**Undetermined**

Bibliographic reference
Balderer G, Borbely AA (1985). Effect of valerian on human sleep. *Psychopharmacology* 87 (4): 406-409.

Trial design
Crossover trial with two parts. One group (*N* = 10) slept at home, whereas the other group (*N* = 8) slept in the laboratory. The home study tested the effects of two doses of valerian (450 mg and 900 mg) compared to placebo. Subjects took medication on a Wednesday or Thursday night of each week for three weeks, and were evaluated based on their sleep that night. The lab study compared 900 mg valerian to placebo. Subjects slept five consecutive nights in the sleep lab. The first night for these patients served as an adaptation night, and the following four nights the patients received placebo (three of the nights) or valerian (one night).

Study duration	Home study: 1 night a week for 3 weeks; lab study: 4 nights
Dose	450 mg or 900 mg valerian extract
Route of administration	Oral

Randomized	Yes
Randomization adequate	No
Blinding	Double-blind
Blinding adequate	Yes
Placebo	Yes
Drug comparison	No
Site description	Home and sleep lab
No. of subjects enrolled	H = 10; L = 8
No. of subjects completed	H = 10; L = 8
Sex	Male and female
Age	H = 24-44 years; L = 21-26 years

Inclusion criteria
Subjects were in apparently good health and did not report major sleep disturbances.

Exclusion criteria
None mentioned.

End points
Sleep was evaluated on the basis of questionnaires, self-rating scales, and nighttime motor activity. In addition, polygraphic sleep recordings and spectral analysis of the sleep EEG were performed in the laboratory group.

Results
Home Study: Sleep latency and wake time after sleep onset were reduced by more than 50 percent after the higher dose, whereas the lower dose had a somewhat smaller effect. A declining trend was also seen for the number of awakenings. Nighttime motor activity was enhanced in the middle of the night and reduced in the last third. The self-rating of sleep quality and of the momentary state in the morning and at noon showed no significant differences between the three treatments. Laboratory Study: No significant differences from placebo were obtained. However the trend of the changes in the subjective and objective measures of sleep latency and wake time after sleep onset, as well as nighttime motor activities, corresponded to that observed under home conditions. There was no evidence for a change in sleep stages and EEG spectra between the valerian night and the three placebo nights.

Side effects
None mentioned.

Authors' comments
The present study, in conjunction with previous experiments, provides evidence for a mild hypnotic action of the aqueous valerian extract.

Reviewers' comments

In this pilot study, inclusion and exclusion criteria were not well defined. The study reported no significant effect of valerian on objective polysomnographic outcome measures in the lab component, although some trends were noted. The subjective home component observed a significant effect on decrease in sleep latency for the valerian group. (3, 4)

Product Profile: Valerian Nighttime™

Manufacturer	**Dr. Willmar Schwabe GmbH & Co., Germany**
U.S. distributor	**Nature's Way Products, Inc.**
Botanical ingredient	**Valerian root extract**
Extract name	None given
Quantity	160 mg
Processing	Plant to extract ratio 4.5:1, aqueous/ ethanolic dried extract
Standardization	A minimum of 0.2% valerenic acid
Botanical ingredient	**Lemon balm leaf extract**
Extract name	None given
Quantity	80 mg
Processing	Plant to extract ratio 5.5:1, aqueous/ ethanolic dried extract
Standardization	No information
Formulation	Tablet

Recommended dose: Take one to two tablets one hour before bedtime. Up to three tablets may be taken.

DSHEA structure/function: Clinically proven to promote restful sleep.

Cautions: If sleeplessness persists for more than two weeks, consult your doctor. Insomnia may be a symptom of serious underlying medical illness. Do not take this product if you are taking sedatives or tranquilizers without first consulting your doctor. Avoid alcohol and do not drive or operate machinary while taking this product.

Other ingredients: Calcium (calcium phosphate 25 mg), cellulose, maltodextrin, modified cellulose, modified cellulose gum, stearic acid, titanium dioxide, gylcerin, silica, riboflavin, carmine.

Comments: Sold as Euvegal® forte in Europe.

Source(s) of information: Product label (© 2000 Nature's Way Products, Inc.); Dressing, Kohler, and Muller, 1996; Dressing et al., 1992.

Clinical Study: Euvegal® forte

Extract name	None given
Manufacturer	Spitzner Arzneimittel GmbH, Germany (Dr. Willmar Schwabe GmbH & Co., Germany)
Indication	**Insomnia**
Level of evidence	**II**
Therapeutic benefit	**Yes**

Bibliographic reference
Dressing H, Kohler S, Muller WE (1996). Improvement of sleep quality with a high-dose valerian/lemon balm preparation: A placebo-controlled, double-blind study. *Psychopharmakotherapie* 3: 123-130.

Trial design
Parallel. The trial was preceded by a one-week, single-blind, placebo run-in phase. Following the two-week placebo-controlled trial, a one-week, single-blind, placebo observation period was conducted.

Study duration	2 weeks
Dose	2 (160 mg valerian and 80 mg lemon balm extract) tablets twice daily
Route of administration	Oral
Randomized	No
Randomization adequate	No
Blinding	Double-blind
Blinding adequate	Yes
Placebo	Yes
Drug comparison	No
Site description	10 general practices
No. of subjects enrolled	68
No. of subjects completed	66
Sex	Male and female
Age	22-86 years (mean: 57)

Inclusion criteria
Patients at least 18 years of age with mild insomnia requiring treatment ac-

cording to the DSM-III-R or ICD-10; subjectively reported falling asleep latency of greater than 30 minutes; subjective sleep duration less than six hours per night or subjective difficulties in continued sleep (at least three interruptions per night).

Exclusion criteria
Exclusion criteria included: schizophrenia and depressive psychoses; conditions of acute cerebral confusion; sleep apnea syndrome; medication, drug, or alcohol abuse; chronic intake of psychotropic medications and potent analgesics within one week prior to the study; pregnancy or breast-feeding; poor patient compliance; simultaneous participation in another clinical study or such participation during the 30 days immediately preceding the study; improvement in sleep quality during the placebo run-in phase; severe liver, kidney, heart, or metabolic diseases; myasthenia gravis; or phases of acute delirium.

End points
Patients were evaluated weekly for major outcome measures: sleep quality (Visuelle Analogskalen morgens [VIS-M] item 2); and either day-to-day well-being (Visuelle Analogskalen abends [VIS-A] item 2) or change in condition of clinical global impression (CGI item 2). In addition, sleep questionnaire B was used. Secondary parameters also included: time to fall asleep; total sleep duration; ability to concentrate; performance; aftereffects of sedation; and anxiolytic effects.

Results
Mean sleep quality during treatment increased in both groups, but the extent of improvement with valerian/balm was significantly greater than with placebo ($p = 0.02$). Motivational status throughout the day also improved relative to placebo ($p = 0.001$). The CGI scale also indicated improvement compared to placebo ($p = 0.05$). Advantages for active treatment compared to placebo were also found in the secondary parameters: time participants required to fall asleep ($p = 0.08$), sleep quality ($p = 0.005$), relaxedness after sleep ($p = 0.0004$), psychosomatic symptoms during the sleep phase ($p = 0.03$), mentally balanced in the evening ($p = 0.06$), and mentally exhausted in the evening ($p = 0.04$). No hangover, discontinuation, or rebound phenomena were observed. Some positive effects of therapy remained during the week following treatment.

Side effects
Thirteen adverse events were reported: eight in the treatment group and five in the placebo group. Adverse events included: stomachache, headache, and cramps in the calves.

Authors' comments
High-dose valerian/lemon balm preparations constitute a therapeutic alter-

native or complement in the treatment of insomnia cases that may be mild, but nevertheless require treatment.

Reviewers' comments
This is a reasonably well-designed and well-reported study. The inclusion and exclusion criteria are well-defined, and there is a nice description of side effects and adverse events. The randomization process was not described. (Translation reviewed) (3, 5)

Clinical Study: Euvegal® forte

Extract name	None given
Manufacturer	Spitzner Arzneimittel GmbH, Germany (Dr. Willmar Schwabe GmbH & Co., Germany)
Indication	**Sleep quality** in healthy volunteers
Level of evidence	**III**
Therapeutic benefit	**Undetermined**

Bibliographic reference
Dressing H, Riemann D, Low H, Schredl M, Reh C, Laux P, Muller WE (1992). Insomnia: Are valerian/balm combinations of equal value to benzo-diazepine? *Therapiewoche* 42 (12): 726-736.

Trial design
Crossover. Volunteers were monitored for a total of nine nights in the sleep laboratory: five nights, followed by a one-week washout period, and then another four nights. The first night was used for adaptation. Using a double dummy approach, one capsule and one tablet containing either placebo or active substance were given every night in the sleep lab. Either the valerian/balm preparation or the benzodiazepine triazolam (0.125 mg) was administered on the third/fourth or on the seventh/eighth night.

Study duration	4 nights
Dose	1 (160 mg valerian and 80 mg lemon balm extract) tablet
Route of administration	Oral
Randomized	Yes
Randomization adequate	No
Blinding	Double-blind
Blinding adequate	No
Placebo	Yes

Drug comparison	Yes
Drug name	Triazolam
Site description	Sleep laboratory
No. of subjects enrolled	20
No. of subjects completed	20
Sex	Male and female
Age	30-50 years (mean: 37.2)

Inclusion criteria
Healthy volunteers ages 30 to 50.

Exclusion criteria
Physical and/or psychiatric conditions, family history of psychiatric diseases.

End points
Sleep EEG was recorded on all nine nights and evaluated for continuity, sleep architecture, and REM sleep parameters. Before, during, and after the trial, well-being (subjective condition status) and other psychopathological variables were recorded, and heart rate was monitored. During the interval week, participants were given stress tests: Concentration Performance Test (CPT) and Labyrinth test.

Results
After ingestion of triazolam, sleep efficiency increased significantly, falling-asleep latency decreased, the awake stage was reduced, Stage 2 was increased, and REM latency was significantly lengthened. No significant effects were established for the valerian/lemon balm preparation until the participants were divided into groups of "good" or "bad" sleepers. The "good" sleepers showed a significant reduction of REM-phase sleep and duration of the first REM phase. The groups of 'bad' sleepers showed a significant increase in sleep efficiency compared to placebo and a tendency to increase deep sleep Stages 3 and 4. There was a tendency toward reduction of REM density. The valerian/balm preparation did not have any influence on concentration or performance of participants. No rebound effect or daytime sedation effect were observed.

Side effects
None reported.

Authors' comments
In the assessment of the "bad" sleepers, the effects of the valerian/balm preparation were comparable to triazolam. The results here obtained demonstrate that plant-based combination preparations, such as high-dosage

valerian/balm combinations, present a thoroughly effective and safe alternative to benzodiazepines in the treatment of specific sleeping disturbances.

Reviewers' comments
This study was limited by several factors: small sample size, inappropriate inclusion/exclusion criteria, and unclear outcome measures. Neither the blinding nor the randomization were adequately described. Overall, this was not a well-described study. (Translation reviewed) (1, 3)

Product Profile: Songha Night®

Manufacturer	**Pharmaton S.A., Switzerland**
U.S. distributor	None
Botanical ingredient	**Valerian root extract**
Extract name	None given
Quantity	120 mg
Processing	Plant to extract ratio 4.5:1
Standardization	No information
Formulation	Tablet
Botanical ingredient	**Lemon balm leaf extract**
Extract name	None given
Quantity	80 mg
Processing	Plant to extract ratio 5:1
Standardization	No information

Source(s) of information: Cerny and Schmid, 1999.

Clinical Study: Songha Night®

Extract name	None given
Manufacturer	Pharmaton S.A., Switzerland
Indication	**Sleep quality** in healthy volunteers
Level of evidence	**II**
Therapeutic benefit	**Undetermined**

Bibliographic reference
Cerny A, Schmid K (1999). Tolerability and efficacy of valerian/lemon balm in healthy volunteers: A double-blind, placebo-controlled, multicenter study. *Fitoterapia* 70 (3): 221-228.

Trial design
Parallel.

Study duration	1 month
Dose	3 (120 mg valerian and 80 mg lemon balm extract) tablets 30 minutes before bed
Route of administration	Oral
Randomized	Yes
Randomization adequate	Yes
Blinding	Double-blind
Blinding adequate	Yes
Placebo	Yes
Drug comparison	No
Site description	3 hospitals, 3 general practices
No. of subjects enrolled	98
No. of subjects completed	95
Sex	Male and female
Age	20-70 years (mean: 34)

Inclusion criteria
Healthy volunteers between the ages of 20 and 70 who were fit for work.

Exclusion criteria
Patients with renal insufficiency, hepatic dysfunction, cardiovascular disease, psychic disorder, drug and alcohol abuse, concomitant treatment with other drugs including herbal sedatives, known hypersensitivity to any of the ingredients of the study drug, pregnancy, lactation, women of childbearing potential who did not use an established contraceptive, and participation in another study within the past 30 days.

End points
Primary parameters were assessment of tolerability and incidence of adverse events. Secondary parameters included laboratory tests, physical examination, and assessments of well-being and sleep quality rated on the 100 mm visual analogue scale (VAS).

Results
Tolerance was acceptable to excellent for both valerian/balm and placebo (no significant difference between groups). There was no significant difference between the two groups in reporting of adverse events and none were severe. The valerian/balm group reported a significantly higher quality of sleep, 33 percent compared to 9 percent of the placebo group ($p = 0.04$).

Analysis of the results of the visual analogue scale showed a slight but nonsignificant improvement in sleep quality. Well-being in both groups remained unchanged. No significant differences were found between groups in terms of physical examination or laboratory tests.

Side effects
About 28 percent in both groups reported adverse events. The two most often reported were sleep disturbances and tiredness (both groups). One patient in each group quit the study because of nausea and sleep disturbances.

Authors' comments
In the present study, sleep quality improved significantly in subjects who received valerian/lemon balm, which was surprising since only healthy volunteers not complaining of insomnia participated. The observed effect has to be considered with caution because it was shown only in the assessment of change and not in the assessment of the actual state by VAS.

Reviewers' comments
This is a fairly well-designed phase I, tolerability study. No difference was observed between the valerian and placebo groups on the secondary outcome measure of sleep quality (subjective rating by visual analogue scale). (5, 5)

Product Profile: Alluna™ Sleep

Manufacturer	**Zeller AG, Switzerland**
U.S. distributor	**GlaxoSmithKline**
Botanical ingredient	**Hops extract**
Extract name	**Ze 91019**
Quantity	60 mg
Processing	Plant to extract ratio 5-7:1
Standardization	No information
Botanical ingredient	**Valerian root extract**
Extract name	**Ze 91019**
Quantity	250 mg
Processing	Plant to extract ratio 4-6:1
Standardization	No information
Formulation	Tablet

Recommended dose: Take two tablets one hour before bedtime with a glass of water. Not habit forming.

DSHEA structure/function: Promotes a healthy sleep pattern. Helps promote calm and relaxation so you can fall asleep naturally and rest through the night. Helps your body maintain its own natural sleep pattern so you wake up refreshed.

Cautions: Contact your doctor before use if you are pregnant or lactating. Driving or operating machinery while using this product is not recommended. Chronic insomniacs should consult their doctor before using this product.

Other ingredients: Microcrystalline cellulose, soy polysaccharide, hydrogenated castor oil, hydroxypropyl methylcellulose. Contains less than 2 percent titanium dioxide, propylene glycol, magnesium sterate, silica, polyethylene glycol (400, 6,000, and 20,000), blue 2 lake, artificial flavoring.

Comments: Sold as IVEL® and ReDormin® in Europe.

Source(s) of information: Product package (© 1999 SmithKline Beecham); Vonderheid-Guth et al., 2000.

Clinical Study: IVEL® or ReDormin®

Extract name	Ze 91019
Manufacturer	Zeller AG, Switzerland
Indication	**Electrophysiological effects** in healthy volunteers
Level of evidence	**III**
Therapeutic benefit	**MOA**

Bibliographic reference
Vonderheid-Guth B, Todorova A, Brattstrom A, Dimpfel W (2000). Pharmacodynamic effects of valerian and hops extract combination (Ze 91019) on the quantitative-topographical EEG in healthy volunteers. *European Journal of Medical Research* 5 (4): 139-144.

Trial design
Crossover. Subjects participated in two trials separated by several months. First trial: low dose (500/120 mg valerian/hops) compared to placebo; second trial: high dose (1,500/360 mg valerian/hops) compared to placebo. In each trial, valerian/hops was compared to placebo on two days with a one-week washout period in between.

Study duration	2 days
Dose	2 or 6 (250 mg valerian and 60 mg hops) pills
Route of administration	Oral
Randomized	Yes
Randomization adequate	No
Blinding	Single-blind
Blinding adequate	No
Placebo	Yes
Drug comparison	No
Site description	Not described
No. of subjects enrolled	12
No. of subjects completed	12
Sex	Male
Age	18-30 years (mean: 24)

Inclusion criteria
Healthy young adults.

Exclusion criteria
Relevant pathological findings.

End points
Quantitative topographical EEG (qEEG) was recorded at baseline and one, two, and four hours after drug intake. Recording conditions were eyes open, eyes closed, and under mental demand (taking the Concentration Performance Test [CPT]).

Results
After administration of low-dose valerian/hops, qEEG power changes remained more or less equivalent to placebo, except for a tendency toward reduction of alpha- and beta1-activity after four hours. The high dose of valerian/hops led to a power increase in the delta region, decreases in alpha-power, and a weak decrease in beta-power. No significant EEG changes were measurable during CPT. A minimal increase in answer time and time for correct answers was observed four hours after administration of low dose and one hour after administration of high dose.

Side effects
None mentioned.

Author's comments
Within four hours after oral administration, the valerian-hops extract combination Ze 91019 produces slight though clear visible EEG power changes in

healthy subjects. These EEG changes have been related to the time after administration and the dose used, whereby the pharmacodynamic response of the target organ (CNS) to Ze 91019 is clearly demonstrated.

Reviewers' comments
This evaluation of 17-channel EEG data following a single dose of drug or placebo has limited methodologic detail for EEG analysis. The EEG data is confounded by large numbers of variables with no statistical adjustment of p values. This results in an uncertain effect on EEG. (0, 3)

2nd Wind™

Ingredients:
  Ginseng (*Panax ginseng* C.A. Meyer) root
  Cordyceps [*Cordyceps sinensis* (Berk.) Sacc.]
  Reishi mushroom [*Ganoderma lucidum* (Curtis: Fr.) P. Karst.]
  Enoki mushroom [*Flammulina velutipes*]
  Siberian ginseng [*Eleutherococcus senticosus* (Rupr. & Maxim.) Maxim.] root
  Tangerine (*Citrus reticulata* Blanco) peel

PREPARATIONS USED IN REVIEWED CLINICAL STUDIES

2nd Wind™ is a proprietary blend of six different ingredients: ginseng (root extract), cordyceps (fermentation), reishi mushroom (fermentation), enoki mushroom (fermentation), Siberian ginseng (root extract), and tangerine (peel extract). It is manufactured and distributed by Botanica BioScience Corporation.

SUMMARY OF REVIEWED CLINICAL STUDIES

2nd Wind is formulated to accelerate recovery after exercise by enhancing the clearance of lactic acid (lactate) from the muscles during

2ND WIND™ SUMMARY TABLE

Product Name	Manufacturer/ U.S. Distributor	Product Characteristics	Dose in Trials	Indication	No. of Trials	Benefit (Evidence Level-Trial No.)
2nd Wind™	Botanica BioScience Corporation/Botanica BioScience Corporation	Blend of six ingredients	1-1.35 g daily	Recovery after exercise	2	Undetermined (III-2)

and after exercise. Lactic acid is produced during exercise, and its accumulation in muscles can result in soreness and fatigue. With intense exercise, lactic acid buildup can reduce blood pH and cause a condition known as acidosis. Thus, enhancing the clearance of lactic acid is a key principle in increasing athletic performance, and is a means to speeding recovery from exercise. Lactate measurements in the blood give an indirect, but reliable indication of lactate levels in muscle cells (Burke, 1996).

2nd Wind

Recovery After Exercise

Two unpublished, placebo-controlled clinical studies were reviewed. In the first study, including 20 healthy young males, 1 g of the formula per day caused a statistically significant increase in the clearance of lactic acid in the blood following exercise after two weeks of treatment compared to baseline measurements. Clearance of lactic acid in the placebo group did not improve (Burke, 1996). The second study, with 12 healthy students given 1.35 g 2nd Wind or placebo daily for five weeks, also reported comparatively less lactic acid in the blood following exercise. The plasma pH following exercise appeared to be more stable in the treatment group as well (Seifert, Burke, and Lahr, 1998). A review by Dr. Mary Hardy found that neither study established therapeutic benefit due to an inadequate description of the methods and results in the trial reports.

ADVERSE REACTIONS OR SIDE EFFECTS

No side effects were reported in either trial.

REFERENCES

Burke ER (1996). Clinical study to evaluate effects of 2nd Wind ARX (athletic recovery x-cclerator) on blood lactate clearance in healthy human subjects. Conducted at Beijing Medical University Sports Research Institute. Unpublished clinical report.

Seifert JG, Burke ER, Lahr J (1998). The effects of herbal intake on clearance of lactic acid and cycling performance. Unpublished report.

DETAILS ON 2ND WIND PRODUCT
AND CLINICAL STUDIES

A profile on the product is followed by details of the clinical studies associated with that product. Clinical studies are grouped by therapeutic indication, in accordance with the order in the Summary Table.

Product Profile: 2nd Wind™

Manufacturer	**Botanica BioScience Corporation**
U.S. distributor	**Botanica BioScience Corporation**
Formula botanicals	***Cordyceps sinensis*** (fermentation); ***Ganoderma lucidum*** (fermentation); ***Flammulina velutipes*** (fermentation); **Siberian ginseng** (*Eleutherococcus senticosus;* std. Root extract); ***Panax ginseng*** (std. Root extract); ***Citrus reticulata*** (extract from peel)
Quantity	450 mg
Processing	See Formula botanicals
Standardization	No information
Formulation	Capsule

Recommended dose: Take two capsules once daily as part of a normal workout regimen. Optimal results have been shown after three to four weeks of continued use.

DSHEA structure/function: Clinically proven to double clearance of lactic acid in the blood. Reduces muscle soreness and fatigue.

Cautions: In case of accidental overdose, seek professional advice immediately. If taking prescription medicine, pregnant, or lactating, consult with a doctor before taking.

Other ingredients: Cellulose, magnesium stearate (vegetable grade), silica.

Source(s) of information: Product package (© 1999 Botanica Bioscience Corporation).

Clinical Study: 2nd Wind™

Extract name	N/A
Manufacturer	Botanica BioScience Corporation
Indication	**Recovery after exercise; lactate clearance**
Level of evidence	**III**
Therapeutic benefit	**Undetermined**

Bibliographic reference
Burke ER (1996). Clinical study to evaluate effects of 2nd Wind ARX (athletic recovery x-celerator) on blood lactate clearance in healthy human subjects. Conducted at Beijing Medical University Sports Research Institute. Unpublished clinical report.

Trial design
Parallel. Subjects were treated with either placebo or 2nd Wind each morning for two weeks. Treatment continued, unblinded, for an additional two weeks in the 2nd Wind group.

Study duration	2 weeks with additional 2-week follow-up
Dose	1 g every morning
Route of administration	Oral
Randomized	Yes
Randomization adequate	No
Blinding	Double-blind
Blinding adequate	Yes
Placebo	Yes
Drug comparison	No
Site description	Sports medicine research institute
No. of subjects enrolled	20
No. of subjects completed	Not given
Sex	Male
Age	Mean: 18.5 years

Inclusion criteria
Healthy students with normal health history, physical examination, and blood liver function tests.

Exclusion criteria
None mentioned.

End points

An exercise challenge test was performed before ingesting the study material, after two weeks of treatment with either 2nd Wind or placebo, and again after four weeks of treatment for the 2nd Wind group. Lactic acid was measured from blood samples obtained from the earlobe taken at rest 30 minutes before exercise, immediately upon finishing exercise as the maximum lactic acid level, and 15 minutes after stopping exercise as the end point level (recovery level).

Results

After treatment with 2nd Wind for two weeks, lactate clearance after exercise recovery increased to 27.4 mg/dl, up from 15.4mg/dl prior to the study. In the placebo group, lactate clearance was 10.1 mg/dl after two weeks compared to 14.3 mg/dl prior to the study. After four weeks of 2nd Wind treatment, lactate clearance in the verum group increased to 31.6 mg/dl.

Side effects

No side effects were reported by the study participants.

Author's comments

These results show a statistically significant improvement in lactate clearance after stopping exercise with the usage of 2nd Wind, as well as a trend of increasing lactate clearance improvement the longer the product is taken.

Reviewer's comments

This trial was double-blinded and randomized, however, the randomization process was not described adequately. Although the outcome measures were defined clearly, the sample size was insufficient to allow full statistical analysis, and no mean or standard deviations were given for the results. (2, 2)

Clinical Study: 2nd Wind™

Extract name	N/A
Manufacturer	Botanica BioScience Corporation
Indication	**Recovery after exercise; lactate clearance**
Level of evidence	**III**
Therapeutic benefit	**Undetermined**

Bibliographic reference
Seifert JG, Burke ER, Lahr J (1998). The effects of herbal intake on clearance of lactic acid and cycling performance. Unpublished report.

Trial design
Parallel.

Study duration	5 weeks
Dose	1,350 mg daily
Route of administration	Oral
Randomized	Yes
Randomization adequate	No
Blinding	Single-blind
Blinding adequate	No
Placebo	Yes
Drug comparison	No
Site description	Not described
No. of subjects enrolled	36
No. of subjects completed	12
Sex	Not given
Age	18-45 years

Inclusion criteria
Active, healthy subjects.

Exclusion criteria
None mentioned.

End points
Prior to the study, subjects were assessed on a ramped cycling performance test in which workload increased every four minutes. At the end of every four-minute interval, a blood sample was taken and analyzed for lactic acid. This test was repeated after five weeks to assess whether fitness levels of subjects had changed over the study period. After the five-week treatment period, subjects cycled at a power output level higher than their lactate threshold for 20 minutes. After this period, subjects were seated, and blood samples were taken every three minutes for 12 minutes during recovery. At 12 minutes, subjects had to cycle as fast as possible to complete 60,000 joules of work. Blood samples were analyzed for lactic acid, blood bicarbonate, and pH.

Results
Compared to placebo, 2nd Wind led to significantly greater change in lactic

acid levels during exercise recovery. Lactic acid values at the end of the 12-minute recovery period were 7 percent below baseline for the 2nd Wind group and 22 percent above baseline for the placebo group. Compared to placebo, the 2nd Wind group had more stability in plasma pH and bicarbonate buffering system. The 2nd Wind group completed the time trial 56.2 seconds faster than the placebo group, although this difference was not statistically significant. No significant differences were observed in the pre- and poststudy fitness levels both within and between groups. Only six subjects in each group were appropriately verified as placebo or treatment product due to administrative difficulties.

Side effects
None mentioned in paper.

Authors' comments
Compared to the placebo group, 2nd Wind led to statistically less lactic acid accumulation following intense cycling, less stress placed upon bicarbonate buffering system, and a strong trend toward improvement in high-intensity cycling performance.

Reviewer's comments
This study was not blinded and the randomization process was not adequately described. The article is poorly referenced and the clinical significance of the results is not clear. The outcome measures were clearly defined. (Publication draft reviewed) (0, 5).

Cystone®

Ingredients:
Shilapushpa (*Didymocarpus pedicellata* R. Br.) leaves
Pasanabheda (*Saxifraga ligulata* Wall.) root
Rough chaff tree (*Achyranthes aspera* L.) seed
Indian madder (*Rubia cordifolia* L.) root
Ash-colored fleabane (*Vernonia cinerea* [L.] Less.) whole
Umbrella's edge (*Cyperus scariosus* R. Br.) tuber
Sedge (*Onosma bracteatum* Wall.) aerial parts
Mineral pitch

PREPARATIONS USED
IN REVIEWED CLINICAL STUDIES

Cystone® tablets contain a combination of seven herbal extracts and mineral pitch, a total of 540 mg per tablet. Current labels suggest a dose of one to two tablets twice daily, for a total quantity of 1.08 to 2.16 g per day. Cystone is manufactured by The Himalaya Drug Company in India, and distributed in the United States by Himalaya USA. Cystone is also available under the name UriCare®. The current Cystone product label lists the ingredients indicated previously. The material used in the clinical study had the same name, but contained an additional ingredient: Hajrul yahood bahsma.

The material used in the clinical trial is described as tablets containing 223 mg of the proprietary blend. The ingredients and their quantities were listed in the trial report as: extracts of *Didymocarpus pedicellata* (65 mg), *Saxifraga ligulata* (49 mg), *Rubia cordifolia* (16 mg), *Cyperus scariosus* (16 mg), *Achyranthes aspera* (16 mg), *Onosma bracteatum* (16 mg), *Vernonia cinerea* (16 mg) and Shilajeet (purified mineral pitch) (13 mg), as well as Hajrul yahood bahsma (16 mg). Hajrul yahood bahsma was prepared with *Ocimum basilicum*, *Tribulus terrestris*, *Mimosa pudica*, *Dolichos biflorus*, *Pavonia odorata*, *Equisetum arvense*, and *Tectona grandis* seed. The

CYSTONE® SUMMARY TABLE

Product Name	Manufacturer/ U.S. Distributor	Product Characteristics	Dose in Trials	Indication	No. of Trials	Benefit (Evidence Level-Trial No.)
Cystone®*	The Himalaya Drug Company, India/ Himalaya USA	Blend of 7 ex- tracts and purified mineral pitch	1.34 g daily	Kidney and bladder stones	1	Undetermined (III-1)

*The product used in the trial was slightly different.

dose used in the study was two tablets three times daily or a total of 1.34 g per day (Misgar, 1982).

SUMMARY OF REVIEWED CLINICAL STUDIES

Cystone is an herbal formula tested in the treatment of kidney and bladder stones. Urinary tract stones form in the bladder and kidney. Human urine is saturated with calcium oxalate, uric acid, and phosphates that normally remain in solution. However dehydration, urinary stasis, pH changes, foreign bodies, and infection can lead to the formation of stones. Stones are hard buildups of mineral composed mostly of calcium salts, uric acid, or struvite (phosphate of magnesium and ammonia). Treatment depends upon differentiation between the various stone types as well as recognition and control of any underlying metabolic diseases or structural abnormalities of the urinary tract (Pizzorno and Murray, 1999).

Cystone

Kidney and Bladder Stones

The effect of Cystone on patients with kidney and bladder stones (nephroureterolithiasis) was studied in a four-arm, open, clinical trial including 100 participants. Two groups were given Cystone (two tablets three times daily) and either encouraged to drink plenty of liquids or given forced diuresis (intravenous liquids). Two control groups were given antispasmodics and also either encouraged to drink plenty of fluids or given forced diuresis. In the Cystone treatment groups, 76 and 80 percent, respectively, of participants were able to pass their stones over a period of one to six months and thereby avoid surgery. In the control groups given antispasmodics, only 20 and 28 percent, respectively, were able to avoid surgery (Misgar, 1982). However, due to poor methodological flaws, including the lack of characterization of the size of the kidney and bladder stones in the various treatment groups, our reviewers, Drs. Elliot Fagelman and Franklin Lowe, found the benefit to be undetermined.

ADVERSE REACTIONS OR SIDE EFFECTS

No adverse effects were reported in a clinical trial in which 50 subjects were given two tablets three times daily for six months (Misgar, 1982).

REFERENCES

Misgar MS (1982). Controlled trial in 100 cases with nephro-ureterolithiasis by cystone—An indigenous drug and other advocated methods. *PROBE* 21 (4): 281-287.

Pizzorno JE, Murray MT, eds. (1999). *Textbook of Natural Medicine,* Second Edition, Volume 2. London: Churchill Livingstone.

DETAILS ON CYSTONE PRODUCT
AND CLINICAL STUDIES

A profile on the product is followed by details of the clinical studies associated with that product. Clinical studies are grouped by therapeutic indication, in accordance with the order in the Summary Table.

Product Profile: Cystone®

Manufacturer	**The Himalaya Drug Company, India**
U.S. distributor	**Himalaya USA**
Formula Botanicals	**Shilapushpa leaves** (*Didymocarpus pedicellata* R. Br.); **pasanabheda root** (*Saxifraga ligulata* Wall.); **rough chaff tree seed** (*Achyranthes aspera* L.); **Indian madder root** (*Rubia cordifolia* L.); **ash-colored fleabane whole** (*Vernonia cinerea* [L.] Less.); **umbrella's edge tuber** (*Cyperus scariosus* R. Br.); **sedge aerial parts** (*Onosma bracteatum* Wall.); **mineral pitch**
Quantity	540 mg
Processing	Blend of 7 extracts and purified mineral pitch
Standardization	No information
Formulation	Tablet

Recommended dose: Take one or two tablets two times per day with meals.

DSHEA structure/function: Natural urinary support. Helps regulate calcium absorption and precipitation for efficient kidney and urinary functions.

Other ingredients: Lime silicate, magnesium stearate, sodium carboxymethyl cellulose, microcrystalline cellulose, crospovidone, aerosil.

Comments: Also sold as UriCare®.

Source(s) of information: Product label; Misgar, 1982.

Clinical Study: Cystone®

Extract name	N/A
Manufacturer	Himalaya Drug Company, India
Indication	**Kidney and bladder stones** (nephroureterolithiasis)
Level of evidence	**III**
Therapeutic benefit	**Undetermined**

Bibliographic reference

Misgar MS (1982). Controlled trial in 100 cases with nephro-uretero-lithiasis by Cystone—An indigenous drug and other advocated methods. *PROBE* 21 (4): 281-287.

Trial design

Parallel. Four groups of 25 each. Group I was given Cystone for two to six months and encouraged to drink plenty of fluids. Group II was given Cystone for two to six months, along with forced diuresis (intravenous fluids). Group III was given antispasmodics and encouraged to drink plenty of fluids; this group was followed for a year. Group IV was put on antispasmodics and forced diuresis; they were followed for a year.

Study duration	2-6 months to 1 year
Dose	2 tablets 3 times daily
Route of administration	Oral
Randomized	No
Randomization adequate	No
Blinding	Open
Blinding adequate	No
Placebo	No
Drug comparison	Yes
Drug name	Antispasmodics
Site description	One surgical department
No. of subjects enrolled	100
No. of subjects completed	100
Sex	Male and female
Age	10-60 years

Inclusion criteria

Patients with nephroureterolithiasis (stones in the kidney and ureter).

Exclusion criteria
None mentioned.

End points
X-rays were taken every four weeks to compare the effectiveness of each method. Patients who passed their stones without surgery within the allotted time frame for that group (six months or one year) were assessed as responders to therapy.

Results
In Group I, 19 of 25 cases showed good response to treatment with Cystone, and thereby averted an operation. Six cases underwent surgery. Of the 19 cases that passed stones, 16 expelled the stones between four to eight weeks, two at the end of 12 weeks, and one after six months. All 19 cases observed remarkable relief in the burning sensation during micturition. In Group II, 20 of 25 cases responded well to the treatment, and five cases had to have surgery. Eighteen cases passed stones at the end of eight weeks, and two cases at the end of 16 and 24 weeks respectively. In Group III, only five cases responded to treatment, and 20 had to have surgery. In Group IV seven cases responded to the treatment and 18 cases underwent surgery.

Side effects
No adverse side effects from Cystone.

Author's comments
Of the four different methods tried in the treatment of nephroureterolithiasis, Cystone tablets gave excellent results as compared to other methods. The present study thus establishes that Cystone has a potent role in early cases of nephroureterolithiasis, and should therefore be used in every such case before resorting to surgical intervention.

Reviewers' comments
This study has several flaws. The subjects were not randomized, and there was no control for kidney stone size. The chance of a stone passing is much greater for a small stone. It is possible that the patients treated with Cystone had smaller stones than the other groups, thus skewing the results in favor of Cystone. (1, 3)

Gastrim®

Ingredients:
Crowfoot (*Aconitum palmatum* D. Don.) root
Black pepper (*Piper nigrum* L.) fruit
False black pepper (*Embelia ribes* Burm. f.) fruit
Ginger (*Zingiber officinale* Rosc.) rhizome
Triphala:
  Amalaki (*Emblica officinalis* Gaertn.) fruit
  Vibhitaka (*Terminalia bellerica* [Gaertn.] Roxb.) fruit
  Haritaki (*Terminalia chebula* Retz.) fruit rind
Mint (*Mentha arvensis* L.) leaves
Lemon (*Citrus limon* [L.] Burm. f.) fruit
Papaya (*Carica papaya* L.) fruit

PREPARATIONS USED IN REVIEWED CLINICAL STUDIES

Gastrim® (previously called Gasex®) is manufactured by the Himalaya Drug Company in India, and distributed in the United States by Himalaya USA. Gastrim is also available under the name GastriCare®. The current product label lists the ten herbal ingredients indicated earlier. Also listed on the label, in the category of other ingredients, are purified conch shell ash and purified cowrie shell ash. The recommended dose is one to two 515 mg tablets, before meals or as needed.

The material used in one of the clinical trials is described as tablets containing 214 mg total ingredients. The dose in the trial was two tablets three times a day, for a total of 1.28 g per day. The ingredients and their quantities were listed in one trial report as *Aconitum palmatum* (65 mg), *Piper nigrum* (19 mg), extract of *Embelia ribes* (22 mg), extract of Triphala (22 mg), extract of *Zingiber officinale* (22 mg), cowrie bhasma (purified cowrie shell ash) (32 mg), and shankh bhasma (purified conch shell ash) (32 mg)—all prepared in the juices

1265

GASTRIM® SUMMARY TABLE

Product Name	Manufacturer/ U.S. Distributor	Product Characteristics	Dose in Trials	Indication	No. of Trials	Benefit (Evidence Level-Trial No.)
Gastrim® (previously Gasex®)	The Himalaya Drug Company, India/ Himalaya USA	Blend of 10 herbs plus purified ash	2 tablets 2-3 times daily	Dyspepsia (indigestion)	1	Undetermined (III-1)
				Postopera- tive gastric distress	1	Undetermined (III-1)

and decoctions of *Mentha arvensis, Moringa pterygosperma, Carica papaya, Citrus limon,* etc. (Chandra et al., 1978). The other clinical trial did not provide a list of product ingredients (Mishra and Singh, 1981). The current product differs from that described in the trial in that *Moringa pterygosperma* is not mentioned on the label.

SUMMARY OF REVIEWED CLINICAL STUDIES

The two studies reviewed here test Gastrim (Gasex) for its ability to relieve gastric complaints. As described in the studies, complaints of indigestion or dyspepsia included symptoms of belching, sour eructations, frequent or excessive passage of gas, abdominal fullness, vague abdominal pain, epigastric burning, nausea, and unsatisfactory evacuation. These symptoms were linked to gas in the abdomen.

Gastrim

Dyspepsia (Indigestion)

A trial included 100 patients with symptoms of dyspepsia (indigestion) who were given either Gasex or placebo for two weeks. The dose of Gasex was two tablets three times daily for one week, and then two tablets twice daily for the second week. Thirty-six of the 50 patients in the placebo group did not have any response after two weeks and were switched to Gasex treatment. Of all the subjects given Gasex, 71 of 86 were judged as having a good to excellent therapeutic response (Mishra and Singh, 1981). Our reviewers, Drs. Karriem Ali and Richard Aranda, commented that the crossing over of the placebo nonresponders to the treatment arm, without any distinction in the reporting of the results, obscures the purpose of having a placebo group.

Postoperative Gastric Distress

Another trial with Gasex studied 150 women recovering from gynecological surgery. Treatment began on the postoperative day at the onset of bowel sounds, with either Gasex (two tablets three times daily) or vitamin B complex tablets as placebo, and continued for one to two weeks. All patients taking Gasex showed considerable improvement in symptoms compared to the controls. In the Gasex group, a good to excellent response was observed in 95 percent of patients with abdominal discomfort, and in 88 percent with flatulence, compared to 14 percent and 4 percent of the control group, respectively (Chandra et al., 1978). The randomization and blinding processes were inadequate, and the use of vitamin B complex as placebo was not explained.

ADVERSE REACTIONS OR SIDE EFFECTS

Neither study observed or mentioned any side effects.

REFERENCES

Chandra R, Agrawal S, Bajaj S, Goel S (1978). A clinical trial of Gasex in gastro-intestinal disorders in post-operative gastro-intestinal symptoms. *PROBE* 17 (4): 330-333.

Mishra DN, Singh T (1981). Clinical trial of Gasex in functional dyspepsias. *PROBE* 20 (3): 208-211.

DETAILS ON GASTRIM PRODUCT
AND CLINICAL STUDIES

A profile on the product is followed by details of the clinical studies associated with that product. Clinical studies are grouped by therapeutic indication, in accordance with the order in the Summary Table.

Product Profile: Gastrim®

Manufacturer	**The Himalaya Drug Company, India**
U.S. distributor	**Himalaya USA**
Formula Botanicals	**Crowfoot root** (*Aconitum palmatum* D. Don.); **black pepper fruit** (*Piper nigrum* L.); **false black pepper fruit** (*Embelia ribes* Burm. f.); **ginger rhizome** *(Zingiber officinale* Rosc.); **Triphala** [including amalaki fruit (*Emblica officinalis* Gaertn.); vibhitaka fruit (*Terminalia bellerica* [Gaertn] Roxb.); haritaki fruit rind (*Terminalia chebula* Retz.); **mint leaves** (*Mentha arvensis* L.); **lemon fruit** (*Citrus limon* [L.] Burm. f.); **papaya fruit** (*Carica papaya* L.)
Quantity	515 mg
Processing	No information
Standardization	No information
Formulation	Tablet

Recommended dose: Take one or two tablets before meals or whenever needed.

DSHEA structure/function: Natural digestive support. Provides support for the whole digestive function, and is an effective antiflatulent that alleviates bloating and relieves upset stomach or occasional heartburn.

Other ingredients: Purified conch shell ash, purified cowrie shell ash, magnesium stearate, sodium carboxymethylcellulose, microcrystalline cellulose, crospovidone, aerosil.

Comments: Previously called Gasex®. Also sold as GastriCare®.

Source(s) of information: Product label.

Clinical Study: Gasex®

Extract name	N/A
Manufacturer	The Himalaya Drug Company, India
Indication	**Dyspepsia** (indigestion)
Level of evidence	**III**
Therapeutic benefit	**Undetermined**

Bibliographic reference
Mishra DN, Singh T (1981). Clinical trial of Gasex in functional dyspepsias. *PROBE* 20 (3): 208-211.

Trial design
Parallel. Patients in the placebo group without significant relief after two weeks were switched to Gasex treatment.

Study duration	2 weeks
Dose	2 tablets 3 times daily for 1 week, then 2 tablets twice daily
Route of administration	Oral
Randomized	Yes
Randomization adequate	No
Blinding	Single-blind
Blinding adequate	No
Placebo	Yes
Drug comparison	No
Site description	Not described
No. of subjects enrolled	100
No. of subjects completed	100
Sex	Male and female
Age	10-80 years

Inclusion criteria
Patients with symptoms of dyspepsia and indigestion, including belching, sour eructations, frequent or excessive passage of flatus, abdominal fullness, vague abdominal pain, epigastric burning, nausea, and unsatisfactory evacuation.

Exclusion criteria
Patients with any organic disease or demonstrable structural abnormalities.

End points
Effectiveness was judged subjectively on weekly visits by the patients.

Results
Thirty-six out of 50 patients started on placebo did not have any response in two weeks time and were subsequently put on Gasex tablets. Ten patients with hyperacidity received significant and sustained relief with Gasex. Fourteen patients had cysts of *Entamoeba histolytica* and were given antiamebic treatment. Gasex gave long-lasting relief to these patients. Fourteen of 50 cases responded to placebo. None of these patients had their illness for more than two weeks. Overall, 71 of 86 (82.6 percent) patients responded to Gasex.

Side effects
No side effects were noted.

Authors' comments
Gasex was found to be effective against dyspepsia in 82.6 percent of cases. The drug also seems to have an antacid property, as concluded from subjective relief obtained in ten cases of hyperacidity. The drug also proved beneficial in 14 cases of chronic mucus passers following amebiasis. The response was poor in the relative minority of cases with deep-seated emotional problems.

Reviewers' comments
This is an unsatisfactory trial of poor design. The stated objectives of the study were not met. Efficacy in the treatment of functional dyspepsia was not determined because there was no comparison between the treatment group and controls, and there was no presentation of the methodology data relevant to the treatment of hyperacidity. The crossing over of the placebo nonresponders to the treatment arm and simply including their data as part of the treatment group without any distinction obscures the entire trial. The statement made that the failure of treatment in certain patients was secondary to emotional problems is conjecture not supported by the data or references. The appropriateness of sample size was not subjected to power analysis, but it would appear adequate. The dosage choice was not discussed in the paper nor was it substantiated by reference(s), and the trial length was inadequate for a functional dyspepsia study. (0, 2)

Clinical Study: Gasex®

Extract name	N/A
Manufacturer	Himalaya Drug Company, India

Indication	**Postoperative gastric distress**
Level of evidence	**III**
Therapeutic benefit	**Undetermined**

Bibliographic reference

Chandra R, Agrawal S, Bajaj S, Goel S (1978). A clinical trial of Gasex in gastro-intestinal disorders in post-operative gastro-intestinal symptoms. *PROBE* 17 (4): 330-333.

Trial design

Parallel. Patients were given treatment for 7 to 15 days starting on the post-operative day when bowel sounds began. One hundred patients received either Gasex, and 50 patients were given vitamin B complex tablets (as placebo).

Study duration	7-15 days
Dose	2 tablets 3 times daily
Route of administration	Oral
Randomized	No
Randomization adequate	No
Blinding	Single-blind
Blinding adequate	No
Placebo	Yes
Drug comparison	No
Site description	Medical college hospital
No. of subjects enrolled	150
No. of subjects completed	150
Sex	Female
Age	21-70 years

Inclusion criteria

Patients in the gynecological section of the hospital recovering from surgery.

Exclusion criteria

None mentioned.

End points

Responses in the patients were subjectively interpreted in terms of the relief of symptoms, with responses of excellent, good, fair, or poor.

Results

One hundred subjects were in the treatment group and 50 were in the control group. All patients taking Gasex showed considerable improvement in their symptoms compared to the controls taking placebo. In the treatment group, a good to excellent response was observed in 95 percent of subjects with abdominal discomfort, compared to only 14 percent in the control group. Good to excellent responses were reported by 88, 40, 88, 56, and 70 percent of those with flatulence, regurgitation, epigastric discomfort, acidity/epigastric pain, and nausea, respectively. The comparative responses in the control group were 4, 20, 10, 25, and 17 percent, respectively.

Side effects
No side effects were observed.

Authors' comments
These observations prove the definite usefulness of Gasex tablets in the postoperative period to relieve symptoms associated with gaseous distension of the abdomen. Gasex is recommended for use until the patient assumes full normal dietary and working routine.

Reviewers' comments
The effect of opiates, given for pain, was noted, but no data were presented regarding other medications taken by the subjects. The dosage choice was not discussed in the paper nor substantiated by reference(s). It appears that the dosage form was "prepared in the juices and decoctions" of various additional plant species. It is unclear whether this reference to preparation is in regard to the procedure implemented in the study site prior to administration of the test agent to study subjects, or whether it is part of the description of the proprietary formulation. The selection of vitamin B complex tablets as placebo also was not discussed in the paper or substantiated by reference(s). As well, their specific composition was not revealed. The treatment length was adequate. (1, 4)

Geriforte®

First nine of a total thirty ingredients (for more information, see the Product Profile):

Chyavanprash concentrate
Cow-itch plant (*Mucuna pruriens* [L.] DC.) seed
Gotukola (*Centella asiatica* [L.] Urb.) leaves
Shatavari (*Asparagus racemosus* Willd.) root
Loosestrife (*Asparagus adscendens* Roxb.) root
Ashwagandha (*Withania somnifera* [L.] Dunal.) root
Arjuna (*Terminalia arjuna* [Roxb. ex. DC.] Wight & Arn.) bark
Elephant creeper (*Argyreia speciosa* [L. f.] Sweet) root
Licorice (*Glycyrrhiza glabra* L.) root

PREPARATIONS USED IN REVIEWED CLINICAL STUDIES

Geriforte® is manufactured by The Himalaya Drug Company in India, and distributed in the United States by Himalaya USA. Each tablet contains 1.005 g of a proprietary herbal blend of thirty ingredients (see the product report for a full list of ingredients). The current recommended dose is one tablet twice a day (Himalaya USA, 2002). A prior formulation of Geriforte, label dated May 1999, also cited 12 mg vitamin C and 40 mg calcium. No details of the product used in the following trial were included in the trial report. Geriforte is also available under the name of GeriCare®.

GERIFORTE® SUMMARY TABLE

Product Name	Manufacturer/ U.S. Distributor	Product Characteristics	Dose in Trials	Indication	No. of Trials	Benefit (Evidence Level-Trial No.)
Geriforte®	The Himalaya Drug Company, India/ Himalaya USA	Formula containing 29 herbal ingredients plus mineral pitch	2 tablets (unknown weight) 3 times daily	Menopausal symptoms	1	Undetermined (III-1)

SUMMARY OF REVIEWED CLINICAL STUDIES

Geriforte

Geriforte is described by the manufacturer as a "unique complex rejuvenative tonic with strong adaptogenic action" that "offers a broad range of health benefits and balances the body's organs and systems for increased mental alertness and greater fitness" (Geriforte label).

Menopausal Symptoms

The benefits of Geriforte were assessed in a small controlled study that included 25 women with postmenopausal depression and symptoms of headache, vague body ache, hot flashes, chest pain, palpitations, personality change, insomnia, loss of appetite, weight loss, and others. The study participants were given placebo for six weeks and then Geriforte (two tablets three times a day) for six weeks. They were evaluated every week during the 12-week period. Geriforte was effective in reducing symptoms of headache, hot flashes, insomnia, and improved self-confidence compared to placebo (Damle and Gore, 1983). However, the study was not well described and appeared to have significant methodological limitations. Thus, according to our reviewer, Dr. Tieraona Low Dog, any potential benefit for menopausal symptoms cannot be determined from this trial.

ADVERSE REACTIONS OR SIDE EFFECTS

No significant side effects were reported and no abnormalities were revealed by laboratory tests. Epigastric distress was reported in six patients (24 percent) in the initial phase of the study. The study report explained that this side effect disappeared with a reduction in dose, but did not give any further details such as how much the dose was reduced (Damle and Gore, 1983).

REFERENCES

Damle VB, Gore AG (1983). A controlled trial of Geriforte in post-meno-pausal depression. *Capsule* 3: 50.

Himalaya USA. GeriCare by Himalaya. <http://www.himalayausa.com>. Accessed November 11, 2002.

DETAILS ON GERIFORTE PRODUCT
AND CLINICAL STUDIES

A profile on the product is followed by details of the clinical studies associated with that product. Clinical studies are grouped by therapeutic indication, in accordance with the order in the Summary Table.

Product Profile: Geriforte®

Manufacturer	**The Himalaya Drug Company, India**
U.S. distributor	**Himalaya USA**
Formula Botanicals	**Chyavanprash concentrate; ashwagandha root** (*Withania somnifera* [L.] Dunal.); **asparagus root** (*Asparagus racemosus* Willd.); **gotukola leaves** (*Centella asiatica* [L.] Urb.); **licorice root** (*Glycyrrhiza glabra* L.); **haritaki fruit rind** (*Terminalia chebula* Retz.); **capers root bark** (*Capparis spinosa* L.), **wild chicory seed** (*Cichorium intybus* L.); **Malabar nut, whole** (*Adhatoda vasica* Nees.); **elephant creeper root** (*Argyreia speicosa* [L. f.] Sweet); **loosestrife root** (*Asparagus adscendens* Roxb.); **tree turmeric root** (*Berberis aristata* DC.); **teri pod seed** (*Caesalpinia digyna* Rottl.); **thistles, whole** (*Eclipta alba* [L.] Hassk.); **cow-itch plant seed** (*Mucuna pruriens* [L.] DC.); **nutmeg seed and mace** (*Myristica fragrans* Houtt.); **Indian long pepper fruit** (*Piper longum* L.); **saffron flower** (*Crocus sativus* L.); **black nightshade, whole** (*Solanum nigrum* L.); **arjuna bark** (*Terminalia arjuna* [Roxb. ex. DC.] Wight & Arn.); **bishop's weed/lovage mericap** (*Carum copticum* Benth. & Hook); **staff tree seed** (*Celastrus paniculatus* Wild.); **turmeric rhizome** (*Curcuma longa* L.); **cardamom fruit** (*Elettaria cardamomum* [L.] Maton.), **cloves, dried flower bud** (*Syzygium aromaticum* Merr. & L. M.

Perry), **yarrow, aerial parts** (*Achillea millefolium* L.); **Negro coffee seed** (*Cassia occidentalis* L.), **tamarisk, whole** (*Tamarix gallica* L.); **mace aril** (*Myristica fragrans* Houtt.); **mineral pitch.**

Quantity	1.005 g
Processing	No information
Standardization	No information
Formulation	Tablet

Recommended dose: Take one tablet twice per day with meals.

DSHEA structure/function: Natural antistress and rejuvenative. Has strong adaptogenic action that helps cope with life's daily stress. Balances all of the body's organs and systems for increased mental alertness and greater physical fitness.

Other ingredients: Biotite ash, zinc oxide, ferric oxide, iron oxide, magnesium stearate, sodium carboxymethylcellulose, microcrystalline cellulose, crospovidone, aerosil.

Comments: Also sold as GeriCare®.

Source(s) of information: Product label.

Clinical Study: Geriforte®

Extract name	N/A
Manufacturer	The Himalaya Drug Company, India
Indication	**Menopausal symptoms**
Level of evidence	**III**
Therapeutic benefit	**Undetermined**

Bibliographic reference
Damle VB, Gore AG (1983). A controlled trial of Geriforte in post-menopausal depression. *Capsule* 3: 50.

Trial design
Parallel. Two-stage study. During Stage I, patients received placebo for six weeks, and in Stage II, patients received Geriforte for six weeks. Patients were then followed for an additional four to six weeks.

Study duration	3 months
Dose	2 tablets 3 times daily

Route of administration	Oral
Randomized	No
Randomization adequate	No
Blinding	Double-blind
Blinding adequate	Yes
Placebo	Yes
Drug comparison	No
Site description	Not described
No. of subjects enrolled	25
No. of subjects completed	25
Sex	Female
Age	35-59 years

Inclusion criteria

Patients with postmenopausal depression. Patients also presented with somatic symptoms, such as headache, vague body ache, hot flashes, chest pain, palpitations, personality change, insomnia, loss of appetite, weight loss, and others.

Exclusion criteria

Patients with hepatic, renal, or cardiac diseases.

End points

Patients were assessed every two weeks in Stage I and every week in Stage II. Patients were followed up for four to six weeks after the trial. Responses to therapy were graded as poor (less than 50 percent improvement), fair (50 to 75 percent improvement), good (75 to 90 percent improvement) and excellent (greater than 90 percent improvement).

Results

Response to Geriforte was mostly good or excellent (64 percent of patients), whereas the response to placebo was mostly poor (68 percent of patients). The symptoms that showed improvement were headache, hot flashes, and insomnia, among others. Six cases regained self-confidence. Six cases showed relapse after discontinuation of therapy. When these six were given repeat treatment with Geriforte, all of them responded again.

Side effects

No significant side effects. Epigastric distress was seen in six cases, but disappeared with reduction in dosage (further details were not given).

Authors' comments

As indicated by the present study, Geriforte could be an important drug in the management of postmenopausal depression.

Reviewer's comments

The trial methodology was described inadequately, and the study was small. Although the study population was described, the inclusion criteria were vague. (3, 1)

Iberogast™

Ingredients:
German chamomile (*Matricaria recutita* L.) flower
Clown's mustard (*Iberis amara* L.) plant
Angelica (*Angelica archangelica* L.) root and rhizome
Caraway (*Carum carvi* L.) fruit
Milk thistle (*Silybum marianum* [L.] Gaertn.) fruit
Lemon balm (*Melissa officinalis* L.) leaf
Celandine (*Chelidonium majus* L.) aerial part
Licorice (*Glycyrrhiza glabra* L.) root
Peppermint (*Menthae × piperita* L.) leaf

PREPARATIONS USED
IN REVIEWED CLINICAL STUDIES

Iberogast™ is named for the herb *Iberis amara* L. (commonly called bitter candytuft or clown's mustard plant), the principal ingredient in this formula containing a total of nine plant extracts. Iberogast, also known as STW 5, is manufactured in Germany by Steigerwald GmbH, and distributed in the United States by Enzymatic Therapy.

SUMMARY OF REVIEWED CLINICAL STUDIES

Iberogast has been tested in several trials for its ability to benefit dyspepsia. Symptoms of dyspepsia include belching, sour eructation, frequent or excessive passage of gas, abdominal fullness, vague abdominal pain, epigastric burning, nausea, and unsatisfactory evacuation. Three different subtypes of functional dyspepsia have been described, attributing the symptoms to ulcers, dysmotility, or some unspecified cause. Symptoms can be rated according to the gastrointestinal symptom (GIS) score, a sum of ten dyspepsia symptoms.

IBEROGAST™ SUMMARY TABLE

Product Name	Manufacturer/ U.S. Distributor	Product Characteristics	Dose in Trials	Indication	No. of Trials	Benefit (Evidence Level-Trial No.)
Iberogast™	Steigerwald GmbH, Germany/ Enzymatic Therapy	Ethanolic extracts of nine botanicals	20 drops after meals	Dyspepsia (indigestion)	2	Trend (I-1, III-1)

Treatments for functional dyspepsia include prokinetic drugs that stimulate gastric motility (e.g., metoclopramide, domperidone, and cisapride) (Hardman et al., 1996).

Iberogast

Dyspepsia (Indigestion)

We reviewed two trials that compared Iberogast with either metoclopramide or cisapride in treatment for functional dyspepsia. A single-blind, drug comparison trial included 77 patients with functional dyspepsia given either Iberogast or metoclopramide (both 20 drops three times daily) after meals for up to two weeks. As a result, an almost parallel improvement in dyspepsia symptoms was observed in both groups. A statistically significant change compared to baseline was reached for symptoms (pressure/pain, nausea, belching, heartburn, stomach cramps, vomiting, fullness, and lack of appetite) between days three and seven (Nicolay, 1984). The trial did not score well in the quality rating because it was single-blind (the two liquids were different colors) and the randomization process was not adequately described.

Another trial, with excellent methodology, compared Iberogast (STW 5, 20 drops three times daily) to another similar research formula (with three fewer herbal ingredients than STW 5, called STW 5-II) and cisapride (10 mg three times daily). The one-month study used a double placebo to ensure double-blinding. Included were 137 participants with a clinical diagnosis of functional dyspepsia of the dysmotility type. As a result of treatment, the mean GIS scores decreased in all groups with no statistical difference between them. For those in all groups who were symptom free at the end of the trial, there was no difference in the relapse rate after six months (Rösch, Vinson, and Sassin, 2002). Our reviewers, Drs. Karriem Ali and Richard Aranda, rated this trial as demonstrating a trend toward efficacy. His reason for doing so is the absence of a placebo group.

Iberogast also demonstrated efficacy for functional dyspepsia in two placebo-controlled studies that we did not review, either because we did not obtain a copy or because we did not obtain an English translation (Buchert, 1994; Madisch et al., 2001). In the latter trial, 60 patients with functional dyspepsia were divided into three groups and given either Iberogast (STW-5), STW 5S (the Iberogast formula minus one botanical ingredient), or placebo for four weeks. Compared to placebo, both extracts showed clinically significant improvement in GIS scores after two and four weeks (Madisch et al., 2001).

ADVERSE REACTIONS OR SIDE EFFECTS

No serious adverse effects were noted in the two trials we reviewed. In one trial, two of 61 patients taking Iberogast reported abdominal cramps, dizziness, and nausea that may have been associated with the medication (Rösch, Vinson, and Sassin, 2002). The formula has been available in Europe for 40 years and has been well tolerated during this time. A postmarketing surveillance study, with 2,267 dyspeptic patients who took Iberogast for one to four weeks, reported only one adverse event that was not related to treatment with Iberogast (Sassin and Buchert, 2000).

REFERENCES

Buchert D (1994). Wirksamkeit und Vertraglichkeit von Iberogast bei patienten mit gesicherter non ulcus dyspepsia. *Zeitschrift für Phytotherapie* 15: 45-46.

Hardman JG, Limbird LE, Molinoff PB, Ruddon RW, Goodman-Gillman A (1996). *Goodman and Gillman's the Pharmacological Basis of Therapeutics,* Ninth Edition. New York: McGraw-Hill.

Madisch A, Melderis H, Mayr G, Sassin I, Hotz J (2001). Ein phytotherpeutikum und seine modifizierte rezeptur bei funktioneller dyspepsia. Ergebnisse einer doppelblinden plazebokontrollierten vergleichsstudie. [Commercially available herbal preparation and its modified dispense in patients with functional dyspepsia, results of a double-blind, placebo-controlled, randomized multicenter trial.] *Zeitschrift für Gastroenterologie* 39 (7): 511-517.

Nicolay K (1984). Functional gastroenteropathies in the therapeutic double blind trial of metoclopramide and the phytopharmaceutical agent Iberogast. *Gastro-Entero-Hepatologie* 2 (4): n.p.

Rösch W, Vinson B, Sassin I (2002). A randomized clinical trial comparing the efficacy of a herbal preparation STW 5 with the prokinetic drug cisapride in patients with dysmotility type of functional dyspepsia. *Zeitschrift für Gastroenterologie* 40 (6): 401-408.

Sassin I, Buchert D (2000). Efficacy and tolerability of the herbal preparation Iberogast in the therapy of functional dyspepsia. *Phytomedicine* 7 (Suppl. II): 91-92.

DETAILS ON IBEROGAST PRODUCT
AND CLINICAL STUDIES

A profile on the product is followed by details of the clinical studies associated with that product. Clinical studies are grouped by therapeutic indication, in accordance with the order in the Summary Table.

Product Profile: Iberogast™

Manufacturer	**Steigerwald Arzneimittel GmbH, Germany**
U.S. distributor	**Enzymatic Therapy**
Formula botanicals	**Clown's mustard plant** (*Iberis amara* L.); **German chamomile flower** (*Matricaria recutita* L.); **angelica root and rhizome** (*Angelica archangelica* L.); **caraway fruit** (*Carum carvi* L.); **milk thistle fruit** (*Silybum marianum* [L.] Gaertn.); **lemon balm leaf** (*Melissa officinalis* L.); **celandine aerial part** (*Chelidonium majus* L.); **licorice root** (*Glycyrrhiza glabra* L.); **peppermint leaf** (*Menthae × piperita* L.)
Quantity	No information
Processing	Ethanolic extracts of the fresh plants
Standardization	No information
Formulation	Liquid

Recommended dose: Adults take 20 drops (1 ml) with a favorite drink (warm water is recommended) three times daily; children 12 and under take ten drops three times daily.

DSHEA structure/function: Dietary supplement for the entire digestive system. Provides synergistic advantages for the entire intestinal tract and digestive system.

Other ingredients: Water, alcohol (31%).

Source(s) of information: Product label; Iberogast product information page <http://www.enzy.com/>.

Clinical Study: Iberogast®

Extract name	STW 5
Manufacturer	Steigerwald Arzneimittel GmbH, Germany
Indication	**Dyspepsia** (indigestion)
Level of evidence	**III**
Therapeutic benefit	**Trend**

Bibliographic reference

Nicolay K (1984). Functional gastroenteropathies in the therapeutic double-blind trial of metoclopramide and the phytopharmaceutical agent Iberogast. *Gastro-Entero-Hepatologie* 2 (4): n.p.

Trial design

Parallel. Trial was single-blind because the two medications differed in color. Patients were given either Iberogast or metoclopramide (20 drops three times daily after meals). Duration of treatment was planned for one to two weeks with discontinuation for cases with a complete lack of symptoms after one week.

Study duration	1-2 weeks
Dose	20 drops 3 times daily (after meals)
Route of administration	Oral
Randomized	Yes
Randomization adequate	No
Blinding	Single-blind
Blinding adequate	No
Placebo	No
Drug comparison	Yes
Drug name	Metoclopramide
Site description	Multicenter
No. of subjects enrolled	94
No. of subjects completed	77
Sex	Male and female
Age	18-60 years

Inclusion criteria

Patients suffering from functional dyspepsia with at least three of the following symptoms: pressure or pain in the abdominal area, stomach cramps, fullness, eructation, nausea, vomiting, pyrosis, or lack of appetite.

Exclusion criteria
Patients suffering from organic diseases of the gastrointestinal tract, as well as patients who were simultaneously treated with H2 histamine receptor blockers, antacids, anticholinergics, psychotropic substances, antibiotics, or antirheumatic agents.

End points
Evaluation by doctors occurred at baseline and on days 3, 7, and 14 of treatment. Doctors evaluated patients with a questionnaire. Patients also took notes in a diary.

Results
A notable, almost parallel improvement of all symptoms was observed in both groups. Between days 3 and 7, statistical significance of almost all the parameters reached $p < 0.01$ compared to baseline. In treating the symptoms of fullness and lack of appetite, Iberogast seems to have a tendency to take effect faster than metoclopramide.

Side effects
Metoclopramide five cases; Iberogast two cases (tiredness after three days, none after seven and 14 days).

Author's comments
In the treatment of nonspecific gastrointestinal symptoms, Iberogast practically does not cause any side effects, and is an alternative of absolutely equal value to the standard substance metoclopramide. Special attention should be paid to the fact that an equal therapeutic effect is achieved without targeting the central nervous system.

Reviewers' comments
The exclusion of organic causes of disease/diagnosis was not well defined. The lack of a placebo arm is a flaw in the study of a nonspecific functional gastrointestinal disorder. The sample size may have been appropriate; but no power calculation was presented. Although the trial length was adequate, the dosage choice was not discussed in the paper nor was it substantiated by reference(s). (Translation reviewed) (1, 4)

Clinical Study: Iberogast®

Extract name	STW 5
Manufacturer	Steigerwald Arzneimittel GmbH, Germany
Indication	**Dyspepsia** (indigestion)
Level of evidence	I
Therapeutic benefit	**Trend**

Bibliographic reference
Rösch W, Vinson B, Sassin I (2002) A randomized clinical trial comparing the efficacy of a herbal preparation of STW 5 with the prokinetic drug cisapride in patients with dysmotility type of functional dyspepsia. *Zeitschrift für Gastroenterologie* 40 (6): 401-408.

Trial design
Parallel. Pretrial washout period of one week. Patients received one of three treatments three times daily: 20 drops STW 5 (Iberogast) plus one tablet placebo; 20 drops STW 5-II (a research formula missing three herbal ingredients present in STW 5) plus one tablet placebo; 20 drops placebo plus one (10 mg) tablet cisapride.

Study duration	1 month
Dose	20 drops 3 times daily
Route of administration	Oral
Randomized	Yes
Randomization adequate	No
Blinding	Double-blind
Blinding adequate	No
Placebo	Yes
Drug comparison	Yes
Drug name	Cisapride, STW 5-II
Site description	Multicenter
No. of subjects enrolled	186
No. of subjects completed	137
Sex	Male and female
Age	Mean: 45 years

Inclusion criteria
Outpatients ages 21 to 70 years; clinical diagnosis of functional dyspepsia of the dysmotility type, relapsing or with symptoms for more than six months; two or more of the symptoms of the Gastrointestinal Symptom Score (GIS) had to be classified as moderate or more (except the symptoms "acidic eructation/heartburn" and "retrosternal pain"); echosonography of upper abdomen and endoscopy of the upper gastrointestinal tract did not show relevant disorders; written and informed consent of the patient.

Exclusion criteria
Known organic disease that could have explained the dyspeptic symptoms: reflux esophagitis, gastrointestinal tumors or findings suspicious of tumors,

gastric or duodenal ulcer, acute erosive gastritis/duodenitis with more than five erosions, Whipple's disease, diverticulitis, polyposis coli, ulcerative colitis, Crohn's disease, diabetic or infectious enteropathy, food allergies, malabsorption, maldigestion; bulbous scars as signs of chronic ulcer; predominance of symptoms of an irritable bowel disease; relevant defecation frequency anomalies; mesenteric vascular disorders; cholecystitis, cholangitis; pancreas tumors, pancreatitis; thyroid disorders; relevant hepatic disease; diseases of the urogenital system; history of abdominal surgery (with exception of appendectomy, hysterectomy, or cholecystectomy, when at least six months before study start, without complications and without connection to dyspeptic symptoms); history of gastrointestinal ulcers; abuse of laxatives, regular intake of nonsteroidal anti-inflammatory drugs; concomitant medication influencing the gastrointestinal tract.

End points
Patients were examined before the pretrial washout, at baseline (day 0), and on days 14 and 28, as well as six months later. The primary efficacy measure was the difference of the GIS sum score between the start and the end of therapy for cisapride compared to STW 5 and STW 5-II. Secondary endpoints included efficacy and tolerability assessments, recurrences and safety parameters.

Results
The mean values of the GIS decreased considerably between day 0 and day 28 for all study groups. The decreases from baseline values for STW 5, STW 5-II, and cisapride were 84 percent, 81 percent, and 75 percent, respectively. Both investigators and patients evaluated the efficacy of three treatments (STW 5, STW 5-II, and cisapride) favorably: investigators rated the treatments as good or excellent for 77 percent, 78 percent, and 62 percent of the patients, respectively. A majority of patients in the three groups also rated the treatments as good or excellent (70 percent, 76 percent, and 58 percent, respectively). No difference in relapse rate for the three groups was observed at the six-month follow-up.

Side effects
No serious adverse effects were noted. Three adverse events were classified as probably or possibly caused by the study medication: two of them were in the STW 5 group (abdominal cramps; dizziness and nausea); one was in the cisapride group (diarrhea).

Authors' comments
The equal efficacy of STW 5 and cisapride in this study indicates that the well-tolerated herbal preparation STW 5 is a potent therapeutical option for the treatment of functional dyspepsia of dysmotility type.

Reviewers' comments

This is an excellent study except that it lacks a placebo arm. Functional dyspepsia typically shows a significant (~20 to 30 percent) placebo response. The dosage is appropriate to the product literature, and the treatment length is appropriate to the disorder. (5, 6)

Padma®

Ingredients:

Bengal quince [*Aegle marmelos* (L.) Corrêa] fruit

Allspice [*Pimenta officinalis* Lindl., syn. *P. dioica* (L.) Merr.] fruit

Colombine (*Aquilegia vulgaris* L.) aerial part

Marigold/calendula (*Calendula officinalis* L.) flower

Cardamom [*Elettaria cardamomum* (L.) Maton] fruit

Clove [*Syzygium aromaticum* (L.) Merr. & L.M. Perry] flower

Costus (Indian) [*Saussurea lappa* (Decne.) C.B. Clarke, syn. *Sassurea costus* (Falc.) Lipsch.] root

Ginger lily (*Hedychium spicatum* Sm.) rhizome

Lettuce (*Lactuca sativa* L.) leaf

Iceland moss (*Cetraria islandica* L. Ach.)

Licorice (*Glycyrrhiza glabra* L.) root

Neem/margosa (*Azadirachta indica* A. Juss., syn: *Melia azadirachta* L.) fruit

Myrobalan (Tropical almond) (*Terminalia chebula* Retz.) fruit

Ribwort/English plantain (*Plantago lanceolata* L.) aerial part

Knotgrass (*Polygonum aviculare* L.) aerial part

Golden cinquefoil (*Potentilla aurea* L.) aerial part

Red sandalwood (*Pterocarpus santalinus* L. f.) heart wood

Country mallow/heartleaved sida (*Sida cordifolia* L.) aerial part

Valerian (*Valeriana officinalis* L.) root

Gypsum/calcium sulfate

Dextro-camphora/natural camphor

Note: This is the ingredient list for Padma® BASIC. Full scientific names have been added where they were missing on the product label.

PADMA® SUMMARY TABLE

Product Name	Manufacturer/ U.S. Distributor	Product Characteristics	Dose in Trials	Indication	No. of Trials	Benefit (Evidence Level-Trial No.)
Padma® 28 (EU), Padma® BASIC (US)	Padma Inc., Switzerland/ EcoNugenics Inc.	Proprietary blend of 19-20 herbs plus camphor and calcium sulfare	1-2 (340-403 mg) capsules/tablets 2-3 times daily	Peripheral arterial occlusion	5	Yes (I-2, II-2) Trend (II-1)
				Angina pectoris	1	Trend (III-1)
				Multiple sclerosis	1	Trend (III-1)
				Respiratory tract infection	1	Undetermined (III-1)

PREPARATIONS USED
IN REVIEWED CLINICAL STUDIES

Padma® 28 (recipe No. 28 of the Padma recipe series) is an herbal remedy consisting of 22 ingredients prepared according to Tibetan medicine principals. The recipe was brought to St. Petersberg, Russia in the middle of the nineteenth century by a physician/monk, Sultim Badma. The original formula has been altered with its entry into Western Europe, in that some of the ingredient plants from Tibet and India have been substituted with plants from Europe. The European version has been tested in numerous clinical studies and is registered as a drug in Switzerland. It is indicated for symptoms of poor circulation, including tingling, formication (feeling of insects crawling on the skin), feeling of heaviness, and tension in the arms and legs, as well as numbness of the hands and feet (Saller and Kristof, 1997).

The formula available in the United States is Padma® BASIC, which is Padma 28 minus one ingredient. The missing ingredient is aconite tuber (*Aconitum napellus* L.), which is considered an "unsafe herb" in the United States, subject to import restriction (CADHS, 1996). Thus, Padma BASIC is a blend of 19 herbs plus camphor and calcium sulfate. Padma BASIC is manufactured in Switzerland by Padma AG, and distributed in the United States by EcoNugenics Inc.

Although Padma 28 and Padma BASIC are not equivalent, their ingredients are very similar, and the products are both made by the same manufacturer. Thus, we decided to include Padma BASIC in this listing. Another product for sale in the United States that is also similar to Padma 28 is Adaptrin, manufactured by Pacific BioLogic. However, we determined that the ingredients in that formula are sufficiently different from Padma 28 and so have decided not to include it here.

Obtaining sufficient information to evaluate the similarity of Padma 28, Padma BASIC, and Adaptrin products was not a trivial task. The ingredient lists often quoted either common names or Latin names, requiring some research on our part. Some common names are distinctive, but others are ambiguous and may refer to more than one plant. Although we had obtained the Latin names of all botanical ingredients in Padma 28 from the clinical literature (Sallon et al., 1998), the Latin names of all ingredients were not included on the Padma Basic label. We therefore had to correlate common names with Latin names to compare the two ingredient lists. In addition, since the formulas are listed as proprietary blends without disclosing the amount of each ingredient, there is no way for us to know whether the ingredients in Padma BASIC and Padma 28 are present in the same amounts.

SUMMARY OF REVIEWED CLINICAL STUDIES

Experimental studies with Padma 28 indicate that it may have antioxidant and anti-inflammatory properties (Saller and Kristof, 1997). We reviewed two trials that included adults with multiple sclerosis or children with recurrent respiratory tract infections. However, the majority of the studies (six) that we reviewed focused on the ability of Padma 28 to treat symptoms of circulatory disorders.

Intermittent claudication is a symptom that occurs when the blood supply is adequate to meet the needs of the exercising muscle. This occurs most commonly due to occlusive arterial disease, also known as peripheral arterial disease, or more commonly known as peripheral arterial occlusion (PAO). PAO is a condition in which narrowing of the arteries, generally caused by atherosclerosis, limits the blood supply to the legs. Early stages of the disease are without symptoms, but later stages are associated with leg pain and muscle cramps upon walking, and ultimately, ischemic ulceration, gangrene, and tissue loss. The stages have been classified in a system according to Fontaine: Stage I represents those who are asymptomatic with isolated arterial stenosis of the lower limb; Stage II is mild to moderately severe leg pain and muscle cramps upon walking; Stage III are those with pain while resting; and Stage IV are those with ulcerations and gangrene (Dicter et al., 2002). The Padma studies included patients with Stage II of the disease. After the subject walks a "pain-free distance," cramplike ischemic pains begin. These pains eventually force the subject to stop walking, determining the "maximal walking distance." Upon rest, the legs recover from deficiencies of blood and oxygen, the pain disappears, and the subject can again walk a certain distance (Schrader, 1985).

Padma 28

Peripheral Arterial Occlusion

Five good-quality, placebo-controlled trials explored the use of Padma 28 in treatment of peripheral arterial disease or peripheral arterial occlusion. A large trial included 93 patients with a diagnosis of PAO of the lower extremities (Fontaine Stage II), given either 760 mg Padma twice daily or placebo for four months. Patients receiving Padma 28 had an increase in maximum walking distance from 95.7 to 205 yards (87.5 to 187.7 m), whereas the placebo group only had an insignificant increase in maximum walking distance. The treatment group also had significant reductions in cholesterol, triglycerides, and total lipid levels, as well as platelet aggregation, compared to baseline (Smulski and Wojcicki, 1995).

Another study of 100 subjects with PAO, Fontaine Stage II, were given either 760 mg Padma 28 twice daily or placebo for four months. With treatment, maximal walking distance was nearly doubled in the treatment group, whereas it did not change in the placebo group. As with the trial mentioned earlier, there were significant reductions in cholesterol, triglycerides, and total lipid levels, as well as platelet aggregation, in the treatment group. These changes were not observed in the placebo group (Samochowiec et al., 1987).

Two smaller trials also reported significant increases in maximal walking distance after four months of treatment, with no change in the placebo groups. In the first trial, including 43 patients with PAO Stage II according to Fontaine, pain-free walking distance also improved compared to the placebo group. However, this difference was not significant. Blood pressure differences between the arm and ankle decreased in the Padma group and increased in the placebo group (Schrader, 1985). In the second trial, with 36 subjects with PAO (Fontaine stage not given), there was a significant increase in pain-free walking distance compared to baseline and placebo. No difference was observed in the blood pressure ratio between the arm and leg (Drabaek et al., 1993).

Another placebo-controlled trial of 59 subjects with PAO (Fontaine stage not given) reported significant improvements in ankle blood pressure and recovery following exercise after six months of treatment compared to baseline levels and the placebo group. This improvement correlated with an increase in pain-free walking distance reported by the patients. No such improvement was observed in the placebo group (Sallon et al., 1998).

Angina Pectoris

One poor-quality study explored the ability of Padma 28 to reduce the number of angina attacks in those with chronic angina, averaging seven or more attacks per week. The study included 50 subjects who were given placebo before and after two weeks of treatment so that each patient served as their own control. As a result, the number of attacks during the treatment decreased by 69 percent compared to the initial two-week control period. Similarly, the demand for nitroglycerin tablets decreased during the treatment period. With treatment, patients were able to exercise longer before developing anginal pain, and the heart rate at peak exercise was reduced. In addition, the threshold for platelet aggregation was increased, and total lipids were significantly reduced (Wojcicki and Samochowiec, 1986). Our reviewer, Dr. Mary Hardy, reported that the strength of the evidence was hard to judge since the trial methods were poorly described in the available translation, and the data were not presented in detail.

Multiple Sclerosis

An open trial with 100 subjects examined the ability of Padma 28 to improve symptoms of multiple sclerosis. For one year, the Padma group was given two tablets three times daily. The control group was treated symptomatically with drugs (not named) to reduce pain, spasticity, and cramps. The authors reported a positive effect in 44 percent of subjects given Padma, with improvement in their general condition, an increase in muscle strength, and a decrease or disappearance of disorders affecting sphincters. In the control group, none felt better, and 40 percent showed a deterioration of symptoms (Korwin-Piotrowska et al.,1992). However, our reviewer determined that the trial methodology was very poor, and it was therefore difficult to evaluate the strength of this study.

Respiratory Tract Infection

A controlled study tested the ability of 19 children, ages two to four, with recurrent infections of the respiratory tract, to improve their capacity to resist infection. Treatment with one tablet Padma 28 three times daily for one month improved spontaneous bactericidal activity in blood samples taken from the children. No such changes were seen in the adults who served as controls (Jankowski et al., 1991). Our reviewer commented that the ex vivo intermediate outcome (bactericidal activity in blood) was not clearly linked to the disease outcome (recurrent infections of the respiratory tract). Thus, the trial was rated as having undetermined efficacy.

ADVERSE REACTIONS OR SIDE EFFECTS

The trials reviewed earlier did not report any major side effects. Minor side effects, such as gastrointestinal complaints and fatigue, were similar in the treatment and placebo groups.

REFERENCES

California Department of Health Services (CADHS) (April 3, 1996). *Common Traditional Chinese Herbal Products That Are Subject to Import Restriction.*

Dicter RS, Chu WW, Pacanowski JP, McBride PE, Tanke TE (2002). The significance of lower extremity peripheral arterial disease. *Clinical Cardiology* 25: 3-10.

Drabaek H, Mehlsen J, Himmelstrup H, Winther K (1993). A botanical compound, Padma 28, increases walking in stable intermittent claudication. *The Journal of Vascular Diseases* 44 (11): 863-867. (The biochemical aspects of this trial were published in Winther K, Kharazmi A, Himmelstrup H, Drabaek H, Mehlsen J [1994]. PADMA-28, a botanical compound, decreases the oxidative burst response of monocytes and improves fabrinolysis in patients with stable intermittent claudication. *Fibrinolysis* 8 [2]: 47-49.)

Jankowski S, Jankowski A, Zielinska S, Walczuk M, Brzosko WJ (1991). Influence of Padma 28 on the spontaneous bactericidal activity of blood serum in children suffering from recurrent infections of the respiratory tract. *Phytotherapy Research* 5: 120-123.

Korwin-Piotrowska T, Nocon D, Stankowska-Chomicz A, Starkiewicz A, Wojcicki J, Samochowiec L (1992). Experience of Padma 28 in multiple sclerosis. *Phytotherapy Research* 6 (3): 133-136.

Saller R, Kristof O (1997). Padma 28: A traditional Tibetan herbal mixture. *Internistische Praxis* 2: 408-412.

Sallon S, Beer G, Rosenfeld J, Anner H, Volcoff D, Ginsberg G, Paltiel O, Berlatzky Y (1998). The efficacy of Padma 28, a herbal preparation, in the treatment of intermittent claudication: A controlled double-blind pilot study with objective assessment of chronic occlusive arterial disease patients. *Journal of Vascular Investigation* 4 (3): 129-136.

Samochowiec L, Wojcicki J, Kosmider K, Dadej R, Smulski H (1987). Clinical test of the effectiveness of Padma 28 in the treatment of patients with chronic arterial occlusion. *Herba Polonica* 33 (1): 29-41.

Schrader R (1985). Effectiveness of PADMA 28 for intermittent claudication in chronic peripheral arterial occlusion: A controlled, double-blind study. Thesis. (Shortened version published in Schrader R [1985]. *Swiss Weekly Medical Review* 115: 752-756.)

Smulski, HS and Wojcicki J (1995). Placebo-controlled, double-blind trial to determine the efficacy of the Tibetan plant preparation Padma 28 for intermittent claudication. *Alternative Therapies* 1 (3): 44-49.

Wojcicki J, Samochowiec L (1986). Controlled double-blind study of Padma-28 in angina pectoris. *Herba Polonica* 32 (2): 107-114.

DETAILS ON PADMA PRODUCT AND CLINICAL STUDIES

A profile on the product is followed by details of the clinical studies associated with that product. Clinical studies are grouped by therapeutic indication, in accordance with the order in the Summary Table.

Product Profile: Padma® BASIC

Manufacturer	**Padma Inc., Switzerland**
U.S. distributor	**EcoNugenics Inc.**
Formula Botanicals	**Iceland moss** (*Cetraria islandica* L. Ach.); **costus root; margosa fruit** (*Azadirachta indica* A. Juss.); **cardamom fruit; red sandalwood heart wood; tropical almond fruit; allspice fruit; Bengal quince fruit** (*Aegle marmelos* [L.] Corrêa); **calcium sulfate; columbine aerial part** (*Aquilegia vulgaris* L.); **English plantain aerial part; licorice root; knotgrass aerial part** (*Polygonum aviculare* L.); **golden cinquefoil aerial part** (*Potentilla aurea* L.); **clove flower; gingerlily rhizome** (*Hedychium spicatum* Sm.); **heartleaved sida aerial part** (*Sida cordifolia* L.); **valerian root, lettuce leaf** (*Lactuca sativa* L.); **calendula flower; natural camphor**
Quantity	402 mg
Processing	No information
Standardization	No information
Formulation	Tablet

Recommended dose: Take two tablets two or three times each day with a full glass of water, preferably on an empty stomach, at least 30 minutes before or approximately two hours after a meal. Maximum dose, two tablets three times daily. It is recommended that the tablets be chewed before swallowing with plenty of water.

DSHEA structure/function: Promotes healthy circulation. Supports the immune system. Supports with antioxidant activity.

Cautions: Check with your health care practitioner before using if you are pregnant or nursing, taking medication, or if you have a medical condition (including allergies or food sensitivities).

Other ingredients: Sorbitol, silicon dioxide.

Comments: This formula plus *Aconitum napellus* L. is sold in Europe as Padma® 28.

Source(s) of information: Product package (© 1999 PADMA Health Products, Inc.); product leaflet (© 1999 PADMA Health Products, Inc.).

Clinical Study: Padma® 28

Extract name	N/A
Manufacturer	Padma Inc., Switzerland
Indication	**Peripheral arterial occlusion**
Level of evidence	I
Therapeutic benefit	**Yes**

Bibliographic reference
Smulski, HS, Wojcicki J (1995). Placebo-controlled, double-blind trial to determine the efficacy of the Tibetan plant preparation Padma 28 for intermittent claudication. *Alternative Therapies* 1 (3): 44-49.

Trial design
Parallel.

Study duration	4 months
Dose	2 (380 mg) capsules twice daily
Route of administration	Oral
Randomized	Yes
Randomization adequate	Yes
Blinding	Double-blind
Blinding adequate	Yes
Placebo	Yes
Drug comparison	No
Site description	Multicenter
No. of subjects enrolled	100
No. of subjects completed	93

Sex   Male and female
Age   35-65 years

Inclusion criteria

Inclusion criteria included: preestablished documented diagnosis of peripheral arterial occlusive (PAO) disease of the lower extremities, Fontaine Stage II, with intermittent claudication; positive anamnesis; positive clinical status with missing or deficient pulse on the back of the foot; maximum walking distance not exceeding 250 m; and minimum six-month duration of disease.

Exclusion criteria

Patients having PAO other than Fontaine Stage II; having a concomitant severe disease or a disease that might impede walking ability such as venous insufficiency, anemia, myocardial infarction within the last 8 months, cardiac insufficiency, severe arthralgia; and deficient steady state of PAO Stage II or manifestations of Stages III or IV. Patients were further excluded from the study if they changed their lifestyle (e.g., starting a walking program); changed medication therapy for concomitant disease; were intolerant to the test medication; had poor compliance; or did not show up to follow-up test sessions.

End points

The main target parameter was maximum walking distance and the secondary parameter was patients' subjective evaluation at the end of the 16-week treatment period. As part of a screening for potential efficacy mechanisms, upper arm blood pressure, blood fats, and platelet aggregation were evaluated. Patients were examined at baseline and 4, 8 ,12, and 16 weeks later.

Results

Patients receiving Padma 28 exhibited on standardized ergometry an increase of maximum walking distance from 87.5 to 187.7 m. The patients receiving placebo showed an insignificant increase of 12.5 m. The increase in walking distance of the group receiving Padma 28 compared with placebo was highly significant after 12 and 16 weeks ($p < 0.01$ and $p < 0.001$, respectively). Subjective evaluation by patients revealed that 82 percent of the Padma 28 group thought that the efficacy was good or very good, compared with only 16 percent of the placebo group. The Padma 28 group had significant reductions in cholesterol, triglyceride, and total lipid levels, as well as platelet aggregation, compared to baseline. No significant change was observed in the placebo group.

Side effects

None observed.

Authors' comments

Padma 28 shows clinically relevant effectiveness in peripheral arterial occlusive disease of the lower extremities, Fontaine II, with intermittent claudication.

Reviewer's comments
The following positive outcomes were seen in the treatment group: an increase in maximum walking distance; and the patients' subjective evaluation favored the treatment. The randomization and double-blinding are well described and adequate, all withdrawals and drop-outs are accounted for, the data are well presented, and the statistical methods were well described and applied. (5, 5)

Clinical Study: Padma® 28

Extract name	N/A
Manufacturer	Padma Inc., Switzerland
Indication	**Peripheral arterial occlusion**
Level of evidence	**II**
Therapeutic benefit	**Yes**

Bibliographic reference
Samochowiec L, Wojcicki J, Kosmider K, Dadej R, Smulski H (1987). Clinical test of the effectiveness of Padma 28 in the treatment of patients with chronic arterial occlusion. *Herba Polonica* 33 (1): 29-41.

Trial design
Parallel. Two-week pretrial run-in period without treatment.

Study duration	4 months
Dose	2 (380 mg) capsules twice daily
Route of administration	Oral
Randomized	Yes
Randomization adequate	No
Blinding	Double-blind
Blinding adequate	Yes
Placebo	Yes
Drug comparison	No
Site description	Not described
No. of subjects enrolled	100
No. of subjects completed	100

Sex   Male and female
Age   Not given

Inclusion criteria
Patients diagnosed with peripheral arterial occlusion, Stage II according to Fontaine, having maximal walking distance on ergometer of less than 150 m, and having had the disease for a minimum of eight months.

Exclusion criteria
Patients having peripheral arterial occlusion other than Fontaine Stage II; concurrent diseases, such as venous disorders, anemia, myocardial infarction within eight months, uncontrollable hypertension, and significant kidney or liver insufficiency.

End points
Patients were examined at inclusion, at the beginning of the treatment period, and after 4, 8, 12, and 16 weeks. An anamnesis, treadmill ergometry, and measurement of upper-arm blood pressure were done every four weeks and after 16 weeks of treatment. Blood serum laboratory tests and hematological tests were conducted before and after treatment.

Results
Patients receiving Padma 28 registered an increase in maximal walking distance of 98 percent ($p < 0.001$). No significant change was observed in the placebo group, and the difference in maximal walking distance between the two groups was significant ($p < 0.001$). The biochemical tests showed that 16 weeks of treatment with Padma 28 led to significant reductions in levels of cholesterol, triglycerides, total lipids, and beta lipoproteins. In the placebo group, beta lipoprotein levels increased significantly. Padma 28 inhibited the thrombocyte aggregation, reducing the tendency of thrombocytes to form plaque deposit on the walls of the blood vessels. In the placebo group these variables remained unchanged.

Side effects
No negative effects were observed.

Authors' comments
The fundamental treatment of chronic peripheral arterial occlusive disease is connected with the regulation of lipid metabolism. Padma 28 represents an effective new therapeutic method of treating peripheral arterial occlusive (PAO) disease.

Reviewer's comments
The following positive outcomes were also reported in this group: a decrease in both systolic and diastolic blood pressure; an increase in walking distance; a decrease in triglycerides, total lipids, and beta lipoproteins; and an increased threshold to adenosine diphosphate (ADP)-induced aggrega-

tion. The blinding in this study was well described, but the randomization was not. No adverse events were reported in the treatment group. The evaluation of the degree of detail of the data and the adequacy of the statistical methods was difficult because the tables were missing in the translation reviewed. (Translation reviewed) (3, 4)

Clinical Study: Padma® 28

Extract name	N/A
Manufacturer	Padma Inc., Switzerland
Indication	**Peripheral arterial occlusion**
Level of evidence	**II**
Therapeutic benefit	**Yes**

Bibliographic reference
Schrader R (1985). Effectiveness of PADMA 28 for intermittent claudication in chronic peripheral arterial occlusion: A controlled, double-blind study. Thesis. (Shortened version published in Schrader R [1985] *Swiss Weekly Medical Review* 115: 752-756.)

Trial design
Parallel. Trial was preceded by a two-week washout phase.

Study duration	4 months
Dose	2 capsules 3 times daily
Route of administration	Oral
Randomized	Yes
Randomization adequate	No
Blinding	Double-blind
Blinding adequate	Yes
Placebo	Yes
Drug comparison	No
Site description	Multicenter
No. of subjects enrolled	53
No. of subjects completed	43
Sex	Male and female
Age	Mean: 69 years

Inclusion criteria
Patients older than 50 years of age diagnosed with atherosclerotic periph-

eral arterial occlusion (PAO) in Stage II according to Fontaine, with an initial walking distance of 250 meters, duration of anamnesis of more than 8 months, and an anamnestic steady state.

Exclusion criteria
Patients with concomitant vasoactive therapy; serious diseases, such as cardiac infarct within the last eight months, cardiac insufficiency, or walking disorder other than claudication; or a wide variance in walking distance or stability of the disease. Subjects were also terminated from the study for the following reasons: strong adverse reaction to the test substance; deterioration of PAO with development of more advanced stages (III or IV); concurrent serious diseases; changes in concomitant medication (e.g., therapy for cardiac insufficiency); change in lifestyle (e.g., beginning walking training); or lack of compliance with study protocol.

End points
Physical examinations were performed at inclusion, at the beginning of treatment, and after 4, 8, 12, and 16 weeks. Efficacy was assessed by anamnesis, treadmill ergometry, measurements of blood pressure in upper arm and ankle arteries, and subjective analysis of treatment by the physician and the patient.

Results
Maximum walking distance significantly increased in the Padma 28 group after 16 weeks of treatment ($p < 0.001$). No statistical improvement was observed in the placebo group, and the difference between the two groups was significant ($p = 0.03$). Pain-free walking distance increased in the Padma 28 group by 66 meters ($p = 0.002$) and by 30 meters ($p < 0.01$) in the placebo group. However, the difference between the two groups was not significant ($p = 0.06$). Pressure differences between arm and ankle blood pressure decreased in the Padma 28 group by 16 mm Hg at rest ($p = 0.03$) and 11 mm Hg after effort. Pressure differences increased by 4 mmHg in the placebo group.

Side effects
Eight patients in each group had minor side effects.

Author's comments
Padma 28 caused an increase in pain-free and maximal walking distances of about 100 percent after four months in Stage II PAO. The positive results provide a basis for regarding Padma 28 as an effective treatment for intermittent claudication.

Reviewer's comments
This trial was fairly well designed and well conducted. Positive outcomes were seen in the average maximal walking distance (clinically relevant),

pain-free walking distance, decrease in the inner arm and ankle pressure difference, and a preference by subjective measure for the verum. However, the randomization process was not adequately described. Some tables were missing from the translation that was reviewed, making it difficult to determine whether the data was present in sufficient detail to permit alternative analysis. (3, 5)

Clinical Study: Padma® 28

Extract name	N/A
Manufacturer	Padma Inc., Switzerland
Indication	**Peripheral arterial occlusion**
Level of evidence	**II**
Therapeutic benefit	**Trend**

Bibliographic reference
Drabaek H, Mehlsen J, Himmelstrup H, Winther K (1993). A botanical compound, Padma 28, increases walking in stable intermittent claudication. *The Journal of Vascular Diseases* 44 (11): 863-867. (The biochemical aspects of this trial were published in Winther K, Kharazmi A, Himmelstrup H, Drabaek H, Mehlsen J [1994]. PADMA-28, a botanical compound, decreases the oxidative burst response of monocytes and improves fibrinolysis in patients with stable intermittent claudication. *Fibrinolysis* 8 [2]: 47-49.)

Trial design
Parallel.

Study duration	4 months
Dose	2 (340 mg) tablets twice daily
Route of administration	Oral
Randomized	Yes
Randomization adequate	No
Blinding	Double-blind
Blinding adequate	Yes
Placebo	Yes
Drug comparison	No
Site description	Not described
No. of subjects enrolled	36
No. of subjects completed	36
Sex	Male and female
Age	44-81 years

Inclusion criteria
Patients with stable peripheral arterial insufficiency in the lower extremities were included if they had a typical intermittent claudication history, clinical steady state for more than six months, a maximal walking distance between 50 and 300 meters, and a ratio lower than 0.85 between systolic blood pressure at the ankle with symptoms and the upper limb. Patients were not allowed to make lifestyle (e.g., diet or exercise) or medication changes during the study.

Exclusion criteria
Patients with symptoms of chronic lung disease, diabetes mellitus, osteoarthrosis in the lower extremities, or other diseases limiting the walking distance.

End points
Patients were assessed at baseline and at each month during the study. Measurements were made of systolic blood pressure at the ankle and the first toe, systemic blood pressure on both upper limbs, walking distance (both pain-free and maximum), and ankle pressure index (ankle systolic pressure/arm systolic pressure). Blood for evaluation of fibrinolytic activity, platelet aggregation, and monocyte oxidative burst reaction was taken before inclusion and after four months of therapy.

Results
After four months of taking Padma 28, patients attained a significant increase in pain-free walking distance (from 52 to 86 meters, $p < 0.05$) and in maximal walking distance (from 115 to 227 meters, $p < 0.05$). The group receiving placebo treatments did not show any significant changes in either parameter. There was no significant change to the ankle pressure index for either group. During treatment with Padma 28, the oxidative burst response of monocytes after stimulation with zymozan decreased, fibrinolytic activity increased, as shown by a shortening of the euglobulin clot lysis time by more than 40 percent, and the level of plasminogen activator inhibitor Type I fell ($p < 0.05$). Again, no such change was observed in the placebo group.

Side effects
None mentioned.

Authors' comments
Treatment with Padma 28 over a period of four months significantly increased the walking distance in patients with stable intermittent claudication of long duration. Whether the augmentation of fibrinolysis and decrease in oxidative burst by monocytes was a direct effect of Padma 28 or an indirect effect of the improved walking capacity is not clear.

Reviewer's comments
The following positive outcomes were seen: increase in pain-free walking distance; increase in maximum walking distance; and no change in ankle pressure index. The blinding, but not the randomization, is adequately described. The small patient population limits the interpretation of this study. (3, 4)

Clinical Study: Padma® 28

Extract name	N/A
Manufacturer	Padma Inc., Switzerland
Indication	**Peripheral arterial occlusion**
Level of evidence	**I**
Therapeutic benefit	**Yes**

Bibliographic reference
Sallon S, Beer G, Rosenfeld J, Anner H, Volcoff D, Ginsberg G, Paltiel O, Berlatzky Y (1998). The efficacy of Padma 28, a herbal preparation, in the treatment of intermittent claudication: A controlled double-blind pilot study with objective assessment of chronic occlusive arterial disease patients. *Journal of Vascular Investigation* 4 (3): 129-136.

Trial design
Parallel.

Study duration	6 months
Dose	2 (403 mg) capsules twice daily
Route of administration	Oral
Randomized	Yes
Randomization adequate	Yes
Blinding	Double-blind
Blinding adequate	Yes
Placebo	Yes
Drug comparison	No
Site description	Outpatient clinic
No. of subjects enrolled	72
No. of subjects completed	59
Sex	Male and female
Age	Mean: 73 years

Inclusion criteria
Outpatients with peripheral arterial occlusive disease (intermittent claudication) according to the following criteria: abnormal wave-form recordings, a preexercise ankle/arm pressure ratio of 0.85 or less, a postexercise drop in the ankle/arm pressure ratio of 15 percent or more, and a depressed systolic ankle pressure during three minutes after exercise.

Exclusion criteria
Exclusion criteria were lower extremity rest pain, ulceration or need for revascularization, previous peripheral arterial surgery, use of the anticoagulant warfarin, active peptic ulcer disease, serious liver or renal disease, mental disease, a significant or serious cardiac condition, carcinoma, and other life-threatening conditions.

End points
Effectiveness of treatment was evaluated by measuring resting ankle/brachial pressure indices, treadmill exercises tests with postexercise ankle pressure measures, hemodynamic tests, self-assessment by patients of perceived changes in walking ability, as well as various parameters of well-being recorded in a questionnaire. Questionnaires were completed at outpatient visits after the first, third, and sixth month. Physical examinations were conducted at the beginning and end of the study.

Results
Padma 28 patients displayed a significant mean improvement of 12.5 percent ($p = .031$) in exercise-induced drop of ankle blood pressure and 0.8 min ($p = .076$) in pressure recovery time compared to pretreatment values. An improvement in pressure drops by more than 15 percent, compared to a deterioration or no change, occurred in 48 percent of Padma 28 patients compared to 22 percent of controls. Calculation of the "ischemic window," a quantitative expression of postexercise hyperemia, showed a significant reduction of 54 percent following treatment with Padma 28 compared to 18.8 percent in controls. Self assessment by patients revealed that perceived improvement in pain-free walking ability in the Padma 28 group correlated significantly with improvement in exercise-induced drop of ankle pressure.

Side effects
Side effects included gastrointestinal complaints and tiredness, similar to those in the placebo group.

Authors' comments
The current pilot study is the first to demonstrate that, following the stress of exercise, changes in ankle systolic pressure and its recovery time are positively affected by Padma 28.

Reviewer's comments
The following positive outcomes were seen in the treatment group: less of a drop in exercise induced ankle/arterial pressure; a decrease in amount of re-covery time; and self assessment by patients favored Padma 28. This was a well-conducted and well-described study with an appropriate sample size. The randomization and blinding were also described adequately. (5, 6)

Clinical Study: Padma® 28

Extract name	N/A
Manufacturer	Padma Inc., Switzerland
Indication	**Angina pectoris**
Level of evidence	**III**
Therapeutic benefit	**Trend**

Bibliographic reference
Wojcicki J, Samochowiec L (1986). Controlled double-blind study of Padma-28 in angina pectoris. *Herba Polonica* 32 (2): 107-114.

Trial design
Crossover. Subjects had a two-week pretrial period with placebo followed by two weeks with Padma 28, and then two subsequent weeks with placebo.

Study duration	2 weeks
Dose	2 (380 mg) capsules twice daily
Route of administration	Oral
Randomized	No
Randomization adequate	No
Blinding	Double-blind
Blinding adequate	No
Placebo	Yes
Drug comparison	No
Site description	Hospital inpatient clinic
No. of subjects enrolled	50
No. of subjects completed	50
Sex	Male and female
Age	40-69 years (mean: 51.2)

Inclusion criteria
Patients with chronic angina (at least six months) that is relatively stable in

duration and severity, which family doctors have been unable to control. Angina attacks averaging seven or more per week.

Exclusion criteria
Patients who were hypertensive, with clinical or radiologic evidence of cardiac enlargement or failure or acute myocardial infarction within the past six months.

End points
Patients were examined at the beginning and at the end of the placebo pretrial period, after two weeks of Padma 28 administration, and again after the two subsequent weeks on placebo. Variables included the clinical response to therapy, exercise tolerance testing, platelet aggregation, and blood lipid levels. Patients kept a record of their daily consumption of nitroglycerin tablets as well as the number of daily angina attacks.

Results
The mean number of anginal attacks was reduced from 37.5 in the two weeks before treatment to 11.5 (by 69 percent) after two weeks of Padma administration ($p < 0.001$), and it was increased to 28.7 during the following two weeks of placebo application. At the same time, the mean number of nitroglycerin tablets decreased from 27.7 before treatment to 7.9 in the two weeks of Padma administration ($p < 0.001$). Patients were able to exercise longer before developing anginal pain after taking Padma. At peak exercise, heart rate was lower during Padma administration than during placebo. The threshold of platelet aggregation was increased by Padma ($p < 0.001$). Total lipids and triglycerides were slightly but significantly reduced after two weeks of Padma administration ($p < 0.05$ and $p < 0.01$, respectively).

Side effects
No side effects were observed.

Authors' comments
Padma 28 can be effective in a considerable percentage of patients with angina. This is probably due to the reduction of platelet aggregation, and may be due to the decrease of myocardial oxygen consumption.

Reviewer's comments
This was a very short study in which patients served as their own control. The report is poorly written, however, and it is very difficult to tell whether this is a case series or a strange kind of crossover trial. The study was double-blinded adequately, but it was not randomized. The sample size was also small, and the data were not described in sufficient detail. (Translation reviewed) (3, 4)

Clinical Study: Padma® 28

Extract name	N/A
Manufacturer	Padma Inc., Switzerland
Indication	**Multiple sclerosis**
Level of evidence	**III**
Therapeutic benefit	**Trend**

Bibliographic reference
Korwin-Piotrowska T, Nocon D, Stankowska-Chomicz A, Starkiewicz A, Wojcicki J, Samochowiec L (1992). Experience of Padma 28 in multiple sclerosis. *Phytotherapy Research* 6 (3): 133-136.

Trial design
Parallel. The control group was treated only symptomatically, receiving drugs to reduce pain, spasticity, and cramps, and to inhibit detrusor contractions.

Study duration	1 year
Dose	2 tablets 3 times daily
Route of administration	Oral
Randomized	Yes
Randomization adequate	No
Blinding	Open
Blinding adequate	No
Placebo	No
Drug comparison	No
Site description	Outpatients clinic
No. of subjects enrolled	100
No. of subjects completed	100
Sex	Male and female
Age	26-60 years

Inclusion criteria
Patients suffering from progressive (and proceeding with attacks) multiple sclerosis.

Exclusion criteria
None mentioned.

End points
The neurological state and visual and auditory evoked potentials were studied prior to the study and during the course of treatment. To evaluate the effi-

cacy of the medication, the following were assessed according to a numerical scale: the number of attacks, the dynamic with which the symptoms regressed after a new attack, the delay in the slowly intensifying course of multiple sclerosis, as well as the diminution in intensity of certain neurological symptoms.

Results
A positive effect of Padma 28 was observed in 44 percent of patients with improvement of their general condition, increase in muscle strength, and a decrease or disappearance of disorders affecting sphincters. In 41 percent of patients with initially abnormal tracing of visual evoked potentials, an improvement or normalization was achieved. Of patients who did not receive Padma 28, none felt better. Moreover, 40 percent showed a deterioration.

Side effects
No side effects were observed.

Authors' comments
The results of this study may be subjective to an extent, in that it is known that multiple sclerosis is characterized by irregular periods of disease activity interspersed by intervals of spontaneous remission. However, Padma 28 may be useful in slowing or arresting the symptoms of chronic multiple sclerosis.

Reviewer's comments
This was an open trial with a mixture of objective and subjective end points. The subjective end points are not described adequately, nor are the statistical methods, the data, or the randomization process. The sample size, however, was adequate. (1, 2)

Clinical Study: Padma® 28

Extract name	N/A
Manufacturer	Padma Inc., Switzerland
Indication	**Respiratory tract infection**
Level of evidence	**III**
Therapeutic benefit	**Undetermined**

Bibliographic reference
Jankowski S, Jankowski A, Zielinska S, Walczuk M, Brzosko WJ (1991). Influence of Padma 28 on the spontaneous bactericidal activity of blood serum

in children suffering from recurrent infections of the respiratory tract. *Phytotherapy Research* 5: 120-123.

Trial design
Parallel. Children (two to four years old) were given Padma 28 for one month, then had a two-week interruption before another two weeks of treatment. During treatment, the children did not receive antibiotics. The control group consisted of ten blood donors (mean age: 23 years) who had not been infected with bacteria such as *Pseudomonas aeruginosa, Salmonella,* or *Escherichia coli.*

Study duration	2 months
Dose	1 tablet 3 times daily
Route of administration	Oral
Randomized	No
Randomization adequate	No
Blinding	Open
Blinding adequate	No
Placebo	No
Drug comparison	No
Site description	Not described
No. of subjects enrolled	19
No. of subjects completed	19
Sex	Male and female
Age	2-4 years

Inclusion criteria
Children suffering from recurrent infections of the respiratory tract were accepted into the study if they had developed at least once a month, for the last nine months, illnesses such as purulent angina, bronchitis, or bronchopneumonia.

Exclusion criteria
None mentioned.

End points
Blood was collected from children and donors before the start of treatment and two months later. The bactericidal activity of the serum was determined using three strains of bacteria: *Salmonella typhimurium* strain 568, and *Escherichia coli* strains 044 and 055.

Results
Results indicate that an increase in spontaneous bactericidal activity (SBA)

in sera of children receiving Padma 28 occurred in almost 85 percent of cases. A considerable increase (bactericidal index less than 2) was observed in 12 children, a lesser increase was seen in four children and no improvement was observed in three children. No change occurred in the SBA in sera of the control blood donors.

Side effects
None mentioned in paper.

Authors' comments
Padma 28 in its multiple modes of action enhances the spontaneous bactericidal activity of the serum of children in comparison with a control group of healthy subjects.

Reviewer's comments
This trial was an ex vivo study without clear clinical significance (i.e., the effect of this intermediate outcome is not clearly linked to the disease studied). The trial was neither randomized nor blinded, the sample size was small, and the data were not described in sufficient detail. (0, 4)

Phytodolor™

Ingredients:
Common ash (European ash) (*Fraxinus excelsior* **L.**) **bark**
Aspen (quaking aspen) (*Populus tremula* **L.**) **bark and leaf**
Goldenrod (European goldenrod) (*Solidago virgaurea* **L.**)
aerial parts

PREPARATIONS USED
IN REVIEWED CLINICAL STUDIES

Phytodolor™ is a formula containing extracts of common ash (*Fraxinus excelsior* L.) bark, aspen (*Populus tremula* L.) bark and leaves, and goldenrod (*Solidago virgaurea* L.) aerial parts. Aspen bark and leaves contain salicylates (Schulz, Hänsel, and Tyler, 2001). Salicylates are perhaps more widely known as constituents of willow bark, and for the synthetic derivative acetylsalicylic acid (known as aspirin). Salicylates are generally known for their ability to reduce inflammation, pain, and fever. Ash preparations contain coumarins that have anti-inflammatory and analgesic properties (Bruneton, 1999). Goldenrod preparations contain flavonoids, saponins, and phenol glycosides. Extracts and individual constituents have demonstrated diuretic, anti-inflammatory, and analgesic activity (Blumenthal, Goldberg, and Brinkmann, 2000).

Phytodolor is a combination of the extracts of common ash bark, aspen bark and leaves, and goldenrod aerial parts in the ratio of 1:3:1. The individual extracts are prepared according to the following plant-to-extract ratios: ash (4.5:1), aspen (4.5:1), and goldenrod (4.8:1). The formula as a whole is standardized to contain salicin (0.75 mg/ml), salicylic alcohol (0.042 mg/ml), isofraxidin (0.015 mg/ml), and rutin (0.06 mg/ml). The recommended dose is 20 drops (1 ml) three to four times daily. Phytodolor is manufactured in Germany by Steigerwald Arzneimittel GmbH and is no longer distributed in the United States.

PHYTODOLOR™ SUMMARY TABLE

Product Name	Manufacturer/ U.S. Distributor	Product Characteristics	Dose in Trials	Indication	No. of Trials	Benefit (Evidence Level-Trial No.)
Phytodolor™	Steigerwald Arzneimittel GmbH, Germany/ None	Extracts of common ash, aspen, and goldenrod	30 to 40 drops three times daily	Arthritis (rheumatoid and degenerative joint diseases)	3	Trend (II-1, III-1) Undetermined (III-1)

SUMMARY OF REVIEWED CLINICAL STUDIES

We reviewed three double-blind, placebo-controlled trials that examined the use of Phytodolor to treat the pain and inflammation associated with various degenerative rheumatic joint diseases or arthritis. The most common degenerative disease is osteoarthritis, caused by wear and tear on the joint. It is characterized by the breakdown of joint cartilage and adjacent bone in the neck, lower back, knees, hips, and/or fingers. The symptoms include pain, stiffness, and swelling in the joints. Degeneration of the joints also occurs with rheumatoid arthritis, an autoimmune disease in which the body's own immune system attacks the membranes surrounding the joints.

Common first-line treatments for relief of symptoms of degenerative joint diseases are the nonsteroidal anti-inflammatory drugs (NSAIDs), which include aspirin and other salicylic acid derivatives, acetaminophen, indomethacin, ibuprofen, and diclofenac (Hardman et al., 1996).

Phytodolor

Arthritis (Rheumatoid and Degenerative Joint Diseases)

A small trial included 38 participants with degenerative rheumatic diseases involving joints or the spinal column, who were given either Phytodolor (30 drops three times daily) or placebo for three weeks. The primary end point was the amount of NSAIDs required by both groups to alleviate symptoms. The Phytodolor group required NSAIDs on three days compared to the placebo group, which required NSAIDs on 47 days. With the combination of treatments, clinical improvements (pain and flexibility) were similar for both groups. For example, the clinical measurements for those whose spinal columns were affected were the finger-to-floor assessment of mobility range and an evaluation of the pain when tapping the spinal column (Huber, 1991). A small crossover trial included 30 subjects with arthritis of the knee, hip, thumb, or shoulder, who were given either Phytodolor (40 drops three times daily) or placebo for one week. The subjects were allowed to take up to six (25 mg) tablets of diclofenac per day if necessary. In both phases of the crossover trial, the group given placebo tended to require more diclofenac than the group given Phytodolor (Schadler, 1988).

A third study compared Phytodolor to both placebo and an inject-able form of indomethacin (Amuno). This was a four-week trial that included 41 subjects with inflammatory or chronic degenerative dis-eases. After one week, mobility improved in the Phytodolor group compared with the placebo group. After two weeks, pain due to movement was improved in the Phytodolor group compared with the placebo group. The indomethacin group showed more relief from pain due to movement and continuous pain than the Phytodolor group after one week, but the improvements were similar after four weeks (Hahn and Hubner-Steiner, 1988).

According to our reviewer, Dr. John Hicks, none of the studies cited previously were large enough to support any definite conclu-sions regarding the benefit of Phytodolor. In addition, the trial meth-odology was deemed moderate to poor according to current stan-dards.

SYSTEMATIC REVIEWS

A systematic review of double-blind, randomized clinical studies on Phytodolor included ten trials. Six trials were placebo-controlled, with three of these trials also including another active medication. Four other studies compared Phytodolor to another active medication without a placebo group. Three of the trials, which we were able to obtain in English or translated into English, were reviewed independ-ently in the previous section. The trials included subjects with muscu-loskeletal problems, including osteoarthritis, epicondylitis, rheuma-toid arthritis, and back pain. The studies evaluated various clinical symptoms, such as pain, grip strength, physical impairment, morning stiffness, swelling, and joint function, as well as the use of rescue medication, as outcome measures. The dose of Phytodolor ranged from 90 to 120 drops per day in liquid form and the equivalent of 200 drops in a tablet form. Treatment lasted from two to four weeks, and the trials ranged in size from 30 to 432 subjects, with a total of 1,135 in the ten trials. The author of the review concluded that Phytodolor is as effective as synthetic drugs (diclofenac, piroxicam, indomethacin) and more effective than placebo in treating musculoskeletal pain. Further, the author commented that data from these trials are supported by nine clinical studies that were not controlled and therefore not included in the review. The limitations of the studies, as stated by the author, were the heterogeneous nature of the patient groups, the use of subjective clinical end points, and the low dose of comparative therapeutic agents. In addition, several of the trial reports were unpublished and therefore not subjected to peer review (Ernst, 1999).

ADVERSE REACTIONS OR SIDE EFFECTS IN CLINICAL STUDIES

Neither the three individual studies nor the systematic review mentioned any significant side effects.

REFERENCES

Blumenthal M, Goldberg A, Brinkmann J, eds. (2000). *Herbal Medicine: Expanded Commission E Monographs.* Austin, TX: American Botanical Council.

Bruneton J (1999). *Pharmacognosy, Phytochemistry, Medicinal Plants,* Second Edition. Trans. CK Hatton. Paris, France: Lavoisier Publishing.

Ernst E (1999). The efficacy of Phytodolor for the treatment of musculoskeletal pain—A systematic review of randomized clinical trials. *Natural Medicine Journal* 2: 14-17.

Hahn S, Hubner-Steiner U (1988). The treatment of painful rheumatic diseases with Phytodolor in comparison to placebo and Amuno treatments. *Rheuma Schmerz & Entzündung* 8 (5): 55-58.

Hardman JG, Limbird LE, Molinoff PB, Ruddon RW, Goodman-Gillman A (1996). *Goodman and Gillman's The Pharmacological Basis of Therapeutics,* Ninth Edition. New York: McGraw-Hill.

Huber B (1991). Therapy of degenerative rheumatic diseases: Requirement for additional analgesic medication under treatment with Phytodolor. *Fortschritte der Medizin* 109 (11): 248-250.

Schadler W (1988). Phytodolor for the treatment of activated arthrosis. *Rheuma: Therapeutic Guidelines Diagnostic Aids* 8: 280-290.

Schulz V, Hänsel R, Tyler VE (2001). *Rational Phytotherapy: A Physicians' Guide to Herbal Medicine,* Fourth Edition. Trans. TC Telger. Berlin: Springer-Verlag.

DETAILS ON PHYTODOLOR PRODUCT AND CLINICAL STUDIES

A profile on the product is followed by details of the clinical studies associated with that product. Clinical studies are grouped by therapeutic indication, in accordance with the order in the Summary Table.

Product Profile: Phytodolor™

Manufacturer	**Steigerwald Arzneimittel GmbH, Germany**
U.S. distributor	**None**
Formula Botanicals	**Common ash bark** (*Fraxinus excelsior* L.) **aspen leaves and bark** (*Populus tremula* L.) **goldenrod aerial parts** (*Solidago virgaurea* L.)
Quantity	Ash
Processing	Fresh plant aqueous alcoholic extracts Plant/extract ratios: ash 4.5:1; aspen 4.5:1; goldenrod 4.8:1
Standardization	Salicin 0.75 mg/ml; salicylic alcohol 0.042 mg/ml; isofraxidin 0.015 mg/ml; rutin 0.06 mg/ml
Formulation	Liquid

Recommended dose: Take 20 drops (1 ml) three to four times daily mixed in water or a favorite drink. For maximum support, double recommendation to 40 drops. Allow two to four weeks for best results.

DSHEA structure/function: Dietary supplement for optimum muscle and joint function.

Cautions: Do not take this product if sensitive to salicylates.

Other ingredients: Water, alcohol (45.6 percent)

Source(s) of information: Product package

Clinical Study: Phytodolor™ N

Extract name	None given
Manufacturer	Steigerwald GmbH, Germany

Indication	**Degenerative rheumatic diseases**
Level of evidence	**II**
Therapeutic benefit	**Trend**

Bibliographic reference

Huber B (1991). Therapy of degenerative rheumatic diseases: Requirement for additional analgesic medication under treatment with Phytodolor. *Fortschritte der Medizin* 109 (11): 248-250.

Trial design

Parallel. Pretrial washout lasting the half-life of the subjects' previous anti-inflammatory medication.

Study duration	3 weeks
Dose	30 drops 3 times daily
Route of administration	Oral
Randomized	Yes
Randomization adequate	Yes
Blinding	Double-blind
Blinding adequate	No
Placebo	Yes
Drug comparison	No
Site description	Not described
No. of subjects enrolled	40
No. of subjects completed	38
Sex	Male and female
Age	50-80 years

Inclusion criteria

Inpatients with at least one rheumatological indication (in degenerative forms) for treatment with anti-inflammatory drugs.

Exclusion criteria

None mentioned.

End points

The condition of the most afflicted joint or the spinal column was measured prior to the study and after one, two, and three weeks. Circumference, maximum flexion in degrees, continuous pain while at rest, and pain during movement were recorded for joints. For the spinal column, finger-to-floor distance, assessment of the mobility range of the spinal column (small and big Schober index), and an evaluation of the pain by tapping on the spinal column were recorded. Patients were given diclofenac (an anti-inflammatory drug) and at times paracetamol, in addition to Phytodolor or placebo, if the analgesic efficacy was insufficient. The amount of additional medication was noted. Laboratory parameters were assessed prior to the study and after three weeks of treatment.

Results
Clinical improvements were almost identical for both groups. Additional medication was required for 2 of 18 in the Phytodolor group, distributed on a total of three days, and 5 of 20 in the control group, distributed on a total of 47 days. The p value of the Wilcoxon test between the two groups was 0.17. Laboratory tests showed a insignificant decrease in leukocyte number in the Phytodolor group.

Side effects
None observed.

Author's comments
When administrating Phytodolor, significantly lower amounts of nonsteroidal anti-inflammatory drugs were required than with placebo. The tolerance of Phytodolor N is clearly better than the tolerance of nonsteroidal anti-inflammatory drugs.

Reviewer's comments
There was a trend toward less need for analgesics while taking Phytodolor. However, the study was not large enough to prove significant effects. Neither the blinding process nor the inclusion/exclusion criteria for the patients were described adequately. (3, 4)

Clinical Study: Phytodolor™

Extract name	None given
Manufacturer	Steigerwald GmbH, Germany
Indication	**Arthritis of various joints**
Level of evidence	**III**
Therapeutic benefit	**Undetermined**

Bibliographic reference
Schadler W (1988). Phytodolor for the treatment of activated arthrosis. *Rheuma: Therapeutic Guidelines Diagnostic Aids* 8: 280-290.

Trial design
Crossover. Patients were allowed to take up to six tablets (25 mg each) diclofenac per day if necessary.

Study duration	1 week
Dose	40 drops 3 times daily
Route of administration	Oral
Randomized	Yes
Randomization adequate	No
Blinding	Double-blind
Blinding adequate	No
Placebo	Yes
Drug comparison	No
Site description	Not described
No. of subjects enrolled	30
No. of subjects completed	30
Sex	Male and female
Age	45-81 years (mean: 66)

Inclusion criteria
Subjects with arthrosis of the knee, hip-joint arthrosis, saddle-joint arthrosis of the thumb, and shoulder-joint arthrosis.

Exclusion criteria
None mentioned.

End points
Amount of diclofenac tablets consumed by each group.

Results
In the first week of treatment, all placebo patients used more diclofenac than during the first day of that treatment, whereas the Phytodolor patients used less. After the crossover, the additional consumption of diclofenac diminished in the Phytodolor group, and the consumption in the placebo group remained the same.

Side effects
No side effects were observed.

Author's comments
The effect of Phytodolor is largely the same as described for "chemical" anti-inflammatory agents. This gives the treating physician several possibilities to use Phytodolor for the benefit of his patients. In numerous cases Phytodolor

alone should be sufficient to improve the complaints of the patient adequately. In other cases, it is possible to reduce consumption of nonsteroidal anti-inflammatory drugs by administering them on an occasional basis.

Reviewer's comments

This study was too small to draw any conclusions. Neither the randomization nor the blinding were described adequately. In addition, the inclusion/exclusion criteria were not described in sufficient detail. (0, 2)

Clinical Study: Phytodolor™

Extract name	None given
Manufacturer	Steigerwald GmbH, Germany
Indication	**Degenerative rheumatic diseases**
Level of evidence	**III**
Therapeutic benefit	**Trend**

Bibliographic reference

Hahn S, Hubner-Steiner U (1988). The treatment of painful rheumatic diseases with Phytodolor in comparison to placebo and Amuno treatments. *Rheuma Schmerz & Entzündung* 8 (5): 55-58.

Trial design

Parallel. Three-arm study. Phytodolor and placebo were packaged in identical form. Amuno (indomethacin) (3 × 1 tsp daily) was administered as suspension. Phytodolor and placebo were double-blind, and administration of Amuno was open.

Study duration	1 month
Dose	30 drops three times daily
Route of administration	Oral
Randomized	Yes
Randomization adequate	No
Blinding	Double-blind
Blinding adequate	Yes
Placebo	Yes
Drug comparison	Yes
Drug name	Amuno
Site description	Medical practice
No. of subjects enrolled	45

No. of subjects completed   41
Sex   Male and female
Age   28-84 years

Inclusion criteria
Patients suffering from inflammatory and chronic degenerative diseases.

Exclusion criteria
Patients with complaints of other causes.

End points
Improvement in disease symptoms after two and four weeks of treatment were compared to symptoms before treatment. Symptoms of pain due to movement, continuous pain, and limited mobility were evaluated on a scale of severe, medium-severe, mild, or nonexistent.

Results
After randomized assignment to treatment groups, the Amuno groups and Phytodolor groups were different in structure with regard to mobility (Amuno group had more pronounced limited mobility than Phytodolor group). Also, patients in the Phytodolor group most often suffered from arthrosis deformans, whereas patients in the Amuno group most often suffered from vertebra syndrome. The disease in the Phytodolor group had most often not persisted for longer than one year, whereas in the Amuno group, most patients had been suffering between one and eight years. After the first week of treatment, reductions in severity of pain due to movement and of continuous pain were more pronounced in the Amuno group than in the Phytodolor group. After four weeks of treatment, Phytodolor and Amuno showed similar success. (These results must be taken with reservations since the two groups were not equal at baseline.) Compared to placebo, the Phytodolor group showed significant improvement in "limited mobility" ($p < 0.01$) after one week and "pain due to movement" after two weeks ($p < 0.05$). In both groups, the symptom "continuous pain" was only mildly pronounced, and statistical differences could not be found.

Side effects
None observed with Phytodolor.

Authors' comments
Phytodolor was significantly more efficient than placebo in the treatment of degenerative and inflammatory rheumatic diseases. Phytodolor and Amuno both showed similar healing effects after a four weeks, though two thirds of the patients treated with indomethacin developed side effects. Because of the insufficient equality between the two patient groups, the results can be compared to a limited degree only.

Reviewer's comments
Compared to placebo, Phytodolor seemed to have more efficacy. However, the flawed randomization and small study size prevents any firm conclusions. No explanations for withdrawal were given for the three subjects who dropped out of the study. (2, 3)

Prostane®

Ingredients:
Salep orchid (*Orchis mascula* L.) tuber
Hygrophila (*Astercantha longifolia* Nees.) seed
Lettuce (*Lactuca scariola* L.) seed
Cow-itch (*Mucuna pruriens* (L.)DC.) seed
Elephant creeper (*Argyreia speciosa* [L. f.] Sweet) root
Small caltrops (*Tribulus terrestris* L.) fruit
Jeevanti (*Leptandenia reticulata* W. & A.) whole
Stone flower [*Parmelia perlata* (Huds.) Ach.] whole

PREPARATIONS USED IN REVIEWED CLINICAL STUDIES

Prostane® is manufactured by The Himalaya Drug Company in India and distributed in the United States by Himalaya USA. Each tablet contains 600 mg of a proprietary blend of eight herbs. Prostane is also sold as ProstaCare®. The product is called "Speman" in the clinical trial we reviewed. Unfortunately that trial did not include any details on the product, so we were unable to compare the material used in the trial to the current product.

SUMMARY OF REVIEWED CLINICAL STUDIES

We reviewed one study with Prostane for treatment of acute and chronic urinary retention due to prostate enlargement. A nonmalignant enlargement of the prostate that is common in men older than 40 years of age is called benign prostatic hyperplasia (BPH). Symptoms of BPH include increased urinary urgency and frequency, urinary hesitancy, intermittency, sensation of incomplete voiding, and decreased force of the urine stream.

PROSTANE® SUMMARY TABLE

Product Name	Manufacturer/ U.S. Distributor	Product Characteristics	Dose in Trials	Indication	No. of Trials	Benefit (Evidence Level-Trial No.)
Prostane®	The Himalaya Drug Company, India/ Himalaya USA	Blend of 8 ingredients	2 tablets 3 times daily	Benign prostatic hyperplasia	1	Undetermined (III-1)

Prostane

Benign Prostatic Hyperplasia

An open, placebo-controlled study with Prostane included 55 men with acute and chronic urinary retention due to prostate enlargement. Forty-seven participants had BPH, six had fibrotic disease, and two had prostate cancer. Forty-five of the patients were treated with Prostane and ten served as controls. Approximately 74 percent (28 of 38) of those in the treatment group with BPH had improved symptoms and decreases in prostate size and urinary congestion after 10 to 14 days of treatment with two tablets three times daily. The other ten in the treatment group with BPH required surgery (prostatectomy). All men that served as controls required surgery (Mukherjee, Ghosh, and De, 1986). The clinical efficacy of Prostane in this study was rated as undetermined due to poor study design.

ADVERSE REACTIONS OR SIDE EFFECTS

No side effects were reported in a clinical trial with 45 subjects given two tablets three times daily for a month (Mukherjee, Ghosh, and De, 1986).

REFERENCES

Mukherjee S, Ghosh TK, De D (1986). Effect of Speman on prostatism— A clinical study. *PROBE* 25 (3): 237-240. (Reprinted from *Indian Medical Journal* 1984; 78: 183.)

DETAILS ON PROSTANE PRODUCT
AND CLINICAL STUDIES

A profile on the product is followed by details of the clinical studies associated with that product. Clinical studies are grouped by therapeutic indication, in accordance with the order in the Summary Table.

Product Profile: Prostane®

Manufacturer	**The Himalaya Drug Company, India**
U.S. distributor	**Himalaya USA**
Formula botanicals	**Salep orchid tuber** (*Orchis mascula* L.); **hydrophila seed** (*Astercantha longifolia* Nees.); **lettuce seed** (*Lactuca scariola* L.); **cow-itch seed** (*Mucuna pruriens* (L.) DC.); **elephant creeper root** (*Argyreia speciosa* [L. f.] Sweet); **small caltrops fruit** (*Tribulus terrestris* L.); **Jeevanti, whole** (*Leptadenia reticulata* W. & A.), **stone flower, whole** [*Parmelia perlata* (Huds.) Ach.]
Quantity	600 mg
Processing	No information
Standardization	No information
Formulation	Tablet

Recommended dose: Take one or two tablets two times per day with meals.

DSHEA structure/function: Natural prostate support. Helps maintain a healthy prostate, and promotes normal urinary flow for optimum comfort.

Other ingredients: Tin sulfide, magnesium stearate, sodium carboxymethylcellulose, microcrystalline cellulose, crospovidone, aerosil.

Comments: Also sold as Speman and ProstaCare®.

Source(s) of information: Product label.

Clinical Study: Speman

Extract name	N/A
Manufacturer	The Himalaya Drug Company, India
Indication	**Benign prostatic hyperplasia; fibrotic disease; prostate cancer**
Level of evidence	**III**
Therapeutic benefit	**Undetermined**

Bibliographic reference

Mukherjee S, Ghosh TK, De D (1986). Effect of Speman on prostatism—A clinical study. *PROBE* 25 (3): 237-240. (Reprinted from *Indian Medical Journal* 1984; 78: 183.)

Trial design

Parallel. Ten patients acted as control and 45 were given Speman for 10 to 14 days. Patients in the study group were continued on Speman for a further 14 days, after which the dose was decreased to one tablet three times daily. Both groups were given antibiotics, antiseptics, and vitamins as necessary. Patients who presented with chronic retention of urine (29 cases) were fitted with a catheter, and the bladder was drained continuously for 10 to 14 days.

Study duration	10 to 14 days
Dose	2 tablets 3 times daily
Route of administration	Oral
Randomized	No
Randomization adequate	No
Blinding	Open
Blinding adequate	No
Placebo	No
Drug comparison	No
Site description	Medical college hospital
No. of subjects enrolled	55
No. of subjects completed	55
Sex	Male
Age	Not given

Inclusion criteria

Patients with prostatism.

Exclusion criteria

None mentioned.

End points
Clinical observations included the magnitude of urinary symptoms (urinary flow and frequency), prostate status (benign, fibrotic, and malignant), and the presence or absence of acute or chronic retention of urine. Efficacy was determined according to whether patients' conditions improved and whether operation was necessary.

Results
Twenty-eight of 38 patients in the treatment group with benign hypertrophy of the prostate improved satisfactorily (decrease urinary frequency both day and night, increased urinary flow, reduction in the size of prostate, and decreased congestion as measured by cystoscopic examination). Of these 38 patients in the treatment group who had benign hypertrophy, only ten needed prostatectomy. In 18 of 29 patients who had been fitted with a catheter, retention of urine recurred after the catheter was removed (14 in Speman group, four in control group). All of these patients were subjected to prostatectomy, in addition to the other six cases from the control group.

Side effects
None mentioned.

Authors' comments
The majority of the patients in the study group who had benign hypertrophy of the prostate had highly satisfactory results with Speman.

Reviewer's comments
Because of the poor study design and confounding factors, little can be determined of the benefits of this agent. Ten to 14 days of treatment is also a short duration. The trial was neither randomized nor blinded. (1, 2)

Resistex™

Ingredients:
Astragalus [*Astragalus membranaceus* (Fisch. ex Link) Bunge] root
Eleuthero (Siberian ginseng) [*Eleutherococcus senticosus* (Rupr. & Maxim.) Maxim.] root
Asian ginseng (*Panax ginseng* C.A. Meyey) root
Stephania (*Stephania tetrandra* S. Moore) root
Echinacea [*Echinacea purpurea* (L.) Moench] root
Barrenwort (*Epimedium grandiflorum* C. Morren) leaf and flower
Dong quai [*Angelica sinensis* (Oliv.) Diels] root

PREPARATIONS USED
IN REVIEWED CLINICAL STUDIES

Resistex® is manufactured and distributed by Botanica BioScience Corporation. Each capsule contains 450 mg of a proprietary blend of *Echinacea purpurea* root and extracts of astragalus, eleuthero (Siberian ginseng), Asian ginseng, stephania, barrenwort, and dong quai.

SUMMARY OF REVIEWED CLINICAL STUDIES

The Resistex formula was developed with the intention of providing resistance to infection with colds or flu. The initial cause of a cold or flu is a viral infection. Colds are caused most commonly by a rhinovirus and less often by a coronavirus. The influenza viruses cause the flu. In theory, bolstering the immune system can prevent disease or reduce symptoms. A number or herbal preparations have been promoted as immunostimulants for this purpose, including those containing echinacea and/or eleuthero (Wagner, 1997). Other herbs have been described as adaptogenic, i.e., substances that assist

RESISTEX® SUMMARY TABLE

Product Name	Manufacturer/ U.S. Distributor	Product Characteristics	Dose in Trials	Indication	No. of Trials	Benefit (Evidence Level-Trial No.)
Resistex™	Botanica BioScience Corporation/Botanica BioScience Corporation	Herbal blend of 7 ingredients	2 (450 mg) tablets per day	Cold and flu (prevention)	1	Undetermined (III-1)

in nonspecific heightened resistance to stress. The adaptogenic properties of these herbs may be due, in part, to antioxidant and/or immunomodulatory activity (Davydov and Krikorian, 2000). Herbs with adaptogenic activity ascribed to them include eleuthero, Asian ginseng, ashwaganda, astragalus, and schisandra (Davydov and Krikorian, 2000; Wagner, Nörr, and Winterhoff, 1992; Wallace, 1998).

Resistex

Cold and Flu (Prevention)

An open, placebo-controlled clinical trial with 61 participants found Resistex to significantly reduce the incidence of colds and flu compared to recall of the previous season. Subjects were divided into three groups and given one or two tablets of Resistex or placebo. Treatment was initially for four weeks, followed by a one-week intermission, which was followed by several two-week treatment periods, each separated by one-week intermissions. The total trial length was four and a half months. As a result, the group that received two tablets Resistex (900 mg daily) had a 67 percent reduction in the incidence of colds and flu compared to the previous season. In comparison, the group that received one tablet (450 mg daily) had a 43 percent reduction, and the placebo group had a 14 percent reduction (Wang, 1998). Methodological flaws, such as the dependence on recall for the previous season's incidence of colds and flu, and lack of detail in the trial report led our reviewer, Dr. Richard O'Connor, to rate the clinical outcome of this trial as undetermined.

ADVERSE REACTIONS OR SIDE EFFECTS

No side effects were reported in a controlled clinical trial with 61 patients that used a dose of 900 mg per day (Wang, 1998).

REFERENCES

Davydov M, Krikorian AD (2000). *Eleutherococcus senticosus* (Rupr. & Maxim.) Maxim. (Araliacaeae) as an adaptogen: A closer look. *Journal of Ethanopharmacology* 72 (3): 345-393.

Wagner H (1997). Herbal immunostimulants for the prophylaxis and therapy of colds and influenza. *The European Journal of Herbal Medicine* 3 (1): 22-30.

Wagner H, Nörr H, Winterhoff H (1992). Drugs with adaptogenic effects for strengthening the powers of resistance. *Zeitschrift für Phytotherapie* 13: 42-54

Wallace EC (1998). Adaptogenic herbs: Nature's solution to stress. *Nutrition Science News* 3 (5): 244-249.

Wang RT (1998). Outcomes study to evaluate the effects of Resistex on colds and flu in humans. China Academy of Preventative Medicine. Unpublished study.

DETAILS ON RESISTEX PRODUCT AND CLINICAL STUDIES

A profile on the product is followed by details of the clniical studies associated with that product. Clinical studies are grouped by therapeutic indication, in accordance with the order in the Summary Table.

Product Profile: Resistex™

Manufacturer	**Botanica BioScience Corporation**
U.S. distributor	**Botanica BioScience Corporation**
Formula Botanicals	***Astragalus membranaceus*** (std. root extract); **Siberian ginseng** (*Eleutherococcus senticosus;* std. root extract); ***Panax ginseng*** (std. root extract); ***Stephania tetrandra*** (extract from root); ***Echinacea purpurea*** (root); ***Epimedium grandiflorum*** (extract from leaves and flowers); ***Angelica sinensis*** (std. root extract).
Quantity	450 mg
Processing	No information
Standardization	No information
Formulation	Capsule

Recommended dose: Take two capsules once a day before or between meals, one week on and one week off. Dosage can be increased up to four capsules, three times a day, at the onset of cold or flu symptoms.

DSHEA structure/function: Cold season defense. Enhances T-cell and antibody production.

Cautions: In case of accidental overdose, seek professional advice immediately. If you are taking prescription medicine or are pregnant or lactating, consult with your doctor before taking.

Other ingredients: Cellulose, magnesium stearate (vegetable grade), silica.

Source(s) of information: Product package (© 1999 Botanica Bio-Science Corporation).

Clinical Study: Resistex™

Extract name	None given
Manufacturer	Botanica Bioscience Corporation
Indication	**Cold and flu** (prevention)
Level of evidence	**III**
Therapeutic benefit	**Undetermined**

Bibliographic reference
Wang RT (1998). Outcomes study to evaluate the effects of Resistex on colds and flu in humans. China Academy of Preventative Medicine. Unpublished study.

Trial design
Parallel. Patients took either Resistex or placebo every day for four weeks, then had a one-week break. This week was followed by two-week periods of taking either Resistex or placebo with one-week intermissions. This pattern was continued for several months. The trial began in November and concluded in March.

Study duration	4.5 months
Dose	1 or 2 (450 mg) tablets per day
Route of administration	Oral
Randomized	Yes
Randomization adequate	No
Blinding	Open
Blinding adequate	No
Placebo	Yes
Drug comparison	No
Site description	Not described
No. of subjects enrolled	61
No. of subjects completed	61
Sex	Male and female
Age	60-80 years

Inclusion criteria
Healthy elderly subjects between the ages of 60 and 80 with normal clinical chemistry profile and physician clearance.

Exclusion criteria
Acute or serious chronic diseases, receiving prescription medication or nonsteroidal anti-inflammatory drugs, taking vitamins or mineral supple-

ments during the least three months, alcohol or drug abuse, marked sleep disturbance, serious allergies, salient emotional or mood problems, or recent history of systemic infection, bone fracture, or surgery.

End points
Comparison of previous season's cold and flu histories with current season after supplementation with Resistex. Prior to random assignment, patients were questioned about their cold and flu history in the preceding year. During the study period, number of times cold or flu occurred and duration of illness were recorded.

Results
Patients in the high-dose treatment group showed a 67 percent reduction in the instance of cold and flu symptoms compared to 43 percent in the low-dose group and 14 percent for the placebo group. The difference between the high-dose group and placebo group was significant ($p < 0.01$).

Side effects
None mentioned.

Author's comments
The results support the comprehensive approach to boosting the body's immune system in the reduction of duration and severity of cold and flu symptoms in the active treatment group compared to the control group.

Reviewer's comments
This is a poorly conceived and poorly conducted study. The trial is apparently unblinded, and patient recalls were used as baseline. The author concludes that the product enhanced the immune system but no tests of immunity were performed. (0, 3)

Sinupret®

Ingredients:
   Gentian (yellow gentian) (*Gentiana lutea* **L.**) **root**
   Cowslip (primrose) (*Primula veris* **L.**) **flower**
   Sorrel (sour dock) (*Rumex acetosa* **L.**) **aerial parts**
   European elder (*Sambucus nigra* **L.**) **flower**
   European vervain (vervain wort) (*Verbena officinalis* **L. ssp.**
      officinalis) **aerial parts**

PREPARATIONS USED
IN REVIEWED CLINICAL STUDIES

Sinupret® is manufactured in Germany by Bionorica Arzneimittel GmbH. It contains a blend of five powdered plant materials: gentian root, European elder flower, European vervain aerial parts, cowslip flower, and sorrel aerial parts. Each tablet contains 78 mg of herbs. Sinupret is also sold in a liquid form: 100 g contains 29 g of aqueous alcoholic extracts (59 percent ethanol) of the herbs mentioned previously. Sinupret is distributed in the United States by Mediceutix, Inc.

SUMMARY OF REVIEWED CLINICAL STUDIES

Sinupret was approved as a drug to treat acute and chronic sinusitis by the federal authorities in Germany in 1997. Sinusitis is characterized by symptoms of nasal obstruction, discharge, postnasal drip, headache, and sore throat. It is often caused by a bacterial infection, and may follow a common cold or flu. Acute sinusitis may last for up to three weeks, but if it lasts for three months, it is considered chronic. Medical treatment is often aimed at eliminating the bacterial infection (if present) and reducing symptoms of sinus congestion and nasal discharge (Behr, 1998).

SINUPRET® SUMMARY TABLE

Product Name	Manufacturer/ U.S. Distributor	Product Characteristics	Dose in Trials	Indication	No. of Trials	Benefit (Evidence Level-Trial No.)
Sinupret®	Bionorica Arzneimittel GmbH, Germany/ Mediceutix, Inc.	Combination of gentian, European elder, European vervain, primrose, and sorrel	2 tablets, or 50 drops liquid, 3 times daily	Sinusitis	2	Yes (II-1) Undetermined (III-1)

Sinupret

Sinusitis

Two double-blind, placebo-controlled clinical studies on patients with acute or chronic sinusitis were reviewed. In a good-quality trial, 160 subjects with acute sinusitis were given either Sinupret (two 78 mg tablets three times daily) or placebo in addition to antibiotic and decongestant therapy. After two weeks, radiographic (X-ray) reports and patients' assessments showed significant improvement with Sinupret compared with placebo (Neubauer and März, 1994).

The other trial, with poor methodological ratings, included 31 subjects with chronic sinusitis and compared treatment with either the liquid or tablet form of Sinupret with two matching placebos. After one week of treatment, radiographic and ultrasound findings showed improvement with both forms of Sinupret compared with placebo. Complete recovery occurred in 12 of 16 subjects in the treatment group and in 6 of 15 subjects in the placebo group (Richstein and Mann, 1999).

Six additional controlled trials were conducted on Sinupret between 1980 and 1992. These trials were not obtained in English in their full form and so were not reviewed for their level of evidence for this book. They were summarized in an unpublished report written on behalf of the manufacturer (Bionorica), as well as in a published review (Behr, 1998; März, Ismail, and Popp, 1999). One study was double-blind and placebo-controlled, including 39 young subjects with asthma. As a result of treatment, radiographic findings showed improvement, and the frequency of asthma attacks was reduced (Lecheler and Mann, 1980). Another study compared Sinupret with antibiotics (doxycycline) to Esberitox (echinacea formula) with antibiotics to antibiotics alone in 90 subjects with acute bacterial sinusitis (Zimmer, 1985). Four other studies, including a total of 594 subjects with acute sinusitis, compared Sinupret to other expectorants: the volatile oil mytrol, acetylcysteine, or ambroxol Mucosolvan® (Kraus and März, 1992; Braum and März, 1990; Simm, Pape, and März, 1991; Wahls and März, 1990). In general the trials were positive, with Sinupret being similar to other active treatments for acute sinusitis.

POSTMARKETING SURVEILLANCE STUDY

A postmarketing surveillance study was conducted with 3,187 patients between 1 and 94 years old, with acute or chronic bronchitis. Sinupret was as effective as other expectorants, following ten days treatment with 150 drops or six tablets per day (Ernst, März, and Sieder, 1997).

ADVERSE REACTIONS OR SIDE EFFECTS

The two studies we reviewed reported no side effects. A small trial with 12 healthy participants, given either the usual or a fivefold dose of either the liquid or the tablet form for six weeks, found no adverse effects in numerous laboratory tests (Strobel, 1984). In a postmarketing surveillance study conducted with 3,187 patients in Germany, side effects were documented in 8 of the 1,013 patients who received Sinupret as their only therapy. The side effects were gastrointestinal intolerance with one instance of dizziness (Ernst, Sieder, and März, 1995).

A retrospective multicenter analysis of one thousand pregnant women who used Sinupret because of sinusitis or bronchitis, reported no evidence of risk for fetal malformations or adverse effects (Becker, Sieder, and März, 1997). Another study of 762 pregnant women also found no indication of teratogenic or embryotoxic effects (Queisser-Luft and Ismail, 2000).

REFERENCES

Becker MKF, Sieder C, März RW (1997). Sinupret in pregnancy—A retrospective study of 1,000 cases: Preliminary results. *Fact: Focus on Alternative and Complementary Therapies* 2 (4): 185. (Presented at the Fourth Annual Symposium on Complementary Healthcare, December 10-12, 1997, Exeter, United Kingdom.)

Behr B (1998). Sinupret: Efficacy and Safety Expert Report 1998. Unpublished.

Braum D, März RW (1990). Randomisierte vergleichsstudie Sinupret Dragees vs Fluimucil (Granulat) bei akuter und chronischer Sinusitis (N=160). Germany: Bericht Bionorica Arzneimittel GmbH, Neumarkt/Opf. Cited in Behr B (1998). Sinupret: Efficacy and Safety Expert Report 1998. Unpublished.

Ernst E, Marz RW, Sieder Ch (1997). Acute bronchitis—Benefits of Sinupret: Comparative post-marketing surveillance study involving 3,187 patients. *Fortschritte der Medizin* 115 (11): 52-53.

Ernst E, Sieder Ch, Marz R (1995). Adverse drug reactions to herbal and synthetic expectorants. *International Journal of Risk and Safety in Medicine* 7: 219-225.

Kraus P, März RW (1992). Randomisierte vergleichsstudie Sinupret Dragees vs. Gelomytol f. bei akuter und chronischer Sinusitis (N=134). Klinischer und biometrischer Bericht, Bionorica GmbH, Neumarkt. Presented at the Fourth National and First International Congress on Phytomedicine, Munich. Cited in Behr B (1998). Sinupret: Efficacy and Safety Expert Report 1998. Unpublished.

Lecheler J, Mann R (1980). Sinupret Doppelblindstudie (bei jugendichen Asthmapatienten; N=39). Germany: Bericht Bionorica Arzneimittel GmbH, Neumarkt/Opf. Cited in Behr B (1998). Sinupret: Efficacy and Safety Expert Report 1998. Unpublished.

März RW, Ismail C, Popp MA (1999). Action profile and efficacy of a herbal combination preparation for the treatment of sinusitis. *Wiener Medezinische Wochenschrift* 149 (8-10): 202-208.

Neubauer N, März RW (1994). Placebo-controlled, randomized double-blind clinical trial with Sinupret sugar-coated tablets on the basis of a therapy with antibiotics and decongestant nasal drops in acute sinusitis. *Phytomedicine* 1 (3): 177-181.

Queisser-Luft A, Ismail Ch (2000). Safety of an herbal combination preparation in pregnancy—An example for using active detection systems for malformations. *Phytomedicine* Supplement II: 12.

Richstein A, Mann W (1999). Treatment of chronic rhino-sinusitis with Sinupret. *Schweizerische Zeitschrift für GanzheitsMedizin* 11 (6): 1-3. (Previously published as Richstein A, Mann W [1980]. Zur Behandlung der chronischen Sinusitis mit Sinupret®. *Therapie der Gegenwart* 119 [9]: 1055-1060.)

Simm KJ, Pape HG, März RW (1991). Doppelblindstudie Sinupret vs. Mucosovan mit/ohne Nasentropfen bei akuter Sinusitis (N=160). Clinical and biometrical report. Germany: Bionorica Arzneimittel GmbH, Neumarkt/Opf. Cited in Behr B (1998). Sinupret: Efficacy and Safety Expert Report 1998. Unpublished.

Strobel W (1984). The tolerance of Sinupret (the influences of long-term medication on clinical/chemical parameters in healthy participants). *Zeitschrift für Phytotherapie* 6: 2-6.

Wahls M, März RW (1990). Randomisierte, kontrollierte Doppelblind-studie Sinupret Tropfen vs Mucosolvan Tropfen bei acuter und chronischer sinusitis (N=160). Germany: Bericht Bionorica Arzneimittel GmbH, Neumarket/Opf. Cited in Behr B (1998). Sinupret: Efficacy and Safety Expert Report 1998. Unpublished.

Zimmer M (1985). Gezielte konservative Therapie der akuten Sinusitis in der HNO-Praxis. *Therapiewoche* 35: 4024-4028. Cited in Behr B (1998). Sinupret: Efficacy and Safety Expert Report 1998. Unpublished.

DETAILS ON SINUPRET PRODUCT AND CLINICAL STUDIES

A profile on the product is followed by details of the clinical studies associated with that product. Clinical studies are grouped by therapeutic indication, in accordance with the order in the Summary Table.

Product Profile: Sinupret®

Manufacturer	**Bionorica Arzneimittel GmbH, Germany**
U.S. distributor	Mediceutix, Inc.
Formula Botanicals	**Gentian root** (*Gentiana lutea* L.) 6 mg; **elder flower** (*Sambucus nigra* L.) 18 mg; **European vervain** aerial parts (*Verbena officinalis* L. ssp. *officinalis*), 18 mg; **cowslip flower** (*Primula veris* L.) 18 mg; **sorrel** aerial parts (*Rumex acetosa* L.), 18 mg
Quantity	78 mg
Processing	Herbs pulverized at low temperature
Standardization	No information
Formulation	Tablet

Other ingredients: Digestible carbohydrates (41.6 percent), and sorbitol (0.1 percent).

Source(s) of information: Neubauer and März, 1994; Physicians' Reference on Sinupret Dragées and Sinupret Drops, Bionorica GmbH Medical Scientific Information, 1991.

Clinical Study: Sinupret®

Extract name	N/A
Manufacturer	Bionorica Arzneimittel GmbH, Germany
Indication	**Acute sinusitis**
Level of evidence	**II**
Therapeutic benefit	**Yes**

Bibliographic reference
Neubauer N, März RW (1994). Placebo-controlled, randomized double-blind clinical trial with Sinupret sugar-coated tablets on the basis of a therapy with antibiotics and decongestant nasal drops in acute sinusitis. *Phytomedicine* 1 (3): 177-181.

Trial design
Parallel. Patients were given Sinupret or placebo in addition to antibiotic therapy, Vibramycin® (doxycycline), and decongestant therapy, Otriven® (xylometazoline).

Study duration	2 weeks
Dose	2 (78 mg) tablets 3 times daily
Route of administration	Oral
Randomized	Yes
Randomization adequate	Yes
Blinding	Double-blind
Blinding adequate	Yes
Placebo	Yes
Drug comparison	No
Site description	Not described
No. of subjects enrolled	177
No. of subjects completed	160
Sex	Male and female
Age	Mean: 24.5 years

Inclusion criteria
Clinical diagnosis of an acute sinusitis in connection with an opacification of the plain sinus radiogram.

Exclusion criteria
Patients with extreme anatomical deviations of the nasal septum were excluded, as well as patients with known intolerance for doxycycline.

End points
Primary outcome criteria were radiographic findings (completely opaque, shadowed, nothing abnormal) and the patients' assessment of the therapy (three categories: asymptomatic, good effect, no effect). Secondary variables were clinical findings (mucosa findings, secretions, patency of the nose, headache). Evaluations took place before and after two weeks of treatment.

Results

Radiographic findings showed that the addition of Sinupret treatment to standard therapy was significantly more effective than standard therapy plus placebo ($p = 0.024$). Patient assessments at the end of therapy also indicated that Sinupret was more effective than placebo. The clinical variables showed that Sinupret was superior to placebo in reducing mucosal swelling, nasal obstruction, headache, and positive trends for nasal patency. No difference regarding secretion was found.

Side effects

None recorded.

Authors' comments

Conventional therapy for acute bacterial sinusitis can be markedly improved by including Sinupret in the therapeutic regimen. Furthermore, it can be deduced from our results that any negative interaction between the herbal preparation and the basic therapy was not observed.

Reviewer's comments

This is a well-described, well-designed study. The only criticism is that no mention is made of blinding the radiologist who interpreted the X-rays, a potential source of bias. This study suggests that the addition of Sinupret to standard therapy may improve therapeutic outcomes. The trial deserves to be replicated with blinding of the radiologist. (5, 5)

Clinical Study: Sinupret®

Extract name	N/A
Manufacturer	Bionorica Arzneimittel GmbH, Germany
Indication	**Chronic sinusitis**
Level of evidence	**III**
Therapeutic benefit	**Undetermined**

Bibliographic reference

Richstein A, Mann W (1999). Treatment of chronic rhino-sinusitis with Sinupret. *Schweizerische Zeitschrift für GanzheitsMedizin* 11 (6): 1-3. (Previously published as Richstein A, Mann W [1980]. Zur Behandlung der chronischen Sinusitis mit Sinupret®. *Therapie der Gegenwart* 119 [9]: 1055-1060.)

Trial design
Parallel. Two formulations (liquid and tablets) of Sinupret were compared with matching placebos.

Study duration	1 week
Dose	2 tablets or 50 drops of liquid formula 3 times daily
Route of administration	Oral
Randomized	Yes
Randomization adequate	No
Blinding	Double-blind
Blinding adequate	No
Placebo	Yes
Drug comparison	No
Site description	Medical school outpatients
No. of subjects enrolled	31
No. of subjects completed	31
Sex	Male and female
Age	6-73 years

Inclusion criteria
Patients suffering from chronic sinusitis, with symptoms such as headache, posterior nasal rhinorrhea, pressure sensation over the affected sinuses, and blocked nose.

Exclusion criteria
Patients for which sinus surgery is indicated as the primary mode of treatment.

End points
Assessment criteria were symptoms, endoscopic, radiologic, and ultrasonographic findings. Assessments were made at the beginning and end of the study, with a follow-up assessment on day 16 (nine days after the end of treatment).

Results
The radiologic (X-ray) and ultrasonographic findings of the paranasal sinuses and the symptoms of the patients showed considerable improvement and even complete recovery in 12 of 16 total patients in the verum group. In the placebo group, only 6 of 15 patients showed improvement. The therapeutic effect did not depend on the formulation (liquid or tablets). Statistical improvement was seen compared to placebo for headache and X-ray analy-

sis (p = 0.025 and p = 0.001, respectively). No difference existed between the two groups in posterior nasal secretion.

Side effects
None mentioned.

Authors' comments
This double-blinded prospective trial study of 31 patients with chronic sinusitis revealed that Sinupret has a positive effect on subjective and objective findings in patients with chronic rhino-sinusitis.

Reviewer's comments
This is a very small trial study whose inclusion criteria are not adequately described. The primary end points are also not described, and no mention of monitoring for adverse events is made. In their introduction, the authors describe a subset of patients who have symptoms but no significant radiologic abnormalities, but then in their inclusion criteria they include patients they describe as having radiologic abnormalities that change with therapy. This appears to be a bit of fuzzy logic. Neither Institutional Review Board (IRB) approval nor informed consent were obtained. Follow-up X-rays were taken with 11 of 16 subjects in the treatment group and 6 of 12 subjects in the placebo group. Neither the randomization nor the blinding were adequately described. (0, 2)

Appendix A

Products Listed by Manufacturer/Distributor

AB Cernelle, Sweden
Cernilton®   Grass pollen

Access Business Group: Home of Nutrilite
Nutrilite® Saw Palmetto
   with Nettle Root   Saw palmetto

Ardeypharm GmbH, Germany
Devil's Claw   Devil's claw

Arkopharma Laboratoires Pharmaceutiques, France
Arkojoint™   Devil's claw
Exolise™   Green tea
Harpadol®   Devil's claw
SPV$_{30}$™   Boxwood

Biofarm S.A., Romania
Silimarina®   Milk thistle

Bioforce AG, Switzerland/Bioforce USA
Aesculaforce   Horse chestnut
Echinaforce®   Echinacea
Geriaforce   Ginkgo
Ginkgoforce   Ginkgo
Hyperiforce   St. John's wort
Venaforce™   Horse chestnut

Bionorica Arzneimittel GmbH, Germany
Mastodynon® N   Chaste tree
Sinupret®   Formula

Bluebonnet Nutrition Corporation
Grape Seed Extract   Grape seed

Botanica BioScience Corporation
2nd Wind™   Formula
Resistex™   Formula

Bruschettini s.r.l., Italy
Procianidol   Grape seed

Chai-Na-Ta Corporation, Canada
American Ginseng   American ginseng

Dalidar Pharma Ltd., Israel
Zintona®   Ginger

Dansk Droge, Denmark
Gerimax Ginseng Extract   Ginseng

Ditta Farmigea S.p.A., Italy
FAR-1   Bilberry

Dr. Loges & Co. GmbH, Germany
Dysto-lux®   St. John's wort

Dr. Willmar Schwabe GmbH & Co., Germany
Crataegutt®   Hawthorn
Euvegal® forte   Valerian
Ginkgold®   Ginkgo
Ginkoba®   Ginkgo
HeartCare™   Hawthorn
Laitan®   Kava
Movana™   St. John's wort
Perika™   St. John's wort
ProstActive®   Saw palmetto
ProstActive® Plus   Saw palmetto
Prostagutt® forte   Saw palmetto
Neuroplant®   St. John's wort
Rökan®   Ginkgo
Tanakan®   Ginkgo
Tebonin® forte   Ginkgo
Valerian Nighttime™   Valerian
Extract: WS 1531   Devil's claw
Extract: WS 1540   Ginger

EcoNugenics Inc.
Padma® BASIC   Formula

Efamol Ltd., UK
Efamol®   Evening primrose

Enzymatic Therapy
Bilberry Extract   Bilberry
Ginkgo Biloba-24%   Ginkgo
Esberitox™   Echinacea
Herpilyn®   Lemon balm
Iberogast™   Formula
Saventaro®   Cat's claw
St. John's Wort Extract   St. John's wort

Essentially Pure Ingredients™
Pure-Gar®   Garlic

Eurovita A/S, Denmark
Eurovita Extract 33   Ginger

General Nutrition Corporation
Bowel Support Formula   Dragon's blood croton
Cycle Balance™   Chaste tree
St. John's Wort Ze 117™   St. John's wort

General Nutrition Research Laboratories
Garlic oil, cold pressed   Garlic

GlaxoSmithKline
Alluna™ Sleep   Valerian
Remifemin®   Black cohosh

Government Pharmaceutical Organization, Thailand
Spray-dried garlic   Garlic

Graminex L.L.C.
Cernilton®   Grass pollen

HBC Protocols, Inc.
Hypericum Perforatum II   St. John's wort

Health from the Sun/Arkopharma
Arkojoint™   Devil's claw
Exolise™   Green tea
SPV$_{30}$™   Boxwood

Hermes Arzneimittel GmbH, Germany
Tegra   Garlic

The Himalaya Drug Company, India/Himalaya USA
Cystone®   Formula
GastriCare®   Formula
Gastrim®   Formula
GeriCare®   Formula
Geriforte®   Formula
ProstaCare®   Formula
Prostane®   Formula
Speman   Formula
UriCare®   Formula

Indena S.p.A., Italy/Indena USA, Inc.
Extract: GinkgoSelect™   Ginkgo
Extract: LeucoSelect™   Grape seed
Leucoselect™-phytosome®   Grape seed
Extract: MirtoSelect™   Bilberry
Extract: PrunuSelect™   Pygeum
Extract: SabalSelect™   Saw palmetto
Extract: Siliphos®   Milk thistle
Extract: St. John Select™   St. John's wort

Inverni della Beffa, Italy (Indena S.p.A., Italy)
Pigenil   Pygeum
Silipide   Milk thistle
Tegens   Bilberry

Laboratoires Fournier, France
Tadenan®   Pygeum

Lichtwer Pharma AG, Germany
Cynara-SL™   Artichoke
Faros® 300   Hawthorn
Ginkai™   Ginkgo
Ginkyo®   Ginkgo
Hepar-SL forte®   Artichoke
Jarsin®   St. John's wort
Jarsin® 300   St. John's wort
Kaveri®   Ginkgo
Kira®   St. John's wort
Kwai®   Garlic
Sedonium™   Valerian

Lomapharm, Rudolf Lohmann GmbH KG, Germany

Herpilyn®	Lemon balm
Lomaherpan®	Lemon balm

Madaus AG, Germany

Agnolyt®	Chaste tree
Echinacin®	Echinacea
Echinagard®	Echinacea
EchinaGuard®	Echinacea
Escin gel	Horse chestnut
Legalon®	Milk thistle

Mitsui Norin Co., Ltd., Japan

Polyphenon E®	Green tea

Natrol, Inc.

Kavatrol™	Kava

Natural Wellness

Maximum Milk Thistle™	Milk thistle
UltraThistle™	Milk thistle

Nature's Way Products, Inc.

EchinaGuard®	Echinacea
Ginkgold®	Ginkgo
HeartCare™	Hawthorn
Perika™	St. John's wort
ProstActive®	Saw palmetto
ProstActive® Plus	Saw palmetto
Sambucol®	Elderberry
Valerian Nighttime™	Valerian

Novartis Consumer Health GmbH, Germany

Valverde Artischocke	Artichoke

Novogen Inc.

Promensil™	Red clover

Novogen Laboratories Pty Ltd., Australia

Promensil™	Red clover

Nutraceutical Corporation

CranActin®	Cranberry

Ocean Spray Cranberries, Inc.
Cranberry Juice Cocktail   Cranberry

Padma Inc., Switzerland
Padma® 28   Formula
Padma® BASIC   Formula

Pharmanex LLC/Pharmanex Natural Healthcare
Cholestin™   Red yeast rice
CordyMax® Cs-4   Cordyceps
JinShuiBao   Cordyceps
Tegreen 97®   Green tea

Pharmaton S.A., Switzerland/Pharmaton Natural Health Products
Gericomplex®   Ginseng
Gincosan®   Ginkgo
Ginkoba®   Ginkgo
Ginkoba M/E™   Ginkgo
Ginsana®   Ginseng
Ginsana® Gold Blend   Ginseng
Extract: GK501™   Ginkgo
Movana™   St. John's wort
Prostatonin®   Pygeum
Songha Night®   Valerian
Venastat™   Horse chestnut
Venostasin® retard   Horse chestnut

Pierre Fabre Médicament, France
Capistan   Saw palmetto
Liberprosta®   Saw palmetto
Permixon®   Saw palmetto
Sereprostat®   Saw palmetto

Razei Bar Industries, Ltd.
Sambucol®   Elderberry

Rexall Sundown, Inc.
St. John's Wort (Ze 117™)   St. John's wort

Sanofi-Synthelabo, France
Endotelon®   Grape seed

Schaper & Brümmer GmbH & Co. KG, Germany
Esberitox™   Echinacea
Remifemin®   Black cohosh
Strogen® uno   Saw palmetto

Scotia Pharmaceuticals Ltd., UK
Efamol Marine   Evening primrose
Epogam®   Evening primrose

Searle, UK
Efamast   Evening primrose

Shaman Pharmaceuticals, Inc./ShamanBotanicals.com
Bowel Support Formula   Dragon's blood croton
Provir™   Dragon's blood croton
SB-Normal Stool Formula™   Dragon's blood croton

Solaray, Inc.
CranActin®   Cranberry

Solvay Arzneimittel GmbH, Germany
Baldrian-Dispert   Valerian
Valdispert®   Valerian

Steigerwald Arzneimittel GmbH, Germany
Iberogast™   Formula
Phytodolor™   Formula

Steiner Arzneimittel, Germany
Extract: STEI 300   St. John's wort

Swanson Health Products
Ginkgo Biloba   Ginkgo

Therabel Pharma, Belgium
Prostaserene®   Saw palmetto

Thomas J. Lipton Co. (now **Unilever Bestfoods, North America**)
Lipton Research Blend   Green tea

Thorne Research
GB24™   Ginkgo
Hyper-Ex®   St. John's wort
O.P.C.-100   Grape seed
Serenoa Gelcaps   Saw palmetto
Vacimyr®   Bilberry

Traditional Medicinals, Inc.
Echinacea Plus®   Echinacea

Wakunaga of America Co., Ltd.
Kyolic® Aged Garlic Extract™,
  HI-PO™ Formula 100   Garlic
Kyolic® Liquid Aged Garlic
  Extract™   Garlic

WBL Peking University Biotech Co. Ltd., China
Zhitai   Red Yeast Rice

Weber & Weber International GmbH & Co. KG, Germany/Weber & Weber USA
Petadolex™   Butterbur, Purple

Wei-Xin Company, China
Xue-zhi-kang   Red yeast rice

Zeller AG, Switzerland
Alluna™ Sleep   Valerian
Cycle Balance™   Chaste tree
Esbericum forte   St. John's wort
IVEL®   Valerian
Rebalance   St. John's wort
ReDormin®   Valerian
Remotiv®   St. John's wort
St. John's Wort (Ze 117™) St. John's wort
St. John's Wort Ze 117™   St. John's wort
Valverde Hyperval   St. John's wort
Extract: ZE 339   Butterbur

Appendix B

Manufacturer/Distributor Contact Information

Corporate addresses and contact information have been verified to the best of the editor's ability. However, some telephone numbers may be incomplete and may require the addition of international dialing codes for the country specified.

AB Cernelle, Sweden
Vegeholm 4320, S-262 94 Engelholm, Sweden
Web site: www.abcernelle.com

Access Business Group: Home of Nutrilite
5600 Beach Boulevard/ P.O. Box 5940, Buena Park, B62 CA 90622-5940
Phone: 714-562-6220
Web site: www.nutrilite.com

Ardeypharm GmbH, Germany
Loerfeldstr. 20, 58313 Herdecke, Germany
Phone: 49-2330-977-677
Fax: 49-2330-977-697
Web site: www.ardeypharm.de

Arkopharma Laboratoires Pharmaceutiques, France
BP 28—06511 CARROS Cedex—France
Phone: 33-4-93-29-11-28
Web site: www.arkopharma.com/english

Biofarm S.A., Romania
Logafat Tantra nr. 99 Street, Sector 3, Bucharest, Romania
Phone: 40-21-3010637, 40-21-3010633, 40-21-3010632
Fax: 40-21-3010605, 40-21-3010631
Web site: www.biofarm.ro

Bioforce AG, Switzerland
CH-9325 Roggwil TG, Switzerland
Phone: 41-71-454-61-61
Fax: 41-71-454-61-62
Web site: www.bioforce.ch/en

Bioforce USA
437 Route 295, Chatham, NY 12037
Phone: 800-641-7555
Fax: 800-798-7555
Web site: www.bioforceusa.com

Bionorica Arzneimittel GmbH, Germany
Kerschensteiner Strasse 11-15, 92318 Neumarkt, Germany / P.O. Box
1851, D-92308 Neumarkt, Germany
Phone: 49-9181-231-90
Fax: 49-9181-231-265
Web site: www.bionorica.de

Bluebonnet Nutrition Corporation
12915 Dairy Ashford, Sugar Lsmf TX, 77478
Phone: 800-580-8866 / 281-240-3332
Fax: 281-240-3535
Web site: www.bluebonnetnutrition.com

Botanica BioScience Corporation
P.O. Box 1477, Ojai, CA 93024
Phone: 805-646-6062
Fax: 805-646-3026
Web site: www.botanica-bioscience.com

Bruschettini s.r.l., Italy
Via Isonzo, 6, 16147 Genova, Italy
Phone: 39-010-381222
Fax: 39-010-3993312
Web site: www.bruschettini.com

Chai-Na-Ta Corporation, Canada
5965 205A Street, Langley, British Columbia, Canada V2A8C4
Phone: 800-406-4668 (Canada & USA)/ 604-533-8883
Fax: 604-8-588-8891
Web site: www.chainata.com

Dalidar Pharma Ltd., Israel
c.o. Bio-Dar Ltd., Yavne Technology Park, P.O. box 344, Yavne 81103, Israel
Phone: 08-9420930
Fax: 08-9420928

Dansk Droge, Denmark
Industrigrenen 10, Ishøj 2635, Denmark
Phone: 435-65656
Fax: 435-65600
Email: info@danskdroge.dk

Ditta Farmigea S.p.A., Italy
No information available

Dr. Loges & Co. GmbH, Germany
P.O. Box 1262/ Schützenstrasse 5, 21423 Winsen, Germany
Phone: 49-4171-707-0
Fax: 49-4171-707-100
Web site: www.loges.de

Dr. Willmar Schwabe GmbH & Co., Germany
Willmar-Schwabe-Strasse 4, 76227 Karlsruhe, Germany
Phone: 49-721-4005-101
Fax: 49-721-4005-202
Web site: www.schwabe.de; www.schwabepharma.com

EcoNugenics Inc.
2208 Northpoint Parkway, Santa Rosa, CA 95407
Phone: 800-308-5518
Fax: 707-526-7689
Web site: www.econugenics.com

Efamol Ltd., UK
No information available

Enzymatic Therapy
825 Challenger Dr., Green Bay, WI 5431-8328
Phone: 920-469-1313/ 800-783-2286
Fax: 920-469-4400
Web site: www.enzy.com

Essentially Pure Ingredients™
21411 Prairie Street, Chatsworth, CA 91311
Phone: 818-739-6046
Fax: 818-739-6042
Web site: www.essentiallypure.com

Eurovita A/S, Denmark
Svejsegangen 4, 2690 Karlslunde, Denmark
Phone: 45-46-15-22-11
Fax: 45-46-15-32-11
Web site: www.eurovita.dk

General Nutrition Corporation
300 Sixth Avenue, Pittsburgh, PA 15222
Phone: 888-462-2548
Web site: www.gnc.com

General Nutrition Research Laboratories
Fargo, North Dakota
No further information available

GlaxoSmithKline Consumer Healthcare
5 Moore Drive, P.O. Box 13398, Research Triangle Park, NC 27709 / One
Franklin Plaza, Philadelphia, PA 19102 / Consumer Healthcare, P.O. Box
1467, Pittsburgh, PA 15230
Phone: 888-825-5249 (Remifemin® adverse events: 800-965-8804)
(Alluna™ Sleep adverse events : 877-725-5862)
Web site: www.gsk.com; www.remifemin.com; www.allunasleep.com

Government Pharmaceutical Organization, Thailand
No information available

Graminex L.L.C.
95 Midland Rd., Saginaw, MI 48603
Phone: 877-472-6469/ 989-797-5502
Fax: 989-799-0020
Web site: www.graminex.com

HBC Protocols, Inc.
8205 Santa Monica Blvd., Suite 472, Los Angeles, CA 90046
Phone: 800-497-3742
Fax: 805-583-7717
Web site: www.hbcstore.com

Health from the Sun/Arkopharma
19 Crosby Drive, Bedford, MA 01730
Phone: 781-276-0505
Fax: 781-276-7335
Web site: www.healthfromthesun.com

Hermes Arzneimittel GmbH, Germany
Georg-Kalb Strasse 5-8, 82049 Grosshesselohe/Munich, Germany
Phone: 49-89-79102-0
Fax: 49-89-79102-280
Web site: www.hermes-arzneimittel.com

The Himalaya Drug Company, India
Makali, Bangalore—562123, India
Phone: 91-80-371-4444/ 91-80-371-4445/91-80-371-4446
Fax: 91-80-371-4468
Web site: www.himalayahealthcare.com

Himalaya USA
10440 Westoffice Drive, houston, Texas 77042
Phone: 713-863-1622/ 800-869-4640
Fax: 713-863-1686/ 800-577-6930
Web site: www.himalayausa.com

IMMODAL Pharmaka GmbH, Austria
Bundesstrasse 44, 6111 Volders/Tirol, Austria
Phone: 43-5224-57678
Fax: 43-5224-57646
Web site: www.immodal.com

Indena S.p.A., Italy
Viale Ortles, 12, 20139 Milano, Italy
Phone: 39-02-574961
Fax: 39-02-57404620
Web site: www.indena.it

Indena USA, Inc.
1001 Fourth Avenue Plaza, Suite 3714, Seattle, WA 98154
Phone: 206-340-6140
Fax: 206-340-0863
Web site: www.indena.com

Inverni della Beffa, Italy
Galleria Passarella 2, 20122 Milano, Italy
Phone: 39-02-574961

Laboratoires Fournier, France
42 re de Longvic, 21300 Chenove, France OR
153 rue de Buzenval, 92380 Garches, France
Phone: 33-3-80-44-70-00
Fax: 33-3-80-44-70-05
Web site: www.groupe-fournier.com

Lichtwer Pharma AG, Germany
Wallenroder Strasse 8-10, 13435 Berlin, Germany
Phone: 49-30-403-70-0
Fax: 49-30-403-70-103
Web site: www.lichtwer.de

Lomapharm, Rudolf Lohmann GmbH KG, Germany
Langes Feld 5, 31860 Emmerthal, Germany
Phone: 49-5155-63-200
Fax: 49-5155-63-240
Web site: www.lomapharm.de

Madaus AG, Germany
Ostmerheimer Strasse 198, D-51109 Köln, Germany
Phone: 49-221-8998-0
Fax: 49-221-8998-701
Web site: www.madaus.de

Mediceutix, Inc.
P.O. Box 21801, Eugene, OR 97402

Mitsui Norin Co., Ltd., Japan
Mitsui-Bekkan, 3-1-20 Muromachi, Nihonbashi, Chuo-ku, Tokyo 103, Japan
Phone: 81-3-3241-3114
Fax: 81-3-3241-6130
Web site: www.mitsui-norin.co.jp/

Natrol, Inc.
21411 Prairie Street, Chatsworth, CA 91311
Phone: 800-326-1520/ 818-739-6000
Fax: 818-739-6001
Web site: www.natrol.com

Natural Wellness
46 Main St./ P.O. Box 1139, Pine Bush, NY 12566
Phone: 800-364-5722
Fax: 845-744-5953
Web site: www.natural-wellness.com, www.liversupport.com

Nature's Way Products, Inc.
10 Mountain Springs Parkway, Springville, UT 84663
Phone: 800-489-1500
Fax: 800-489-1700
Web site: www.naturesway.com

Novartis Consumer Health GmbH, Germany
Zielstattstrasse 40, 81379 Munich, Germany
Phone: 49-89-7877-0
Fax: 49-89-7877-250
Web site: www.novartis-consumerhealth.de

Novogen Inc.
1 Landmark Square, Suite 240, Stamford, CT 06901
Phone: 203-327-1188
Fax: 203-327-0011
Web site: www.novogen.com

Novogen Laboratories Pty Ltd., Australia
140 Wicks Road, North Ryde NSW 2113, Australia
Phone: 61-2-9878-0088
Fax: 61-2-9878-0055
Web site: www.novogen.com

Nutraceutical Corporation
1400 Kearns Boulevard, Park City, UT 84060
Phone: 800-669-8877
Fax: 800-767-8514
Web site: www.nutraceutical.com

Ocean Spray Cranberries, Inc.
Ocean Spray Consumer Affairs Department, Ocean Spray Cranberries,
Inc., One Ocean Spray Drive, Lakeville-Middleboro, MA 02349
Phone: 800-662-3263
Web site: www.oceanspray.com

Padma Inc., Switzerland
Wiesenstrasse 5, CH-8603 Schwerzenbach, Switzerland
Phone: 41-0-1-887-00-00
Web site: www.padma.ch/en/

Pharmanex, LLC
75 West Center Street, Provo, UT 84601
Phone: 801-345-1000
Fax: 801-345-9899
Web site: www.pharmanex.com

Pharmaton Natural Health Products
P.O. Box 368/ 900 Ridgebury Road, Ridgefield, CT 06877-0368
Phone: 800-451-6688
Fax: 203-798-5771
Web site: www.pharmaton.com

Pharmaton S.A., Switzerland
P.O. Box 6903 Lugano, Switzerland
Phone: 41-91-610-32-11
Fax: 41-91-610-32-09

Pierre Fabre Médicament, France
45, Place Abel Gance, 92654 Boulogne, France
Phone: 33-01-49-10-80-00
Web site: www.pierre-fabre.com

Razei Bar Industries, Ltd.
P.O. Box 8625, Jerusalem 91086, Israel

Rexall Sundown, Inc.
6111 Broken Sound Parkway, N.W., Boca Raton, FL 33487-3693
Phone: 888-776-5383/ 800-327-0908
Web site: www.rexallsundown.com

Sanofi-Synthelabo, France
174, av. De France, 75013 Paris, France
Phone: 33-1-5377-4000
Fax: 33-1-5377-4265
Web site: http://en.sanofi-synthelabo.com

Schaper & Brümmer GmbH & Co. KG, Germany
HRA 11133, Amtsgericht Braunschweig, 38251 Salzgitter, Germany
Phone: 49-5341-307-0
Fax: 49-53410307-124
Web site: www.schaper-bruemmer.de

Scotia Pharmaceuticals Ltd., UK
No information available

Searle, UK
No information available

ShamanBotanicals.com
Shaman.com, 213 E. Grand Avenue, South, San Francisco, CA 94080
Phone: 650-952-7070
Fax: 208-247-2533
Web site: www.shamanbotanicals.com

Solaray, Inc.
1400 Kearns Boulevard, Park City, UT 84060
Phone: 800-669-8877
Fax: 800-767-8514
Web site: www.nutraceutical.com

Solvay Arzneimittel GmbH, Germany
Hans-Böckler-Allee 20, D-30177 Hannover, Germany
Phone: 49-511-857-2400
Fax: 49-511-857-3120
Web site: www.solvay-arzneimittel.de

Steigerwald Arzneimittel GmbH, Germany
Havelstrasse 5, D-64295 Darmstadt, Germany/ P.O. Box 10 13 45,
D-64231 Darmstadt, Germany
Phone: 49-6151-3305-0
Fax: 49-6151-3305-410
Web site: www.steigerwald.de

Steiner Arzneimittel, Germany
P.O. Box 45020, 12175 Berlin, Germany
Web site: www.steinerarznei-berlin.de

Swanson Health Products
P.O. Box 2803, Fargo, ND 58108-2803
Phone: 800-437-4148/ 800-603-3198
Fax: 800-834-7197
Web site: www.swansonvitamins.com

Therabel Pharma, Belgium
Rue Egide Van Ophem 108, B-1180 Brussels, Belgium
Phone: 32-2-370-46-11
Fax: 32-2-370-46-90
Web site: www.therabel.com

Thomas J. Lipton Co. (now **Unilever Bestfoods, North America**)
Phone: 800-697-7887
Web site: www.lipton.com

Thorne Research
P.O. Box 25/ 25820 Highway 2 West, Dover, ID 83825
Phone: 208-263-1337
Fax: 208-265-2488
Web site: www.thorne.com

Traditional Medicinals, Inc.
4515 Ross Road, Sebastopol, CA 95472
Phone: 800-543-4372
Fax: 707-823-1599
Web site: www.traditionalmedicinals.com

Wakunaga of America Co., Ltd.
23501 Madero, Mission Viejo, CA 92691-2774
Phone: 800-421-2998/ 949-855-2776
Fax: 949-458-2764
Web site: www.kyolic.com

WBL Peking University Biotech Co. Ltd., China
No information available

Weber & Weber International GmbH & Co. KG, Germany
Herrchinger Str. 33, 82263 Inning/Ammersee, Germany
Phone: 49-8143-927-0
Fax: 49-8143-927-110
Web site: www.weber-weber.net

Weber & Weber USA
1245 Glen Heather
Windermere, FL 34786
Phone: 888-301-1084/ 888-989-3237
Web site: www.webernweber.com

Wei-Xin Company, China
No information available

Zeller AG, Switzerland
Seeblickstrasse 4, CH-8590 Romanshorn 1, Switzerland
Phone: 41-71-466-0500
Fax: 41-71-463-5007
Web site: www.zellerag.ch

Index

Page numbers followed by the letter "t" indicate tables.